ECG Success
Exercises in ECG Interpretation

Shirley A. Jones, MS Ed, MHA, EMT-P, RN

Emergency Medical Services Educator
Arrhythmia Instructor
Riverview Hospital
Noblesville, Indiana
Basic Life Support Instructor
American Heart Association
Advanced Cardiac Life Support Instructor
American Heart Association

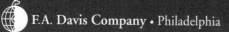
F.A. Davis Company • Philadelphia

F. A. Davis Company
1915 Arch Street
Philadelphia, PA 19103
www.fadavis.com

Printed in the United States of America

Last digit indicates print number: 10 9 8 7 6

Acquisitions Editor: Lisa B. Deitch
Project Editor: Ilysa Richman, Padraic J. Maroney
Director of Content Development: Darlene D. Pedersen
Art and Design Manager: Carolyn O'Brien

As new scientific information becomes available through basic and clinical research, recommended treatments and drug therapies undergo changes. The author(s) and publisher have done everything possible to make this book accurate, up to date, and in accord with accepted standards at the time of publication. The author(s), editors, and publisher are not responsible for errors or omissions or for consequences from application of the book, and make no warranty, expressed or implied, in regard to the contents of the book. Any practice described in this book should be applied by the reader in accordance with professional standards of care used in regard to the unique circumstances that may apply in each situation. The reader is advised always to check product information (package inserts) for changes and new information regarding dose and contraindications before administering any drug. Caution is especially urged when using new or infrequently ordered drugs.

Library of Congress Cataloging-in-Publication Data

Jones, Shirley A.
ECG success : exercises in ECG interpretation / Shirley A. Jones.
   p. ; cm.
  ISBN-13: 978-0-8036-1577-9
  ISBN-10: 0-8036-1577-9
  1. Electrocardiography—Interpretation—Problems, exercises, etc.   I. Title.
  [DNLM: 1. Electrocardiography—methods—Problems and Exercises.   2. Arrhythmia—diagnosis—Problems and Exercises. WG 18.2 J76e 2007]
RC683.5.E5J575 2007
616.1'2075470076—dc22   2007017019

Dedication

To the memory of my father George Francis Jones who was and still is my hero in life. And, to my sister Virginia Kelleher, MD, for all her love and support. Also to my best buddies who have always given me unconditional love, Zachary, Chelsea, Little Zachary, Darby, Spirit, and Francis.

Shirley A. Jones

Preface

No one is born knowing how to read ECG strips. We learn to do many things in a lifetime, and nearly all of them get better with practice. If you're planning to use this book, ECG isn't completely new to you—you have a good idea of what's involved in generating and interpreting a tracing.

ECG Success covers all the information you will need—anatomy and physiology, practice, and case scenarios, and relevant emergency care—to help you feel competent and in control, whether the situation involves an emergency or just a nonthreatening ECG. This book has staying power. You will find its content useful across a spectrum of situations, from classroom study through clinical experience and later in actual practice.

Pattern recognition lies at the heart of ECG interpretation. This skill develops with experience, gained through repetition and variety. You need to see the same patterns over and over again, but you also need to see as great a diversity as possible. In *ECG Success* you'll find more than 550 ECG tracings.

The book is organized into four units. First, two introductory chapters review the background information you need for working with ECG. Chapter One discusses heart anatomy and physiology, including biomechanics and electrophysiology. Chapter Two gives you the basics of ECG: limb and chest leads, electrode placement, cable connections, components of a tracing, rhythm strip analysis, and more.

In Unit Two, seven chapters explain and illustrate the different types of rhythm, some dangerous, others merely troublesome, and a few even normal. Each of these chapters gives you a group of nine practice strips to analyze, with the answers given at the end of the chapter. All types of arrhythmias are discussed and illustrated: sinus, atrial, junctional, and ventricular; atrioventricular and bundle branch blocks; artifact; and artificial pacemaker rhythm. The section ends with a chapter on myocardial infarction and the 12-lead ECG.

The chapter practice strips will warm you up for Unit Three, the working core of the book. You'll find four test chapters with a total of 300 strips and the answers given at the end of each chapter so you can check your work. In case you're hungry for more, the two chapters in Unit Four comprise eleven real-life case studies, followed by multiple-choice questions and illustrated by more ECG strips. Four appendices round out the book: Healthcare Provider Guidelines for Cardiopulmonary Resuscitation, Advanced Cardiac Life Support Protocols, Emergency Medications, and Emergency Medical Skills.

As you page through this book you'll find some special features to guide you. In Units One and Two, frequent Clinical Tips provide valuable information on how an arrhythmia can affect the patient. Hints on rhythm interpretation appear throughout the first practice strip chapter.

I couldn't have written this book without building up a track record of my own ECG successes. The secret: I had a good instructor who was patient and explained everything in detail. She kept emphasizing that we had to follow every step when analyzing a rhythm; shortcuts are dangerous because you can miss critical details on the rhythm strip. Then we had to practice, practice, practice. That repetition, combined with careful attention to every step, was the real key to my success.

Take your time now, and use *ECG Success* to improve your skills. Once you run into a genuine emergency you will have only minutes, or less, to interpret the ECG correctly and ensure the right treatment for the patient.

Shirley A. Jones

Consultants

Dawn McKay, RN, MSN, CCRN
Critical Care Instructor
Assistant Professor of Nursing
Liberty University
Lynchburg, Virginia
Basic Life Support Instructor,
    American Heart Association
Advanced Cardiac Life Support Instructor, American
    Heart Association
Trauma Nursing Core Course Instructor, Emergency
    Nurses Association
Fundamental Critical Care Support Instructor, Society
    of Critical Care Medicine

Carmen J. Petrin, MS, APRN, BC
Nurse Practioner
New England Heart Institute at
    Catholic Medical Center
Manchester, New Hampshire
Former Critical Care Educator
Catholic Medical Center
Manchester, New Hampshire
Basic Life Support Instructor,
    American Heart Association
Advanced Cardiac Life Support Instructor,
    American Heart Association
Pediatric Advanced Life Support Instructor,
    American Heart Association
National Advanced Cardiac Life Support
    Faculty, American Heart Association
Pediatric Advanced Life Support Training
    Center Faculty, American Heart Association
Basic Life Support Training Center
    Faculty, American Heart Association

Shirley A. Jones has worked in the field of emergency medical services for more than 30 years. She received her Master of Science in Education and her Master of Health Administration degrees from Indiana University. She has been awarded five first-place honors in tri-state and state-wide advanced life support competitions, served on the faculty of national conferences, and won honors from the Medical Writers Association for two textbooks. She is an accomplished writer and educator in the fields of electrocardiology and pharmacological and mechanical therapy. She welcomes the comments, criticisms, and ideas of readers for the improvement of future editions.

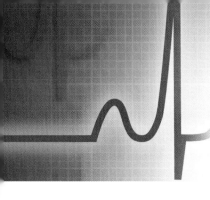

Reviewers

Lori Baker, RN
Surgical Nurse Educator
Lions Gate Hospital
North Vancouver, Canada

Carole Berube, MA, MSN, RN
Professor Emerita in Nursing
Bristol Community College
Fall River, Massachusetts

Daryl Boucher, MSN, RN
Flight Nurse/Nursing and Allied
    Health Faculty
Aroustook Medical Center/Northern
    Maine Community College
Presque Isle, Maine

Carmen Carpenter, RN, MS, CMA
Department Chair, Allied Health
    Sciences and Medical Assisting
South University
West Palm Beach, Florida

**Barbara Chamberlain,
    MSN, APRN, BC**
Critical Care Clinical Nurse
    Specialist
Kennedy Health System
Turnersville, New Jersey

Pam Chambers, MPH, PA-C
Associate Professor, Physician
    Assistant Program
Des Moines University
Des Moines, Iowa

Julie Chew, RN, MS, PhD
Clinical Educator
Sacred Heart Medical Center
Eugene, Oregon

Jeff Chianfagna, BS, MA, PA
Clinical Physician Assistant and
    Academic Instructor/Faculty
Pace Lenox Hill Hospital Physician
    Assistant Program
New York, New York

Nancy Edge, RN, BSN
Clinical Educator, Cardiac Surgery
Vancouver General Hospital
Vancouver, Canada

Sue Ellen Edrington, RN, MSN
Clinical Educator
AHA Training Center Coordinator
Riverview Hospital
Noblesville, Indiana

Linda Latham, RN, BSN, MA
Lead Instructor
Forsyth Technical Community
    College
Winston-Salem, North Carolina

Cindy Light, RN, MSN, CEN
Nursing Instructor
Baker University School of Nursing
Topeka, Kansas

Susan Moore, PhD, RN
Professor of Nursing
New Hampshire Community
    Technical College
Manchester, New Hampshire

Deborah Opacic, EdD, PA-C
Professor, Clinical Educator
Duquesne University
Pittsburgh, Pennsylvania

Patricia Richards, RN, MSN, CCRN
Faculty, Nursing Department
Central Maine Community College
Auburn, Maine

Catherine Richmond, RN, BSN, MSN
Professor, Nursing
SUNY Alfred State College
Alfred, New York

Robert Spears, MPAS, PA-C
Assistant Professor
The University of Findlay
Findlay, Ohio

Walt Stoy, PhD
Director of Education
Center for Emergency Medicine
Pittsburgh, Pennsylvania

Debbie Sullivan, PhD, PA-C
Assistant Professor/PA Program
    Faculty/Interim Director
Midwestern University
Glendale, Arizona

Rita Tomasewski, MSN, ARCNP
Cardiovascular Clinical Nurse
    Specialist
St. Francis Health Center
Topeka, Kansas

Marilyn Turner, RN, CMA
Medical Assisting Program Director
Ogeechee Technical College
Statesboro, Georgia

Contents

Heart Structure and Electrical Activity

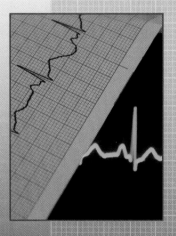

Chapter 1

Anatomy and Physiology of the Heart

OVERVIEW

Cardiovascular disease is a common cause of medical problems. Patients may present with symptoms ranging from chest pain to sudden collapse. You should already be familiar with the most important causes of cardiovascular emergencies: angina, congestive heart failure, acute myocardial infarction, pulmonary edema, cardiogenic shock, arrhythmias, hypertensive emergency, and cardiac arrest. This chapter reviews the anatomy, physiology, and electrical conduction system of the heart.

◼ ANATOMY OF THE HEART

The heart, located in the mediastinum, is the central structure of the cardiovascular system. It is protected by the bony structures of the sternum anteriorly, the spinal column posteriorly, and the rib cage (FIG. 1-1).

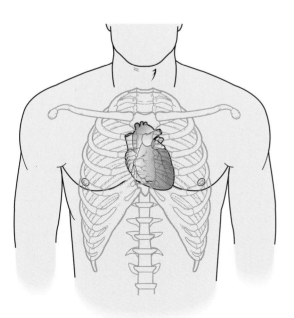

Figure 1.1 ◼ Location of the heart.

This fist-sized muscular organ is roughly conical. The base of the cone is at the top of the heart and the apex (the pointed part) is at the bottom. The heart is rotated slightly counterclockwise, with the apex tipped anteriorly so that the back surface of the heart actually lies over the diaphragm.

♡ Clinical Tip:

The cone-shaped heart has its tip (apex) just above the diaphragm to the left of the midline. This is why we may think of the heart as being on the left side—the strongest beat can be heard or felt there.

LAYERS OF THE HEART

The heart is composed of several different layers of tissue (FIG. 1-2). Surrounding the heart itself is a protective sac called the pericardium. This double-walled sac has an inner, serous (visceral) layer and an outer, fibrous (parietal) layer. Between these layers is the pericardial cavity, which contains a small amount of lubricating fluid to prevent friction during heart contraction. The layers of the heart wall itself include the epicardium, or outermost layer; the myocardium, the thick middle layer of cardiac muscle; and the endocardium, the smooth layer of connective tissue that lines the inside of the heart.

Myocardial tissue is a special type of contractile tissue found only in the heart. Although it is similar in appearance to skeletal muscle tissue, myocardial tissue has some unique structural and electrical properties. These properties are described more fully in the discussion of electrophysiology.

HEART VALVES

To prevent the backflow of blood during cardiac contraction, the atria and ventricles are separated from

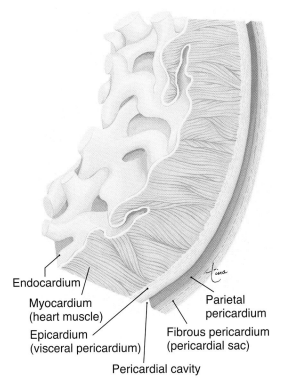

Figure 1.2 ■ Layers of the heart.

cle. The tricuspid valve, which is between the right atrium and ventricle, derives its name from its construction of three feathery leaflets, or cusps. The left AV valve, which has only two cusps, is called the mitral valve. The AV valves open to allow ventricular filling when the intra-atrial pressure exceeds the intraventricular pressure during atrial contraction. The onset of ventricular contraction creates pressure to close the AV valves.

The other set of valves, called semilunar valves, functions by similar pressure changes and prevents the flow of blood back into the ventricles after contraction. The two semilunar valves are the pulmonic valve, located in the outflow tract from the right ventricle to the pulmonary artery, and the aortic valve, between the left ventricle and the aorta.

HEART CHAMBERS AND GREAT VESSELS

The heart is a hollow muscle with an internal skeleton of connective tissue that creates four separate chambers (FIG. 1-4). The superior chambers of the heart are the right and left atria. These chambers primarily collect blood as it enters the heart and help fill the lower chambers.

The more thickly muscled lower chambers of the heart are called ventricles. These are the primary pumping chambers, the left having a thicker myocardial layer than the right. Vertical walls, composed of connective and muscle tissue, separate the two atria and the two ventricles. These walls are called the interatrial septum and the interventricular septum, respectively.

The pulmonary artery, the aorta, the superior and inferior vena cava, and the pulmonary veins are the largest blood vessels in the heart and are often referred to collectively as the great vessels (FIG. 1-4).

each other by two sets of valves composed of endocardial and connective tissue (FIG. 1-3). The fibrous connective tissue prevents enlargement of valve openings and anchors valve flaps.

The first set of heart valves, the atrioventricular (AV) valves, is located between each atrium and ventri-

CORONARY VESSEL CIRCULATION

The coronary arteries and veins provide the blood supply to the heart muscle and the electrical conduction

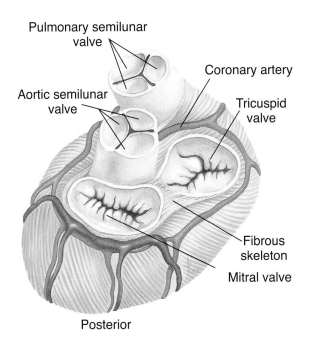

Figure 1.3 ■ Valves of the heart. The atria have been removed in this superior view.

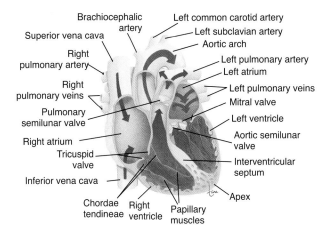

Figure 1.4 ■ Heart chambers and great vessels.

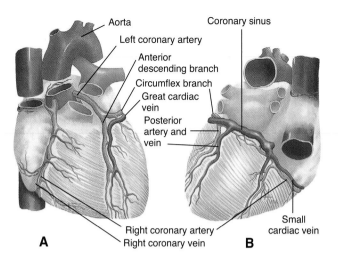

Figure 1.5 ■ Coronary vessels. (A) Coronary vessels in anterior view. (B) Coronary vessels in posterior view.

system. The coronary arteries, left and right, are the first to branch off the aorta, just above the leaflets of the aortic valve (FIG. 1-5). The left coronary artery has two major branches. The anterior descending branch runs along the anterior surface of the heart, while the circumflex branch courses in the groove between the left atrium and ventricle to the posterior surface of the heart. These two branches supply arterial blood to the left ventricle, interventricular septum, part of the right ventricle, and certain electrical conduction structures in those areas.

The right coronary artery arises from the aorta and courses along the right AV groove to the posterior surface of the heart. This artery supplies the right atrium, right ventricle, and part of the left ventricle, in addition to certain electrical conduction structures. The heart's arterial anatomy provides the left ventricle with a dual blood supply, from both coronary arteries.

The coronary veins correspond in distribution to the coronary arteries. They drain venous blood into the right atrium. The largest of these veins, the coronary sinus, provides venous drainage of the left ventricle.

> ♥ *Clinical Tip:*
>
> A protective feature of the coronary vessels is that many interconnections, or anastomoses, exist between the arterioles of the coronary arteries, allowing for development of collateral circulation, if needed.

■ ANATOMY OF THE CARDIOVASCULAR SYSTEM

The cardiovascular system is a closed system consisting of blood vessels and the heart. Arteries and veins are connected by smaller structures in which electrolytes are exchanged across cell membranes.

BLOOD VESSEL STRUCTURES

The systemic, or peripheral, circulation is composed of a circuit of blood vessels that transport substances needed for cellular metabolism to body systems and remove the waste products of metabolism from those same tissues. With the exception of the interconnecting capillaries, the anatomy of all blood vessel walls is a similar three-layer design (FIG. 1-6). The tunica intima is the smooth single-cell layer that lines the inside of all blood vessel walls. The middle layer of elastic fibers and muscle, the tunica media, gives strength and recoil. Contraction or relaxation of this muscle layer varies the diameter of the blood vessel lumen, the cavity through which blood flows. Finally, the tunica externa, a tough outer layer of fibrous tissue, protects the blood vessel from damage.

ARTERIAL CIRCULATION

Arteries carry blood away from the heart and, with the exception of the pulmonary artery, transport oxygenated blood. Arteries carry blood under high pressure and, therefore, are equipped with a much thicker medial layer than other blood vessels. Major arteries of the body to recognize include the aorta and the subclavian, internal and external carotid, axillary, brachial, radial, common iliac, and femoral arteries (FIG. 1-7).

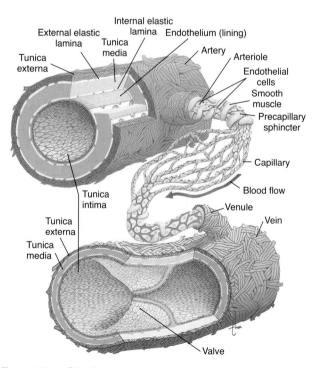

Figure 1.6 ■ Blood vessel structures.

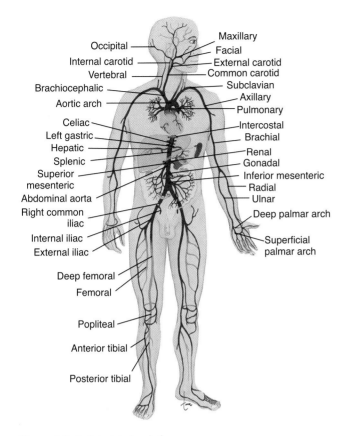

Figure 1.7 ■ Arterial circulation.

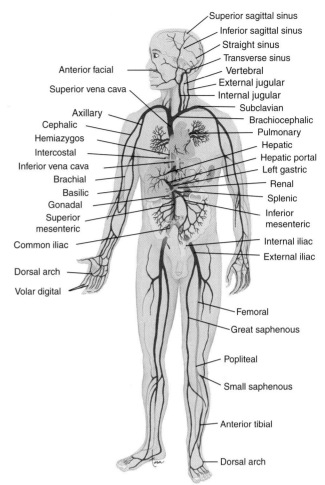

Figure 1.8 ■ Venous circulation.

VENOUS CIRCULATION

With the exception of the pulmonary veins, veins carry blood that is low in oxygen and high in carbon dioxide content. Veins carry blood under much lower pressure than arteries. Movement of this low-pressure blood, often against gravity, is aided by the "milking" action of large muscles that surround veins, particularly in the legs, and a series of intermittent one-way valves in the veins to prevent backflow of blood between heart contractions. Major veins of the body include the superior and inferior vena cava and the internal and external jugular, subclavian, axillary, iliac, and femoral veins (FIG. 1-8).

■ PHYSIOLOGY OF THE HEART

Normal blood flow through the heart begins at the right atrium, which receives systemic venous blood from the superior and inferior venae cavae (see Fig. 1-4). Blood passes from the right atrium, across the tricuspid valve, to the right ventricle. It is then pumped across the pulmonary valve into the pulmonary artery.

Outside the heart, the two branches (left and right) of the pulmonary artery distribute blood to the lungs for gas exchange in the pulmonary capillaries. Oxygenated blood returns to the heart's left atrium through four pulmonary veins. After passing across the mitral valve, blood enters the left ventricle, where it is pumped across the aortic valve and then enters the coronary arteries and the peripheral circulation through the aorta.

MECHANICAL PHYSIOLOGY

The complete cycle of mechanical pumping of blood through the heart and pulmonary circulation is referred to as the cardiac cycle. In this cycle, the right and left atria contract just before the beginning of right and left ventricular contraction. Much of the blood flow from the atria to the ventricles occurs by gravity, but atrial contraction is necessary to fill the ventricles to maximum capacity. The right and left ventricles contract simultaneously while the atria relax. The resulting pressure closes the AV valves, opens the aortic and pulmonary valves, and propels blood into the pulmonary and systemic circulation.

The contraction phase of the cardiac cycle is called systole, which generally refers to ventricular contraction versus atrial contraction. Diastole is the relaxation phase of the cardiac cycle, when the ventricles are filling (Fig. 1-9). This phase lasts much longer than systole.

 Clinical Tip:

Increases in heart rate reduce the length of diastole more significantly than that of systole. The duration of the diastolic phase is important, as this is when about 70% of the coronary artery flow occurs and complete filling of the ventricles takes place.

The amount of blood ejected from either ventricle with a single contraction is called the stroke volume. Stroke volume is determined and affected by three factors: preload, afterload, and cardiac contractility.

Preload can be thought of as the pressure under which the ventricle fills. This pressure is influenced by the amount of venous blood return. A feature of myocardial muscle is that the more it is stretched (up to a limit), the greater its force of contraction. Therefore, stroke volume can be increased considerably by increasing the blood volume that fills the ventricles and thus increasing the amount of myocardial muscle fiber stretch. This concept is known as Starling's law of the heart. Afterload, or the resistance against which the ventricles contract, also influences stroke volume. Afterload is determined by systemic arterial resistance. Cardiac contractility is the third major determinant of stroke volume. It is the intrinsic state of the heart muscle's force of contraction, also called the heart's contractile, or inotropic, state.

Stroke volume (SV) times heart rate (HR) determines the heart's cardiac output (CO), the amount of blood pumped through the circulatory system per minute:

$$CO = SV \times HR$$

An increase in stroke volume alone can improve the cardiac output. However, heart rate also has great impact. Rate increases in the healthy heart can improve the cardiac output up to threefold.

ELECTROPHYSIOLOGY

Automaticity

Arrhythmia interpretation is based on an understanding of the normal anatomy and physiology of electrical conduction in the heart. Myocardial fibers possess

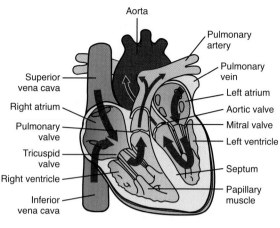

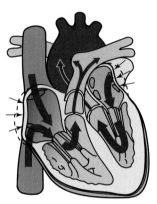

Atrial systolic phase

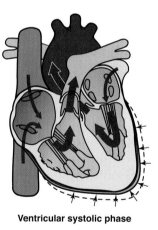

Ventricular systolic phase

Figure 1.9 ■ Systolic and diastolic phases in the heart.

highly specialized electrical properties, in addition to the mechanical property of contractility. Automaticity is the ability to generate an electrical impulse independently of stimulation by the nervous system or any other source. This property is unique to certain cardiac cells called pacemaker cells.

Excitability and Conductivity

Two other electrical properties, excitability and conductivity, are shared by all myocardial cells. Excitability is the ability of cells to respond to electrical stimulation. Conductivity is the ability to pass or propagate an electrical impulse from cell to cell through the heart. These three properties are constantly involved in the electrical conduction system of the heart.

The heart's electrical conduction system is a network of structures that allows electrical impulses to spread through the heart much faster than if they had to spread through muscle cells alone. The structures of the conduction system, in sequence of normal electrical conduction, are shown in Figure 1-10 and listed below:

Sinoatrial (SA) node. This node is the dominant pacemaker of the heart, located in the upper portion of the right atrium. Intrinsic rate is 60–100 bpm.

Internodal pathways. These cells direct electrical impulses between the SA and AV nodes and spread them across the atrial muscle.

Atrioventricular (AV) node. This node is part of an area called AV junctional tissue, which includes some surrounding tissue plus the connected bundle of His. Although AV junctional tissue contains pacemaker cells, none are thought to exist in the AV node itself. The AV node slows conduction, creating a slight delay before electrical impulses are carried to the ventricles. Intrinsic rate is 40–60 bpm.

Bundle of His. Located at the top of the interventricular septum, this bundle of fibers extends directly from the AV node and connects the atria and ventricles electrically.

Bundle branches. The bundle of His splits into two conduction paths called the right and left bundle branches. These bundles carry electrical impulses at high speed to the tissue of the interventricular septum, and to each ventricle simultaneously.

Purkinje system. The bundle branches terminate with this network of fibers, which spread electrical impulses rapidly throughout the ventricular walls. Intrinsic rate is 20–40 bpm.

The creation of electrical impulses and the spread of impulses through the electrical conduction system occur through a process called depolarization. Chemical pumps in the cell walls alter the precise concentration of electrolytes maintained inside and outside the cell. During depolarization, the electrical charge of a cell is changed by the electrolyte concentration shift on either side of the cell membrane. This change in electrical charge stimulates the muscle fiber to contract. A resting, or "polarized," cell is normally more electrically negative on the inside of the cell wall than on the outside (Fig. 1-11).

Electrical stimulation, however, changes the permeability of the cell wall and allows positively charged ions, particularly sodium (Na^+), to move into the cell. The rush of sodium, along with the slower influx of calcium (Ca^{++}), causes the inside of the cell to change from negative to positive. The cell is then said to be depolarized. The response of the muscle to this electrical charge is contraction. Because of conductivity, this process of depolarization moves rapidly from cell to cell in the conduction pathway and throughout the muscle cells of the heart (Fig. 1-12).

After depolarization, myocardial cells must return to their resting state of internal negativity for further depolarization to occur. The proper distribution of electrolytes is re-established by the cell wall chemical pumps, which pump sodium (Na^+) out of the cell and return potassium (K^+) into the cell. This process of re-establishing the internal negative charge of the cell is called repolarization.

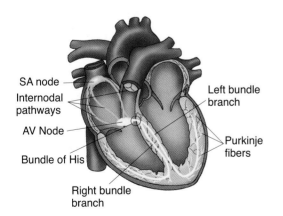

SA node
Internodal pathways
AV Node
Bundle of His
Right bundle branch
Left bundle branch
Purkinje fibers

Figure 1.10 ■ Conduction system of the heart.

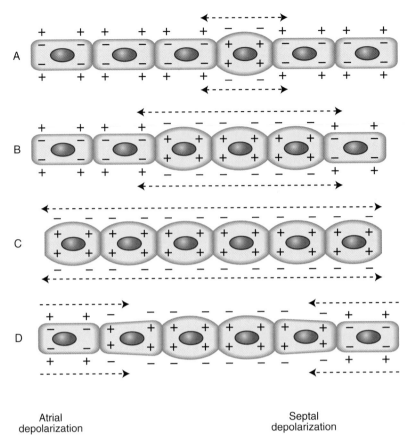

Figure 1.11 ■ The depolarization process. (A) A single cell has depolarized. (B) A wave propagates from cell to cell (C) until all are depolarized. (D) Repolarization than restores each cell's normal polarity.

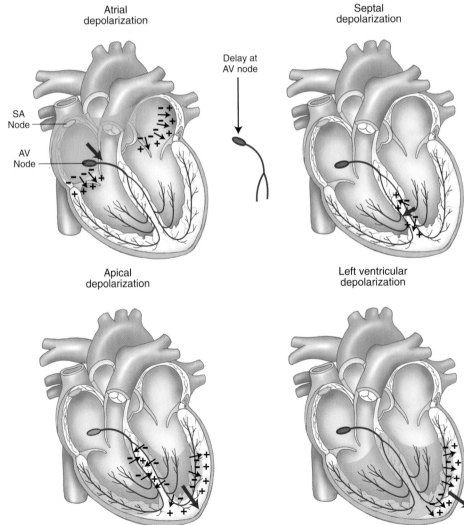

Figure 1.12 ■ Progression of depolarization through the heart.

Chapter 2

The Electrocardiogram

OVERVIEW

In Chapter 1 you learned that movement of electrolytes across the membranes of myocardial cells (depolarization and repolarization) produces a flow of electrical current and creates an electrical field. Depolarization and repolarization can be seen on the electrocardiogram (ECG) (Fig. 2-1).

 Clinical Tip:

It is important to keep in mind that the ECG shows only electrical activity; it tells us nothing about how well the heart is working mechanically.

The body acts as a giant conductor of electrical current. Electrical activity that originates in the heart can be detected on the body's surface through an electrocardiogram (ECG). Electrodes are applied to the skin to measure voltage changes in the cells between the electrodes. These voltage changes are amplified and visually displayed on an oscilloscope and graph paper. This chapter focuses on the ECG and its analysis and interpretation.

The following summarizes a basic ECG:

- An ECG is a series of waves and deflections recording the heart's electrical activity from a certain "view."
- Many views, each called a lead, monitor voltage changes between electrodes placed in different positions on the body.
- Leads I, II, and III are bipolar leads, which consist of two electrodes of opposite polarity (positive and negative). The third (ground) electrode minimizes electrical activity from other sources.
- Leads aVR, aVL, and aVF are unipolar leads and consist of a single positive electrode and a reference

point (with zero electrical potential) that lies in the center of the heart's electrical field.
- Leads V_1 through V_6 are unipolar leads and consist of a single positive electrode with a negative reference point, found at the electrical center of the heart.
- Voltage changes are amplified and visually displayed on an oscilloscope and graph paper.
- An ECG tracing looks different in each lead because the recorded angle of electrical activity changes with each lead.

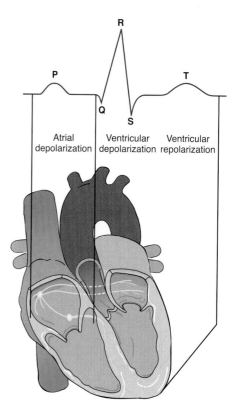

Figure 2.1 ■ Correlation of depolarization and repolarization with the ECG.

- Several different angles allow a more accurate perspective than a single one would.
- The ECG machine can be adjusted to make any skin electrode positive or negative. The polarity depends on which lead the machine is recording.
- A cable attached to the patient is divided into several different-colored wires: three, four, or five for monitoring purposes, or ten for a 12-lead ECG.
- Incorrect placement of electrodes may turn a normal ECG tracing into an abnormal one.

 Clinical Tip:

Patients should be treated according to their symptoms, not merely their ECG tracing.

Clinical Tip:

To obtain a 12-lead ECG, four wires are attached to each limb and six wires are attached at different locations on the chest. The total of ten wires provides 12 views (12 leads).

LIMB LEADS

Electrodes are placed on the right arm (RA), left arm (LA), right leg (RL), and left leg (LL). With only four electrodes, six leads are viewed (FIG. 2-2). These leads include the standard leads—I, II, and III—and the augmented leads—aVR, aVL, and aVF.

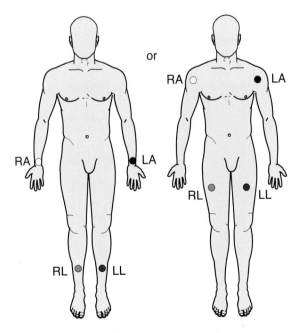

Figure 2.2 ■ Standard limb lead electrode placement.

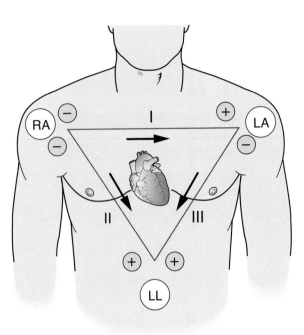

Figure 2.3 ■ Standard leads: I, II, and III.

Table 2.1 ■ **ELEMENTS OF STANDARD LEADS**

Lead	Positive Electrode	Negative Electrode	View of Heart
I	LA	RA	Lateral
II	LL	RA	Inferior
III	LL	LA	Inferior

Standard Leads

Leads I, II, and III make up the standard leads. If electrodes are placed on the right arm, left arm, and left leg, three leads are formed (FIG. 2-3). If you draw an imaginary line between each of these electrodes, an axis is formed between each pair of leads. The axes of these three leads form an equilateral triangle with the heart in the center (Einthoven's triangle). TABLE 2-1 shows the composition of the standard leads.

Augmented Leads

Leads aVR, aVL, and aVF make up the augmented leads (FIG. 2-4). Each letter of an augmented lead refers to a specific term: a = augmented, V = voltage, R = right arm, L = left arm, F = foot (the left foot). TABLE 2-2 shows the composition of the augmented leads.

STANDARD CHEST LEADS

The chest leads are identified as V_1, V_2, V_3, V_4, V_5, and V_6 (FIG. 2-5). Each electrode placed in a "V" position is positive. TABLE 2-3 shows the composition of the chest leads.

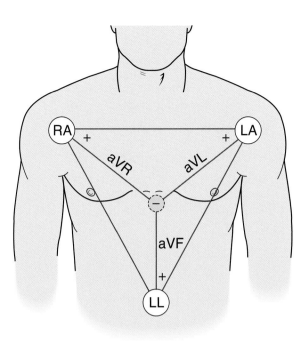

Figure 2.4 ■ Augmented leads: aVR, aVL, and aVF.

Table 2.2 ■ ELEMENTS OF AUGMENTED LEADS

Lead	Positive Electrode	View of Heart
aVR	RA	None
aVL	LA	Lateral
aVF	LL	Inferior

Table 2.3 ■ ELEMENTS OF CHEST LEADS

Lead	Positive Electrode Placement	View of Heart
V_1	Fourth intercostal space to right of sternum	Septum
V_2	Fourth intercostal space to left of sternum	Septum
V_3	Directly between V_2 and V_4	Anterior
V_4	Fifth intercostal space at left midclavicular line	Anterior
V_5	Level with V_4 at left anterior axillary line	Lateral
V_6	Level with V_5 at left midaxillary line	Lateral

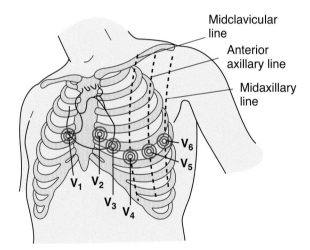

Figure 2.5 ■ Chest leads: V_1, V_2, V_3, V_4, V_5, and V_6.

Table 2.4 ■ MONITORING CABLE CONNECTIONS

U.S.	Connect to	Europe
White	Right arm	Red
Black	Left arm	Yellow
Red	Left leg	Green
Green	Right leg	Black
Brown	Chest	White

CABLE CONNECTIONS

Before you attach the cable to the patient, you need to know whether the cable is an American or European cable. Improper placement of the connections can give incorrect ECG recordings. The colors of the wires differ as shown in TABLE 2-4.

ELECTRODE PLACEMENT USING A THREE-WIRE CABLE

A three-wire patient cable is used to monitor the standard leads, I, II, and III (FIG. 2-6).

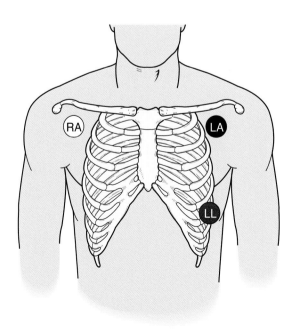

Figure 2.6 ■ Three-wire patient cable.

Clinical Tip:

Lead II is commonly called a monitoring lead. It provides information on heart rate, regularity, conduction time, and ectopic beats. The presence or location of an acute myocardial infarction (MI) should be further diagnosed with a 12-lead ECG.

ELECTRODE PLACEMENT USING A FIVE-WIRE CABLE

A five-wire patient cable is used to monitor the standard leads, I, II, and III; augmented leads, aVR, aVL, aVF; and one chest lead, usually V_1 (FIG. 2-7).

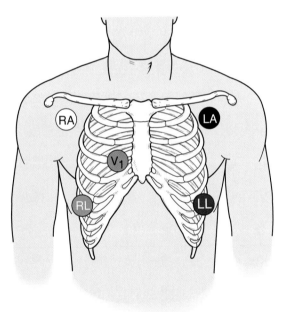

Figure 2.7 ■ Five-wire patient cable.

Clinical Tip:

Five-wire telemetry units are commonly used to monitor leads I, II, III, aVR, aVL, aVF, and V_1 in critical care settings.

MODIFIED CHEST LEADS

Modified chest leads (MCL) are useful in detecting bundle branch blocks and premature beats. Lead MCL_1 simulates chest lead V_1 and views the ventricular septum (FIG. 2-8). Lead MCL_6 simulates chest lead V_6 and views the lateral wall of the left ventricle (FIG. 2-9).

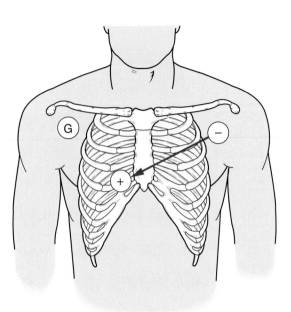

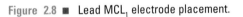

Figure 2.8 ■ Lead MCL_1 electrode placement.

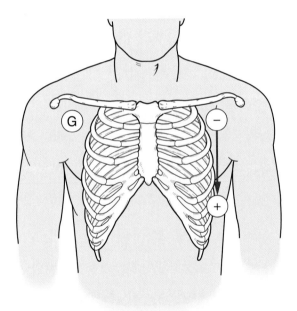

Figure 2.9 ■ Lead MCL_6 electrode placement.

Clinical Tip:

Write on the rhythm strip which simulated lead was used.

THE RIGHT-SIDED 12-LEAD ECG

Other chest leads that are not part of a standard 12-lead ECG may be used to view specific surfaces of the heart. In a right-sided 12-lead ECG, the limb leads are placed

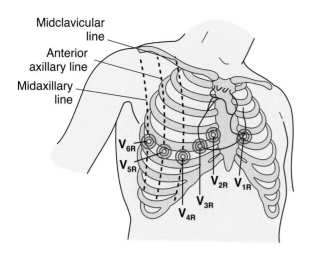

Figure 2.10 ■ The right-sided chest lead placement.

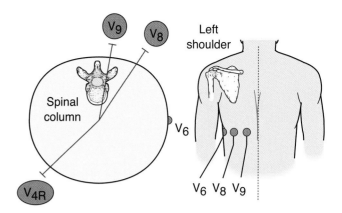

Figure 2.11 ■ Electrode placement for V_{4R}, V_8, and V_9.

as usual, but the chest leads are a mirror image of the standard chest lead placement (FIG. 2-10). The ECG machine cannot recognize that the leads have been reversed. It will still print "V_1–V_6" next to the tracing. Be sure to cross this out and write the new lead positions on the ECG paper. TABLE 2-5 shows the placement of the right-sided chest leads.

Table 2.5 ■ THE RIGHT-SIDED CHEST LEAD PLACEMENT

Chest Leads	Position
V_{1R}	Fourth intercostal space to left of sternum
V_{2R}	Fourth intercostal space to right of sternum
V_{3R}	Directly between V_{2R} and V_{4R}
V_{4R}	Fifth intercostal space at right midclavicular line
V_{5R}	Level with V_{4R} at right anterior axillary line
V_{6R}	Level with V_{5R} at right midaxillary line

Clinical Tip:

Patients with an acute inferior MI should have right-sided ECGs to assess for possible right ventricular infarction.

THE 15-LEAD ECG

Areas of the heart that are not well visualized by the six chest leads include the wall of the right ventricle and the posterior wall of the left ventricle. A 15-lead ECG, which includes the standard 12 leads plus leads V_{4R}, V_8, and V_9, increases the chance of detecting an MI in these areas (FIG. 2-11). TABLE 2-6 shows the chest lead placement for the 15-lead ECG.

Table 2.6 ■ CHEST LEAD PLACEMENT FOR A 15-LEAD ECG

Chest Leads	Electrode Placement	View of Heart
V_{4R}	Fifth intercostal space in right anterior midclavicular line	Right ventricle
V_8	Posterior fifth intercostal space in left mid-scapular line	Posterior wall of left ventricle
V_9	Directly between V_8 and spinal column at posterior fifth intercostal space	Posterior wall of left ventricle

Clinical Tip:

Use a 15-lead ECG when the 12-lead tracing is normal but the history still suggests an acute infarction.

RECORDING OF THE ECG

Paper tracings of the ECG patterns from a monitoring lead, inscribed on graph paper, are called rhythm strips. Rhythm strips are valuable because they permit analysis of the ECG in detail. Several different factors can be measured and compared because the graph paper moves past a heated stylus at a standard, constant speed, usually 25 mm/sec (FIG. 2-12).

The vertical lines on the graph paper measure time—one small box equals 0.04 sec and one large box equals 0.20 sec. Therefore these boxes are useful in measuring the duration of various events. Horizontal lines on the graph paper measure voltage, 0.10 mV per each small box. Voltage measurement, however, is only relevant to calibrated tracings, such as a 12-lead or 15-lead ECG produces.

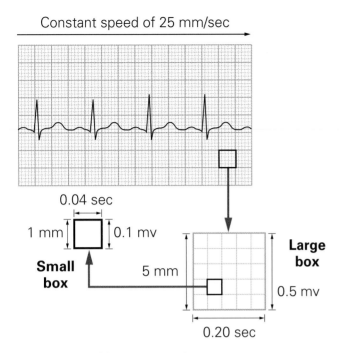

Figure 2.12 ■ ECG graph paper values.

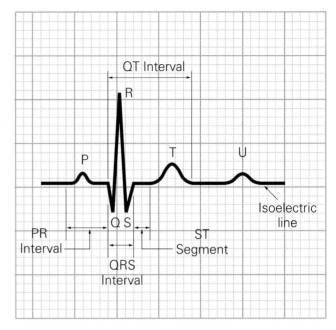

Figure 2.13 ■ The electrical pattern of the cardiac cycle shows waves and intervals.

COMPONENTS OF AN ECG TRACING

An ECG tracing specifically reflects electrical activity in the heart. A single cardiac cycle inscribes various deflections on the graph paper. This electrical activity is described as:

Wave: A deflection, either positive or negative, away from the baseline (isoelectric line) of the ECG tracing

Complex: Several waves

Segment: A straight line between waves or complexes

Interval: A segment and a wave

♥ | *Clinical Tip:*

Between waves and cycles, the ECG records a baseline (isoelectric line), which indicates the absence of net electrical activity (FIG. 2-13).

The various patterns described in Figure 2-13 are derived from electrical impulses that originate in the SA node and spread throughout the heart. These electrical components are described as:

P Wave: First wave seen. Small, rounded, and upright (positive); indicates atrial depolarization (and contraction).

PR Interval: Distance between beginning of P wave and beginning of QRS complex. Measures time during which a depolarization wave travels from the atria to the ventricles.

QRS Complex: Three deflections following P wave. Indicates ventricular depolarization (and contraction).

  Q WAVE: First negative deflection

  R WAVE: First positive deflection

  S WAVE: First negative deflection after R wave

ST Segment: Distance between end of S wave and beginning of T wave. Measures time between ventricular depolarization and beginning of repolarization.

T Wave: Rounded, upright (positive) wave following QRS complex. Represents ventricular repolarization.

QT Interval: Measured from beginning of QRS complex to end of T wave. Represents total ventricular activity.

U Wave: Small, rounded, upright wave following T wave. Most easily seen with a slow heart rate. Indicates repolarization of Purkinje fibers.

METHODS FOR CALCULATING HEART RATE

Heart rate is calculated as the number of times the heart beats per minute (bpm). On an ECG tracing the bpm is usually calculated as the number of QRS complexes. Included are extra beats such as premature ventricular contractions (PVC), premature atrial contractions

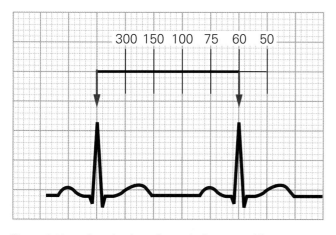

Figure 2.14 ■ Counting large boxes for heart rate. The rate is 60 bpm.

Table 2.7 ■ METHODS 1 AND 2 FOR CALCULATING HEART RATE			
Number of Large Boxes	Rate/Min	Number of Small Boxes	Rate/Min
1	300	2	750
2	150	3	500
3	100	4	375
4	75	5	300
5	60	6	250
6	50	7	214
7	43	8	186
8	38	9	167
9	33	10	150
10	30	11	136
11	27	12	125
12	25	13	115
13	23	14	107
14	21	15	100
15	20	16	94

(PAC), and premature junctional contractions (PJC). The rate is measured from the R-R interval, the distance between one R wave and the next. If the atrial rate (the number of P waves) and the ventricular rate (the number of QRS complexes) vary, the analysis may show them as different rates, one atrial and one ventricular.

Method 1: Count Large Boxes

Regular rhythms can be quickly determined by counting the number of large graph boxes between two R waves (FIG. 2-14). That number is divided into 300 to calculate beats per minute. The rates for the first one to six large boxes can be easily memorized.

Remember: 60 sec/min divided by 0.20 sec/large box = 300 large boxes/min. This method usually gives an approximate heart rate but is not as accurate as method 2, explained below.

Method 2: Count Small Boxes

The most accurate way to measure a regular rhythm is to count the number of small boxes between two R waves. That number is divided into 1500 to calculate

bpm. Remember: 60 sec/min divided by 0.04 sec/small box = 1500 small boxes/min.

Examples: If there are three small boxes between two R waves, 1500/3 = 500 bpm. If there are five small boxes between two R waves, 1500/5 = 300 bpm.

TABLE 2-7 describes methods 1 and 2 for calculating the heart rate.

♡ *Clinical Tip:*

The approximate rate per minute is rounded to the next-highest number.

Method 3: Six-second ECG Rhythm Strip

The best method for measuring irregular heart rates with varying R-R intervals is to count the number of R waves in a 6-second (sec) strip (including extra beats such as PVCs, PACs, and PJCs) and multiply by 10 (FIG. 2-15). This gives the average number of beats per minute.

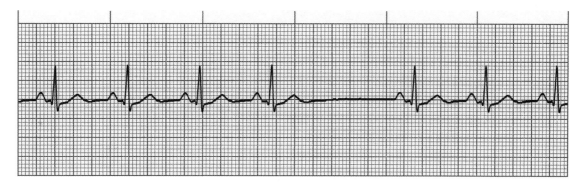

Figure 2.15 ■ Using 6-sec ECG rhythm strip to calculate heart rate: 7 × 10 = 70 bpm.

Clinical Tip:

If a rhythm is extremely irregular, it is best to count the number of R-R intervals per 60 sec (1 min).

RHYTHM STRIP ANALYSIS

Arrhythmia interpretation is easiest when you use a consistent analytical approach. Each of the many possible arrhythmias can be described according to the chosen format, and the "rules" for known arrhythmias can be used as a comparison for analyzing an unknown arrhythmia. Although you can use many formats, try to use one approach consistently, and perform all steps in the analysis process to avoid interpretation errors.

Using the format in this text, we begin by analyzing rate, regularity, P waves, PR interval, QRS interval, and QT interval. Next, we check for dropped beats,

pauses, or both. Finally, we look for any grouping of QRS complexes (TABLE 2-8).

INSTRUCTIONS FOR ANALYZING ECG PRACTICE AND TEST STRIPS

Use the following guidelines when analyzing the ECG practice and test strips in this book. They apply to Unit II (Chaps. 3-10) and Unit III (Chaps. 11-14).

• All of the ECG strips were recorded in lead II.
• All ECG strips are 6 sec in length. Notice the 1-sec marks across the top of each strip.
• Rate is determined by the methods you learned in this chapter. Method 2, the small-box method (p 15), is used to measure the rate for regular rhythms. Method 3, the 6-sec method (p 15), is used to determine the rate for irregular rhythms. With a few exceptions, the ventricular rate (R-R interval) is the rate given in the answer section.

Table 2.8 ■ ANALYZING AN ECG RHYTHM

Component	Characteristic
Rate	The bpm is commonly the ventricular rate. If atrial and ventricular rates differ, as in a third-degree block, measure both rates. Normal: 60–100 bpm Slow (bradycardia): <60 bpm Fast (tachycardia): >100 bpm
Regularity	Measure R-R intervals and P-P intervals. Regular: Consistent intervals Regularly irregular: Repeating pattern Irregular: No pattern
P Waves	If present: Same in size, shape, position? Does each QRS have a P wave? Normal: Upright (positive) and uniform Inverted: Negative Notched: P′ None: Rhythm is junctional or ventricular.
PR Interval	Constant: Intervals are the same. Variable: Intervals differ. Normal: 0.12–0.20 sec and constant
QRS Interval	Normal: 0.06–0.10 sec Wide: >0.10 sec None: Absent
QT Interval	Beginning of QRS to end of T wave Varies with HR. Normal: Less than half the R-R interval
Dropped beats	Occur in AV blocks. Occur in sinus arrest.
Pause	Compensatory: Complete pause following a PAC, PJC, or PVC Noncompensatory: Incomplete pause following a PAC, PJC, or PVC
QRS Complex grouping	Bigeminy: Repeating pattern of normal complex followed by a premature complex Trigeminy: Repeating pattern of 2 normal complexes followed by a premature complex Quadrigeminy: Repeating pattern of three normal complexes followed by a premature complex Couplets: 2 consecutive premature complexes Triplets: 3 consecutive premature complexes

PAC = premature atrial contraction; PJC = premature junctional contraction; PVC = premature ventricular contraction.

Remember to include any extra beats such as PVCs, PACs, or PJCs.

- To determine rhythm, use calipers or an ECG ruler to measure the distance between R-R intervals. If the distance is the same throughout the ECG strip the rhythm is regular. In an irregular rhythm, the R-R intervals are not spaced evenly. Measure each R-R interval on the entire 6-sec ECG strip to make an accurate interpretation of a regular or irregular rhythm.

- Identify and examine the P waves. Notice whether they are normal, absent, or retrograde. Also see whether a pacemaker spike precedes them. Remember, there can be variations of the P wave in each ECG strip.

- Measure the PR intervals. Notice whether each interval is the same or varies in time. If the PR interval is not present, indicate "none."

- Measure the QRS complexes. Indicate whether they appear notched, as in a bundle branch block. Also notice whether a pacemaker spike precedes them.

- Interpret the tracing in detail. Identify any extra, dropped, or grouped complexes or other important features.

- Check your answers against the answer key at the end of the chapter.

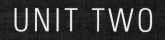

Rhythms and Their Analysis

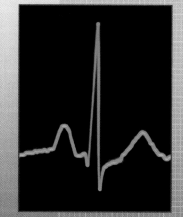

Chapter 3

Sinoatrial Node Arrhythmias

Sinus rhythms all originate in the sinoatrial (SA) node. The ECG features common to all of them are upright P waves, all similar in appearance; normal-duration PR intervals; and normal-duration QRS complexes if no ventricular conduction disturbances are present. Sinus rhythms described here, in addition to normal sinus rhythm, are sinus bradycardia, sinus tachycardia, sinus arrhythmia, sinus pause (sinus arrest), and SA block. All ECG strips, including the practice strips, were recorded in lead II.

NORMAL SINUS RHYTHM (NSR)

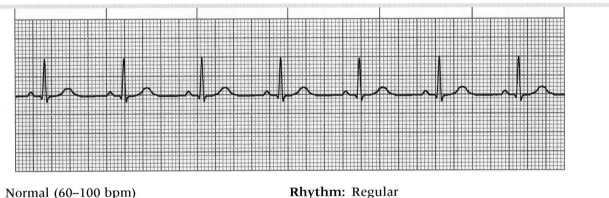

Rate: Normal (60–100 bpm)   **Rhythm:** Regular

P Waves: Normal (upright and uniform)   **PR Interval:** Normal (0.12–0.20 sec)   **QRS:** Normal (0.06–0.10 sec)

♡ *Clinical Tip:*

A normal ECG does not exclude heart disease.

♡ *Clinical Tip:*

This rhythm is generated by the sinus node and its rate is within normal limits (60–100 bpm).

SINUS BRADYCARDIA

- The SA node discharges more slowly than in NSR.

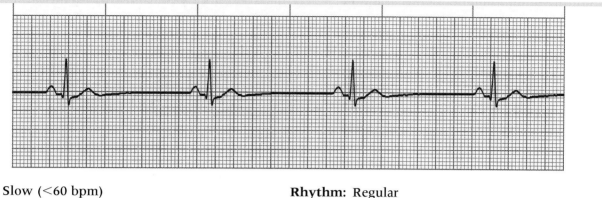

Rate: Slow (<60 bpm)   **Rhythm:** Regular

P Waves: Normal (upright and   **PR Interval:** Normal (0.12–0.20 sec)   **QRS:** Normal (0.06–0.10 sec)
uniform)

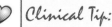 *Clinical Tip:*

Sinus bradycardia is normal in athletes and during sleep. In acute MI, it may be protective and beneficial or the slow rate may compromise cardiac output. Certain medications, such as beta blockers, may also cause sinus bradycardia.

SINUS TACHYCARDIA

- The SA node discharges more frequently than in NSR.

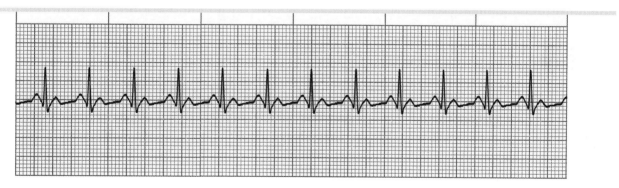

Rate: Fast (>100 bpm)   **Rhythm:** Regular

P Waves: Normal (upright and   **PR Interval:** Normal (0.12–0.20 sec)   **QRS:** Normal (0.06–0.10 sec)
uniform)

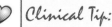 *Clinical Tip:*

Sinus tachycardia may be caused by exercise, anxiety, fever, hypoxemia, hypovolemia, or cardiac failure.

SINUS ARRHYTHMIA

- The SA node discharges irregularly.
- The R-R interval is irregular.

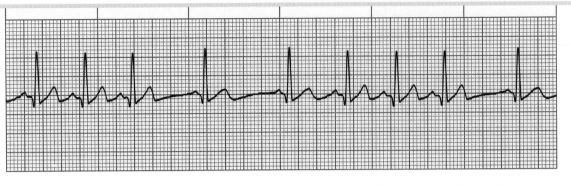

Rate: Usually normal (60–100 bpm); frequently increases with inspiration and decreases with expiration; may be < 60 bpm

Rhythm: Irregular; varies with respiration; difference between shortest R-R and longest R-R intervals is > 0.12 sec

P Waves: Normal (upright and uniform)

PR Interval: Normal (0.12–0.20 sec)

QRS: Normal (0.06–0.10 sec)

Clinical Tip:

The pacing rate of the SA node varies with respiration, especially in children and elderly people.

SINUS PAUSE (SINUS ARREST)

- The SA node fails to discharge and then resumes.
- Electrical activity resumes either when the SA node resets itself or when a lower latent pacemaker begins to discharge.
- The pause (arrest) time interval is not a multiple of the normal P-P interval.

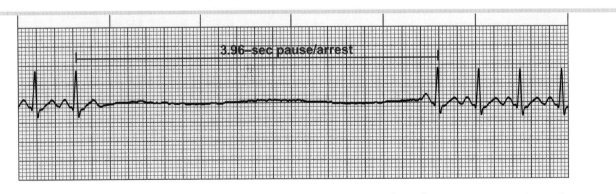

3.96–sec pause/arrest

Rate: Normal to slow; determined by duration and frequency of sinus pause (arrest)

Rhythm: Irregular whenever a pause (arrest) occurs

P Waves: Normal (upright and uniform) except in areas of pause (arrest)

PR Interval: Normal (0.12–0.20 sec)

QRS: Normal (0.06–0.10 sec)

Clinical Tip:

Cardiac output may decrease, causing syncope or dizziness.

SINOATRIAL (SA) BLOCK

- The block occurs in some multiple of the P-P interval.
- After the dropped beat, cycles continue on time.

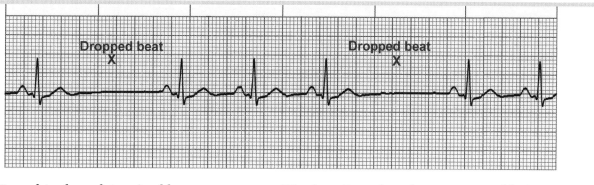

Rate: Normal to slow; determined by duration and frequency of SA block

Rhythm: Irregular whenever an SA block occurs

P Waves: Normal (upright and uniform) except in areas of dropped beats

PR Interval: Normal (0.12–0.20 sec)

QRS: Normal (0.06–0.10 sec)

Clinical Tip:

Cardiac output may decrease, causing syncope or dizziness.

ECG PRACTICE STRIPS

For instructions on analyzing these practice strips, please see the guidelines given at the end of Chapter 2.

ECG 3•1

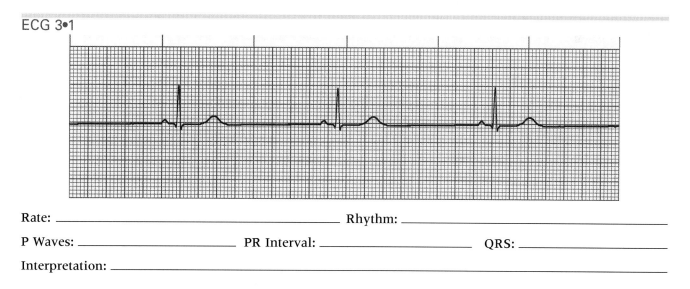

Rate: _____   Rhythm: _____

P Waves: _____   PR Interval: _____   QRS: _____

Interpretation: _____

ECG 3•2

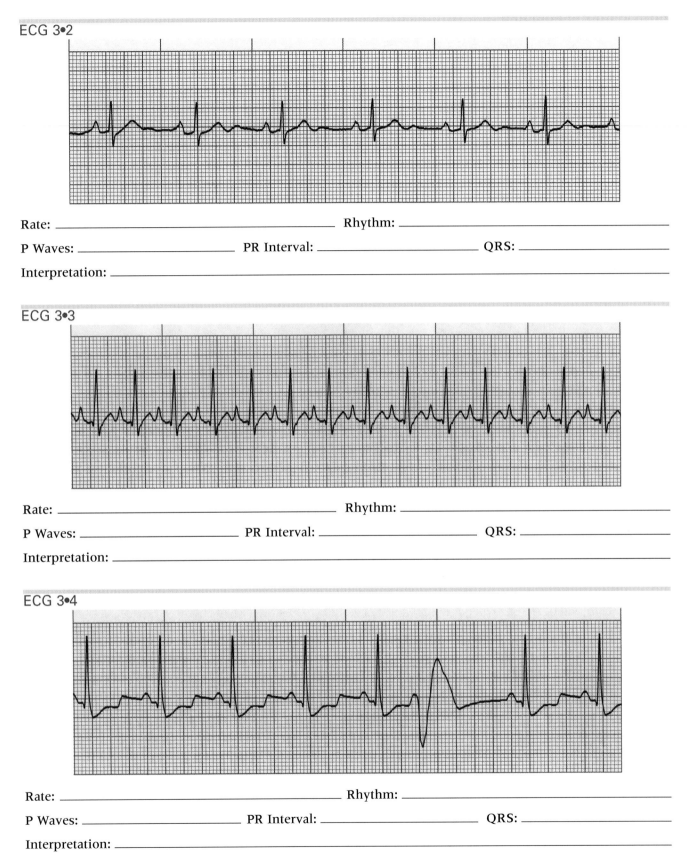

Rate: _____   Rhythm: _____

P Waves: _____   PR Interval: _____   QRS: _____

Interpretation: _____

ECG 3•3

Rate: _____   Rhythm: _____

P Waves: _____   PR Interval: _____   QRS: _____

Interpretation: _____

ECG 3•4

Rate: _____   Rhythm: _____

P Waves: _____   PR Interval: _____   QRS: _____

Interpretation: _____

ECG 3•5

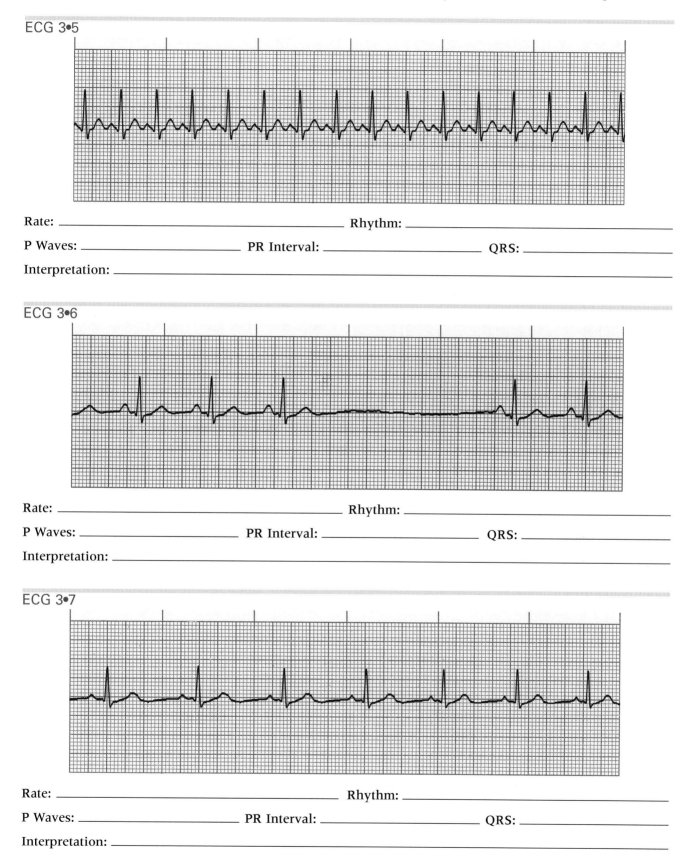

Rate: _____ Rhythm: _____

P Waves: _____ PR Interval: _____ QRS: _____

Interpretation: _____

ECG 3•6

Rate: _____ Rhythm: _____

P Waves: _____ PR Interval: _____ QRS: _____

Interpretation: _____

ECG 3•7

Rate: _____ Rhythm: _____

P Waves: _____ PR Interval: _____ QRS: _____

Interpretation: _____

ECG 3•8

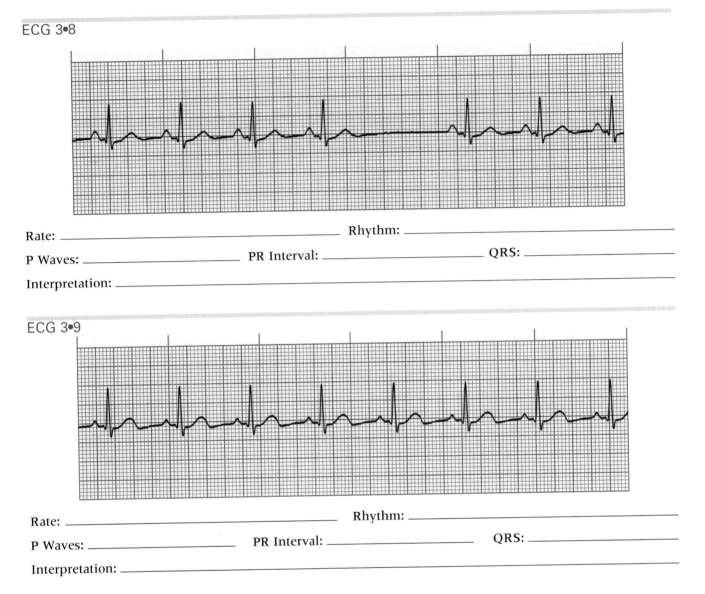

Rate: _____   Rhythm: _____

P Waves: _____   PR Interval: _____   QRS: _____

Interpretation: _____

ECG 3•9

Rate: _____   Rhythm: _____

P Waves: _____   PR Interval: _____   QRS: _____

Interpretation: _____

Answers to Chapter 3
ECG PRACTICE STRIPS ▪

▪ ECG 3•1
Rate: 35 bpm
Rhythm: Regular
P Waves: Normal
PR Interval: 0.16 sec
QRS: 0.08 sec
Interpretation: Sinus bradycardia

▪ ECG 3•2
Rate: 63 bpm
Rhythm: Regular
P Waves: Normal
PR Interval: 0.20 sec
QRS: 0.10 sec
Interpretation: Normal sinus rhythm with U wave

▪ ECG 3•3
Rate: 136 bpm
Rhythm: Regular
P Waves: Normal
PR Interval: 0.16 sec
QRS: 0.10 sec
Interpretation: Sinus tachycardia

▪ ECG 3•4
Rate: 80 bpm
Rhythm: Irregular
P Waves: Normal
PR Interval: 0.16 sec
QRS: 0.10 sec
Interpretation: Sinus rhythm with
    ST segment depression and one
    PVC at beat 6

■ ECG 3•5
Rate: 150 bpm
Rhythm: Regular
P Waves: Normal
PR Interval: 0.12 sec
QRS: 0.10 sec
Interpretation: Sinus tachycardia

■ ECG 3•6
Rate: 50 bpm
Rhythm: Irregular
P Waves: Normal
PR Interval: 0.16 sec
QRS: 0.10 sec
Interpretation: Sinus pause (sinus arrest)

■ ECG 3•7
Rate: 70 bpm
Rhythm: Irregular
P Waves: Normal
PR Interval: 0.16 sec
QRS: 0.10 sec
Interpretation: Sinus arrhythmia

■ ECG 3•8
Rate: 70 bpm
Rhythm: Irregular
P Waves: Normal
PR Interval: 0.16 sec
QRS: 0.10 sec
Interpretation: Sinoatrial block

■ ECG 3•9
Rate: 75 bpm
Rhythm: Regular
P Waves: Normal
PR Interval: 0.16 sec
QRS: 0.10 sec
Interpretation: Normal sinus rhythm

Chapter 4

Atrial Arrhythmias

Atrial rhythms originate in the atria. Their common ECG features are P waves that differ in appearance from sinus P waves, and normal-duration QRS complexes if no ventricular conduction disturbances are present. Atrial rhythms to be described here are wandering atrial pacemaker (WAP), multifocal atrial tachy-cardia (MAT), premature atrial contractions (PAC), atrial tachycardia, supraventricular tachycardia (SVT), paroxysmal supraventricular tachycardia (PSVT), atrial flutter (A-flutter), atrial fibrillation (A-fib), and Wolff-Parkinson-White (WPW) Syndrome. All ECG strips, including the practice strips, were recorded in lead II.

WANDERING ATRIAL PACEMAKER (WAP) ▪

- The pacemaker site transfers from the SA node to other latent pacemaker sites in the atria and the AV junction and then moves back to the SA node.

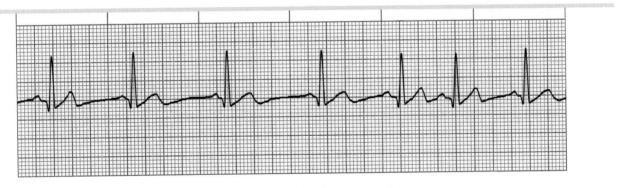

Rate: Normal (60–100 bpm)

P Waves: At least three different forms, determined by focus in atria

Rhythm: Irregular

PR Interval: Variable; determined by focus

QRS: Normal (0.06–0.10 sec)

♥ *Clinical Tip:*

Wandering atrial pacemaker may occur in normal hearts as a result of fluctuations in vagal tone. It may also be seen in patients with heart disease or COPD.

MULTIFOCAL ATRIAL TACHYCARDIA (MAT)

- This form of WAP is associated with a ventricular response of >100 bpm.
- MAT may be confused with atrial fibrillation (A-fib); however, MAT has a visible P wave.

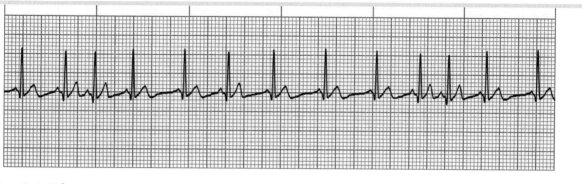

Rate: Fast (>100 bpm)   **Rhythm:** Irregular

P Wave: At least three different   **PR Interval:** Variable; determined   **QRS:** Normal (0.06–0.10 sec)
forms, determined by focus in atria   by focus

 Clinical Tip:

MAT is commonly seen in patients with chronic obstructive pulmonary disease but may also occur in acute MI.

PREMATURE ATRIAL CONTRACTION (PAC)

- A single contraction occurs earlier than the next expected sinus contraction.
- After the PAC, sinus rhythm usually resumes.

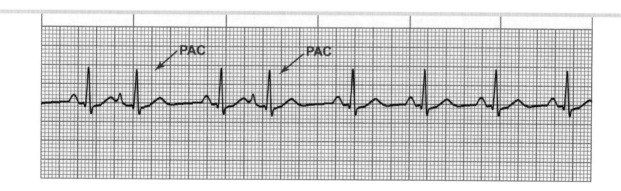

Rate: Depends on rate of underlying rhythm   **Rhythm:** Irregular whenever a PAC occurs

P Waves: Present; in the PAC,   **PR Interval:** Varies in the PAC;   **QRS:** Normal (0.06–0.10 sec)
may have a different shape   otherwise normal (0.12–0.20 sec)

Clinical Tip:

In patients with heart disease, frequent PACs may precede PSVT, A-fib, or A-flutter.

ATRIAL TACHYCARDIA ▨

- A rapid atrial rate overrides the SA node and becomes the dominant pacemaker.
- Some ST wave and T wave abnormalities may be present.

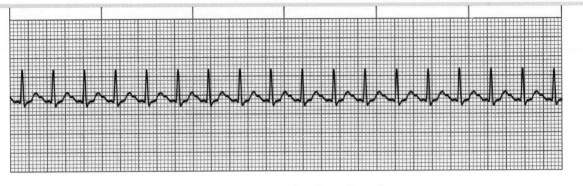

Rate: 150–250 bpm   **Rhythm:** Regular

P Waves: Normal (upright and uniform) but differ in shape from sinus P waves

PR Interval: May be short (<0.12 sec) in rapid rates

QRS: Normal (0.06–0.10 sec) but can be aberrant at times

SUPRAVENTRICULAR TACHYCARDIA (SVT) ▨

- This arrhythmia has such a fast rate that the P waves may not be seen.

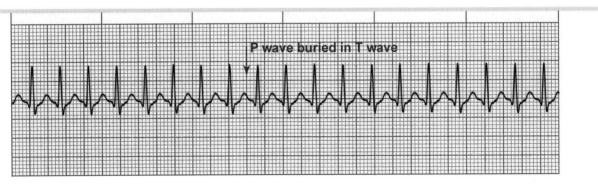

P wave buried in T wave

Rate: 150–250 bpm   **Rhythm:** Regular

P Waves: Frequently buried in preceding T waves and difficult to see

PR Interval: Usually not possible to measure

QRS: Normal (0.06–0.10 sec) but may be wide if abnormally conducted through ventricles

 Clinical Tip:

SVT may be related to caffeine intake, nicotine, stress, or anxiety in healthy adults.

Clinical Tip:

Some patients may experience angina, hypotension, light headedness, palpitations, and intense anxiety.

PAROXYSMAL SUPRAVENTRICULAR TACHYCARDIA (PSVT) ▪

- PSVT is a rapid rhythm that starts and stops suddenly.
- For accurate interpretation, the beginning or end of the PSVT must be seen.
- PSVT is sometimes called paroxysmal atrial tachycardia (PAT).

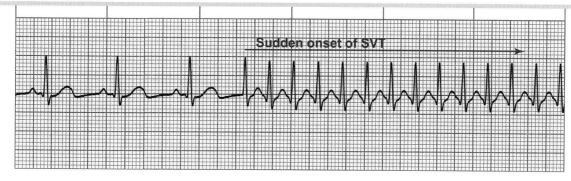

Rate: 150–250 bpm

Rhythm: Irregular

P Waves: Frequently buried in preceding T waves and difficult to see

PR Interval: Usually not possible to measure

QRS: Normal (0.06–0.10 sec) but may be wide if abnormally conducted through ventricles

💙 *Clinical Tip:*

The patient may feel palpitations, dizziness, lightheadedness, or anxiety.

ATRIAL FLUTTER ▪

- The AV node conducts impulses to the ventricles at a 2:1, 3:1, 4:1, or greater ratio (rarely 1:1).
- The degree of AV block may be consistent or variable.

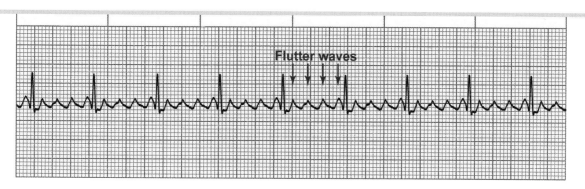

Rate: Atrial: 250–350 bpm; ventricular: variable.

Rhythm: Atrial: regular; ventricular: variable

P Waves: Flutter waves have a saw-toothed appearance; some may not be visible, being buried in the QRS

PR Interval: Variable

QRS: Usually normal (0.06–0.10 sec), but may appear widened if flutter waves are buried in QRS

💙 *Clinical Tip:*

The presence of A-flutter may be the first indication of cardiac disease.

💙 *Clinical Tip:*

Signs and symptoms depend on the ventricular response rate.

ATRIAL FIBRILLATION ▨

- Rapid, erratic electrical discharge comes from multiple atrial ectopic foci.
- No organized atrial depolarization are detectable.

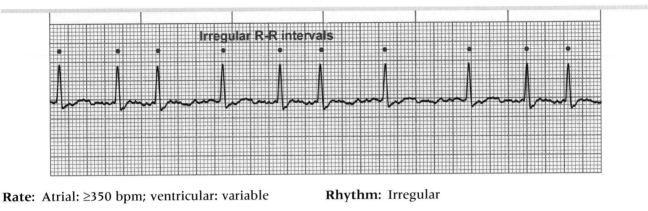

Rate: Atrial: ≥350 bpm; ventricular: variable   **Rhythm:** Irregular

P Waves: No true P waves; chaotic   **PR Interval:** None   **QRS:** Normal (0.06–0.10 sec)
atrial activity

♥ | *Clinical Tip:*

Atrial fibrillation is often a chronic arrhythmia associated with underlying heart disease.

♥ | *Clinical Tip:*

Signs and symptoms depend on the ventricular response rate.

WOLFF-PARKINSON-WHITE (WPW) SYNDROME ▨

- In WPW an accessory conduction pathway is present between the atria and the ventricles. Electrical impulses may be rapidly conducted to the ventricles.
- These rapid impulses create a slurring of the initial portion of the QRS; the slurred effect is called a delta wave.

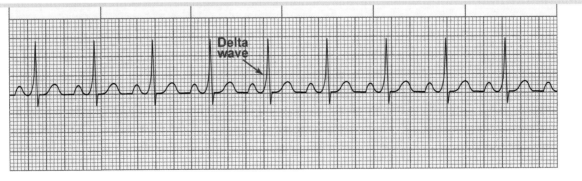

Rate: Depends on rate of underlying rhythm   **Rhythm:** Regular unless associated with A-fib

P Waves: Normal (upright and   **PR Interval:** Short (<0.12 sec)   **QRS:** Wide (>0.10 sec); delta
uniform) unless A fib is present   wave present

♥ | *Clinical Tip:*

WPW is associated with narrow-complex tachycardias, including A-flutter and A-fib.

ECG PRACTICE STRIPS ◾

For instructions on analyzing these practice strips, please see the guidelines given at the end of Chapter 2.

ECG 4•1

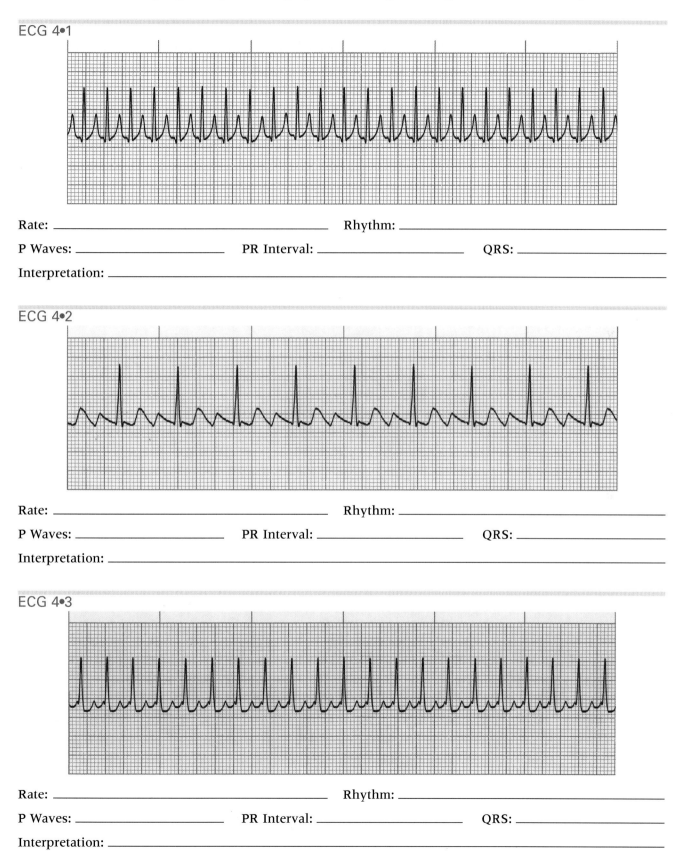

Rate: _____ Rhythm: _____

P Waves: _____ PR Interval: _____ QRS: _____

Interpretation: _____

ECG 4•2

Rate: _____ Rhythm: _____

P Waves: _____ PR Interval: _____ QRS: _____

Interpretation: _____

ECG 4•3

Rate: _____ Rhythm: _____

P Waves: _____ PR Interval: _____ QRS: _____

Interpretation: _____

ECG 4•4

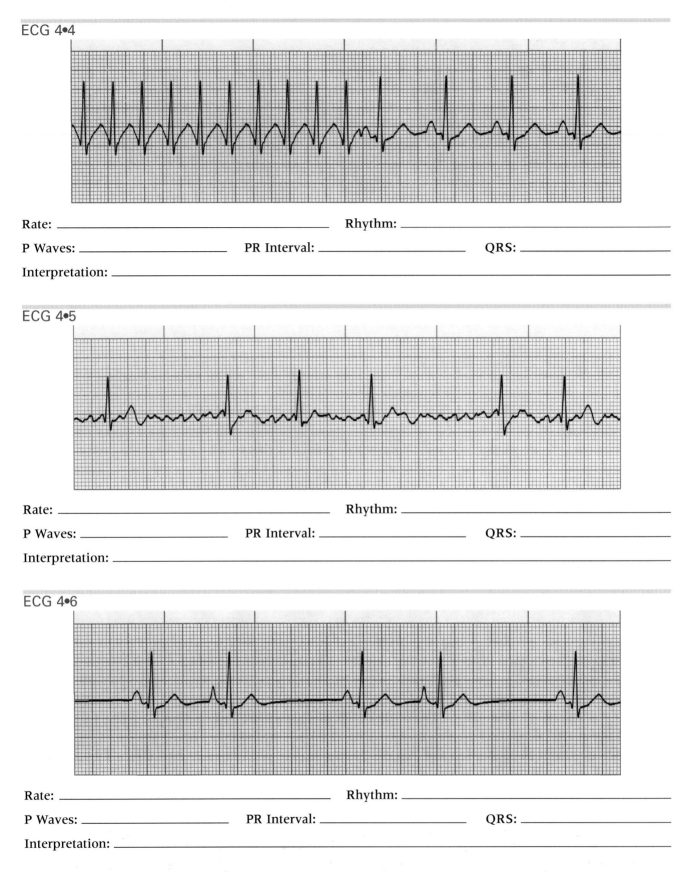

Rate: _____   Rhythm: _____

P Waves: _____   PR Interval: _____   QRS: _____

Interpretation: _____

ECG 4•5

Rate: _____   Rhythm: _____

P Waves: _____   PR Interval: _____   QRS: _____

Interpretation: _____

ECG 4•6

Rate: _____   Rhythm: _____

P Waves: _____   PR Interval: _____   QRS: _____

Interpretation: _____

ECG 4•7

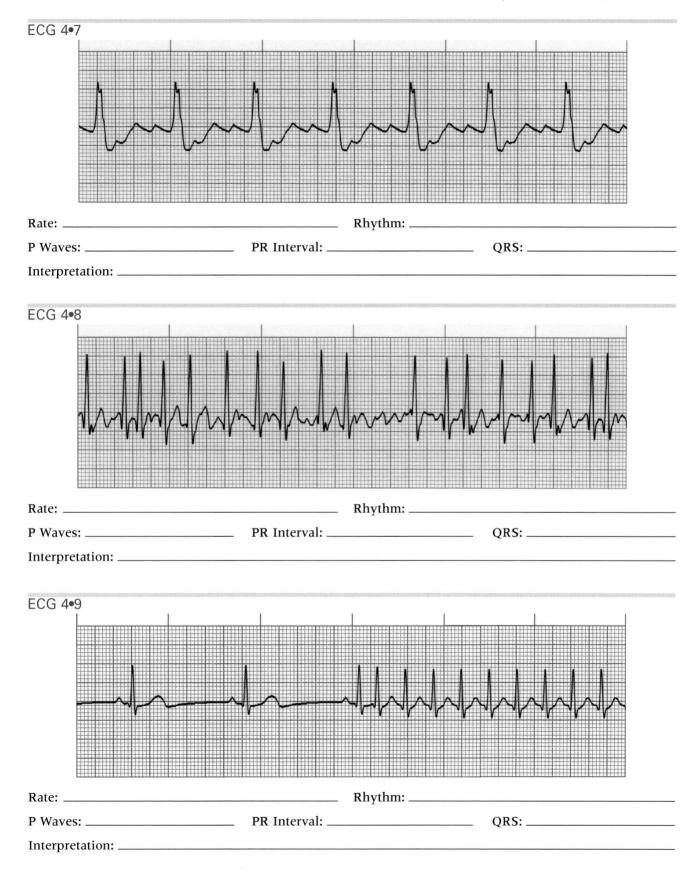

Rate: _____ Rhythm: _____

P Waves: _____ PR Interval: _____ QRS: _____

Interpretation: _____

ECG 4•8

Rate: _____ Rhythm: _____

P Waves: _____ PR Interval: _____ QRS: _____

Interpretation: _____

ECG 4•9

Rate: _____ Rhythm: _____

P Waves: _____ PR Interval: _____ QRS: _____

Interpretation: _____

Answers to Chapter 4

ECG PRACTICE STRIPS ■

■ ECG 4•1
Rate: 214 bpm
Rhythm: Regular
P Waves: Buried in T waves
PR Interval: Not possible to measure
QRS: 0.08 sec
Interpretation: Supraventricular tachycardia

■ ECG 4•2
Rate: 94 bpm
Rhythm: Regular
P Waves: Flutter waves
PR Interval: Not possible to measure
QRS: 0.10 sec
Interpretation: Atrial flutter with 3:1 block (every third flutter wave is buried in the QRS)

■ ECG 4•3
Rate: 214 bpm
Rhythm: Regular
P Waves: Not clearly visible
PR Interval: Not measurable
QRS: 0.08 sec
Interpretation: Supraventricular tachycardia with ST segment depression

■ ECG 4•4
Rate: 140 bpm
Rhythm: Irregular
P Waves: Buried in T waves in beats 1 through 10, normal in beats 11 through 14
PR Interval: None in beats 1 through 10, 0.16 sec in beats 11 through 14
QRS: 0.10 sec
Interpretation: Paroxysmal supraventricular tachycardia (supraventricular tachycardia converting to normal sinus rhythm)

■ ECG 4•5
Rate: 60 bpm
Rhythm: Irregular
P Waves: None
PR Interval: None
QRS: 0.10 sec
Interpretation: Atrial fibrillation

■ ECG 4•6
Rate: 50 bpm
Rhythm: Irregular
P Waves: Normal
PR Interval: 0.20 sec
QRS: 0.08 sec
Interpretation: Sinus bradycardia with two PACs at beats 2 and 4

■ ECG 4•7
Rate: 68 bpm
Rhythm: Regular
P Waves: Flutter waves
PR Interval: Not possible to measure
QRS: 0.20 sec with notched appearance
Interpretation: Atrial flutter with a bundle branch block

■ ECG 4•8
Rate: 180 bpm
Rhythm: Irregular
P Waves: None
PR Interval: None
QRS: 0.08 sec
Interpretation: Atrial fibrillation

■ ECG 4•9
Rate: 120 bpm
Rhythm: Irregular
P Waves: Normal in first three beats
PR Interval: 0.16 sec in first three beats
QRS: 0.10 sec
Interpretation: Paroxysmal supraventricular tachycardia (sinus bradycardia converting to supraventricular tachycardia)

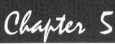

Chapter 5

Junctional Arrhythmias

The internodal pathways in the heart merge with the cells of the atrioventricular (AV) junction, which include the AV node. The AV junction is the origin of junctional rhythms. Because it has pacemaker capabilities, it can act as a back-up to the SA node. The ECG features common to all junctional rhythms include P waves that are absent, inverted, buried in the QRS, or retrograde (after the QRS). A junctional rhythm can also have a PR interval that is absent, short, or retrograde. The rhythms described here are junctional and accelerated junctional rhythms, junctional tachycardia, junctional escape beat, and premature junctional contraction (PJC). All ECG strips, including the practice strips, were recorded in lead II.

JUNCTIONAL RHYTHM ■

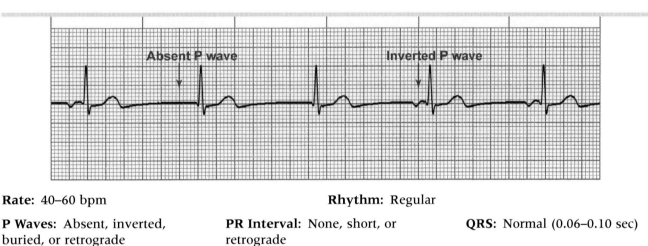

Rate: 40–60 bpm

Rhythm: Regular

P Waves: Absent, inverted, buried, or retrograde

PR Interval: None, short, or retrograde

QRS: Normal (0.06–0.10 sec)

♡ *Clinical Tip:*

The presence of sinus node disease that is causing an inappropriate slowing of the sinus node may exacerbate this rhythm. Young healthy adults, especially those with increased vagal tone during sleep, are often noted to have periods of junctional rhythm that is completely benign, not requiring intervention.

ACCELERATED JUNCTIONAL RHYTHM ▦

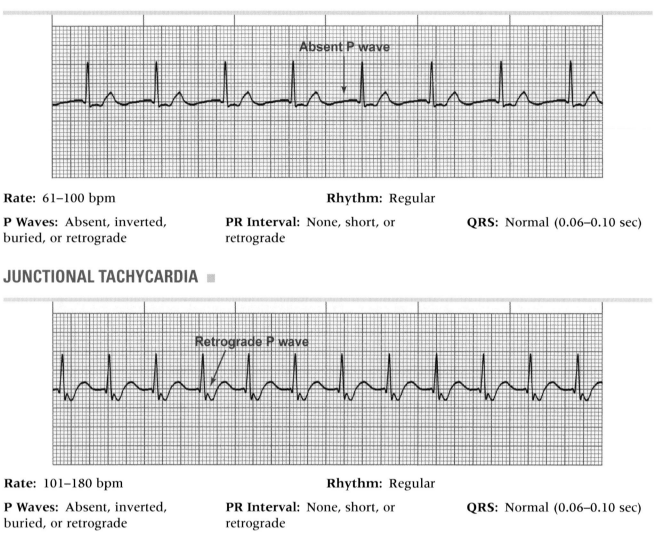

Rate: 61–100 bpm   **Rhythm:** Regular

P Waves: Absent, inverted,   **PR Interval:** None, short, or   **QRS:** Normal (0.06–0.10 sec)
buried, or retrograde   retrograde

JUNCTIONAL TACHYCARDIA ▦

Rate: 101–180 bpm   **Rhythm:** Regular

P Waves: Absent, inverted,   **PR Interval:** None, short, or   **QRS:** Normal (0.06–0.10 sec)
buried, or retrograde   retrograde

💗 | *Clinical Tip:*

Signs and symptoms of decreased cardiac output may be seen in response to the rapid rate.

JUNCTIONAL ESCAPE BEAT ▦

• An escape complex comes later than the next expected sinus complex.

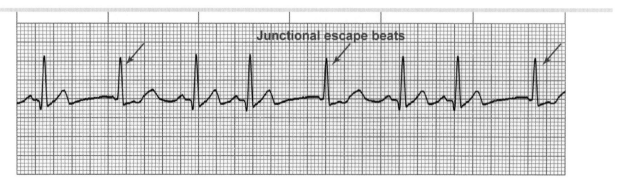

Rate: Depends on rate of underlying rhythm   **Rhythm:** Irregular whenever an escape beat occurs

P Waves: None, inverted, buried,   **PR Interval:** None, short, or   **QRS:** Normal (0.06–0.10 sec)
or retrograde in the escape beat   retrograde

38

PREMATURE JUNCTIONAL CONTRACTION (PJC) ▪

- Enhanced automaticity in the AV junction produces PJCs.

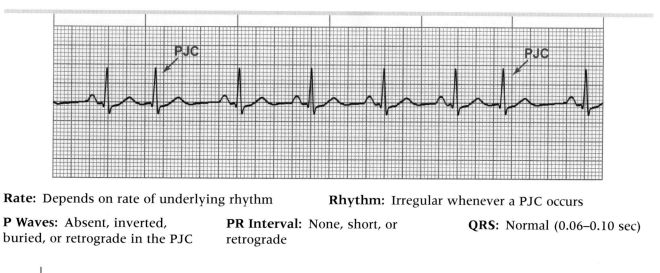

Rate: Depends on rate of underlying rhythm

Rhythm: Irregular whenever a PJC occurs

P Waves: Absent, inverted, buried, or retrograde in the PJC

PR Interval: None, short, or retrograde

QRS: Normal (0.06–0.10 sec)

Clinical Tip:

Before deciding that isolated PJCs are insignificant, consider the cause.

ECG PRACTICE STRIPS ▪

For instructions on analyzing these practice strips, please see the guidelines given at the end of Chapter 2.

ECG 5•1

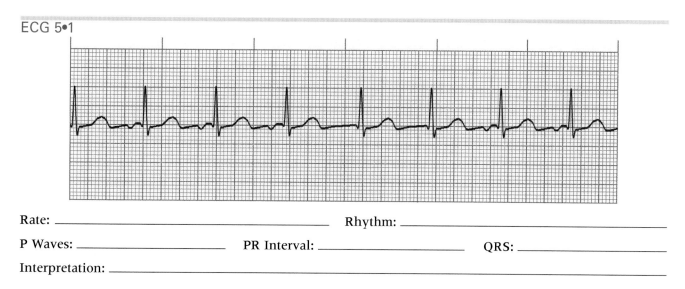

Rate: _____   Rhythm: _____

P Waves: _____   PR Interval: _____   QRS: _____

Interpretation: _____

ECG 5•2

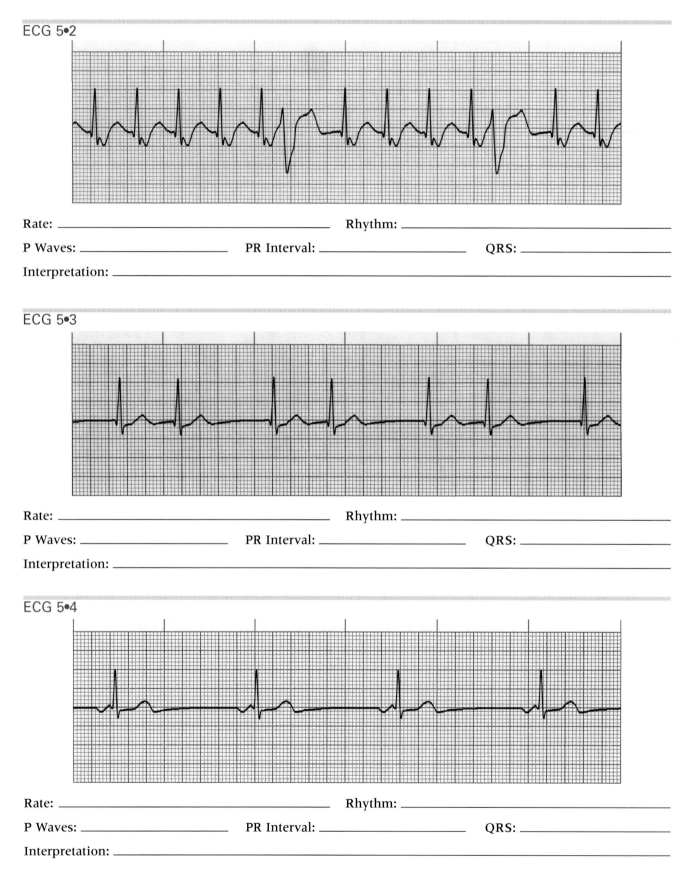

Rate: _____   Rhythm: _____

P Waves: _____   PR Interval: _____   QRS: _____

Interpretation: _____

ECG 5•3

Rate: _____   Rhythm: _____

P Waves: _____   PR Interval: _____   QRS: _____

Interpretation: _____

ECG 5•4

Rate: _____   Rhythm: _____

P Waves: _____   PR Interval: _____   QRS: _____

Interpretation: _____

ECG 5•5

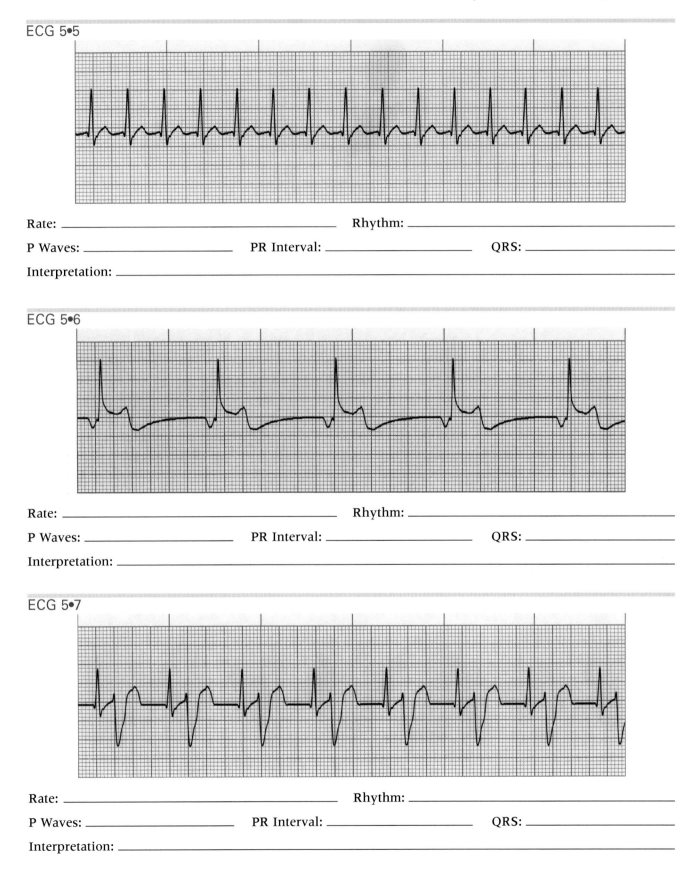

Rate: _____ Rhythm: _____

P Waves: _____ PR Interval: _____ QRS: _____

Interpretation: _____

ECG 5•6

Rate: _____ Rhythm: _____

P Waves: _____ PR Interval: _____ QRS: _____

Interpretation: _____

ECG 5•7

Rate: _____ Rhythm: _____

P Waves: _____ PR Interval: _____ QRS: _____

Interpretation: _____

ECG 5•8

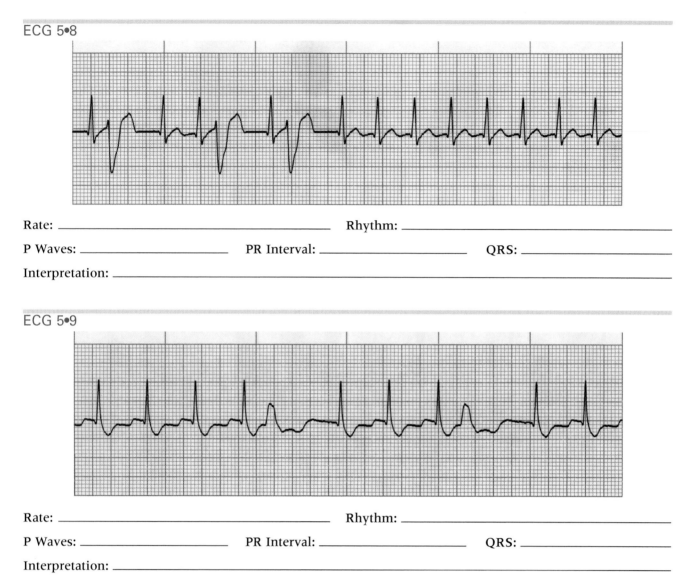

Rate: _____   Rhythm: _____

P Waves: _____   PR Interval: _____   QRS: _____

Interpretation: _____

ECG 5•9

Rate: _____   Rhythm: _____

P Waves: _____   PR Interval: _____   QRS: _____

Interpretation: _____

Answers to Chapter 5

ECG PRACTICE STRIPS ▨

▨ ECG 5•1
Rate: 75 bpm
Rhythm: Regular
P Waves: Inverted or absent
PR Interval: 0.16 sec with inverted P waves
QRS: 0.10 sec
Interpretation: Accelerated junctional rhythm

▨ ECG 5•2
Rate: 130 bpm
Rhythm: Irregular
P Waves: Retrograde
PR Interval: None
QRS: 0.10 sec
Interpretation: Junctional tachycardia with two uni-
form PVCs at beats 6 and 11

▨ ECG 5•3
Rate: 70 bpm
Rhythm: Irregular
P Waves: None
PR Interval: None
QRS: 0.10 sec
Interpretation: Junctional rhythm
with bigeminal PJCs at beats 2, 4,
and 6

▨ ECG 5•4
Rate: 38 bpm
Rhythm: Regular
P Waves: Inverted
PR Interval: 0.16 sec
QRS: 0.10 sec
Interpretation: Junctional rhythm

■ ECG 5•5

Rate: 150 bpm
Rhythm: Regular
P Waves: None
PR Interval: None
QRS: 0.10 sec
Interpretation: Junctional tachycardia

■ ECG 5•6

Rate: 47 bpm
Rhythm: Regular
P Waves: Inverted
PR Interval: 0.10 sec
QRS: 0.10 sec
Interpretation: Junctional rhythm with
    ST segment elevation

■ ECG 5•7

Rate: 160 bpm
Rhythm: Irregular
P Waves: None
PR Interval: None
QRS: 0.10 sec
Interpretation: Accelerated junctional rhythm with
    bigeminal uniform PVCs (R on T phenomenon*)

■ ECG 5•8

Rate: 150 bpm
Rhythm: Irregular
P Waves: None
PR Interval: None
QRS: 0.10 sec
Interpretation: Junctional tachycardia with
    uniform PVCs (R on T phenomenon*) at
    beats 2, 5, and 7

■ ECG 5•9

Rate: 110 bpm
Rhythm: Irregular
P Waves: None
PR Interval: None
QRS: 0.10 sec
Interpretation: Junctional tachycardia with
    ST segment depression and uniform PVCs
    at beats 5 and 9

---

*R on T phenomenon is discussed in Chapter 6.

Chapter 6

Ventricular Arrhythmias

All arrhythmias that originate in the ventricles depolarize the ventricles abnormally and at a slower speed. For this reason, the ECG feature common to all ventricular rhythms is a QRS complex wider than 0.10 sec in duration. The P waves are either absent or, if visible, have no consistent relationship to the QRS interval (the length of the QRS complex). The ventricular rhythms discussed are idioventricular and accelerated idioventricular rhythm, premature ventricular contraction (PVC), monomorphic ventricular tachycardia (VT), polymorphic VT, torsade de pointes, ventricular fibrillation (VF), pulseless electrical activity (PEA), and asystole. All ECG strips, including the practice strips, were recorded in lead II.

IDIOVENTRICULAR RHYTHM ■

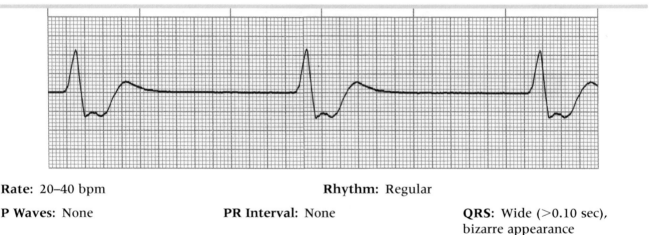

Rate: 20–40 bpm

P Waves: None

Rhythm: Regular

PR Interval: None

QRS: Wide (>0.10 sec), bizarre appearance

Clinical Tip:

Diminished cardiac output is expected because of the slow heart rate. An idioventricular rhythm may be called an agonal rhythm when the heart rate drops below 20 bpm. An agonal rhythm is generally a terminal event and is usually the last rhythm before asystole.

ACCELERATED IDIOVENTRICULAR RHYTHM

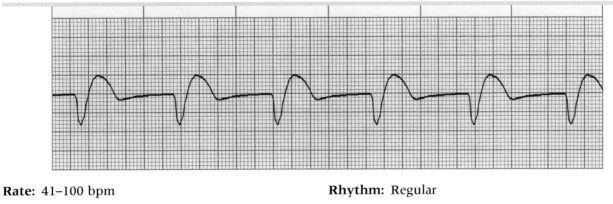

Rate: 41–100 bpm   **Rhythm:** Regular

P Waves: None   **PR Interval:** None   **QRS:** Wide (>0.10 sec), bizarre appearance

💟 *Clinical Tip:*

Idioventricular rhythms appear when supraventricular pacing sites are suppressed or absent.

PREMATURE VENTRICULAR CONTRACTION (PVC)

- PVCs result from an irritable ventricular focus.
- PVCs may be uniform (same form) or multiform (different forms).
- Usually a PVC is followed by a full compensatory pause because the sinus node timing is not interrupted. Normally the sinus rate produces the next sinus impulse on time. In contrast, a PVC may be followed by a noncompensatory pause if the PVC enters the sinus node and resets its timing; this enables the following sinus P wave to appear earlier than expected.

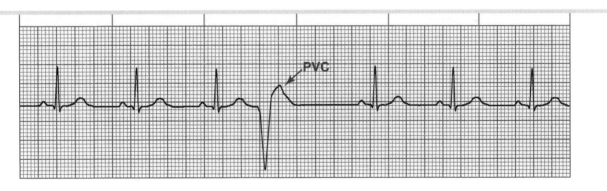

Rate: Depends on rate of underlying rhythm   **Rhythm:** Irregular whenever a PVC occurs

P Waves: None associated with the PVC   **PR Interval:** None associated with the PVC   **QRS:** Wide (>0.10 sec), bizarre appearance

💟 *Clinical Tip:*

Patients may sense the occurrence of PVCs as skipped beats. Because the ventricles are only partially filled, the PVC frequently does not generate a pulse.

PREMATURE VENTRICULAR CONTRACTION: UNIFORM ▪

(ECG strip)

PREMATURE VENTRICULAR CONTRACTION: MULTIFORM ▪

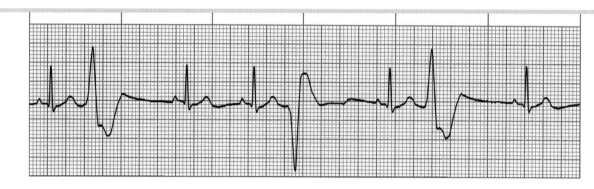

PREMATURE VENTRICULAR CONTRACTION: VENTRICULAR BIGEMINY ▪

- In ventricular bigeminy, the PVC occurs with every other beat.

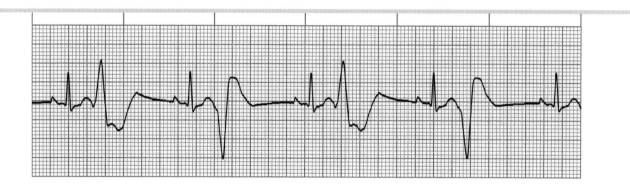

PREMATURE VENTRICULAR CONTRACTION: VENTRICULAR TRIGEMINY ▪

- In ventricular trigeminy, the PVC occurs with every third beat.

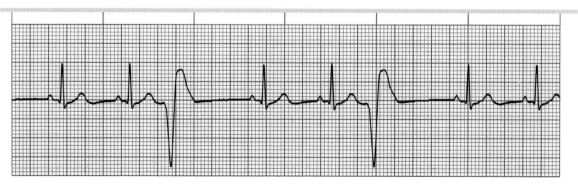

PREMATURE VENTRICULAR CONTRACTION: VENTRICULAR QUADRIGEMINY

- In ventricular quadrigeminy, the PVC occurs with every fourth beat.

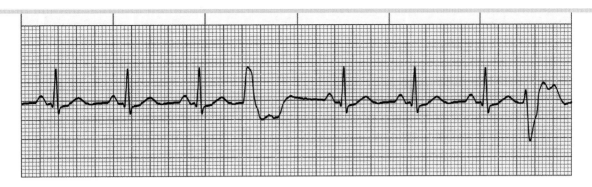

PREMATURE VENTRICULAR CONTRACTION: COUPLETS

- In a rhythm with PVC couplets, the PVCs occur in pairs.

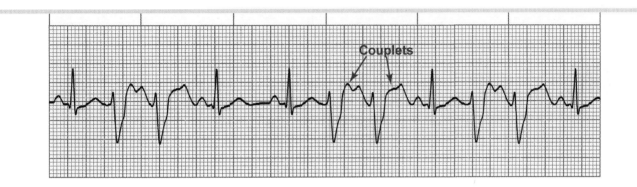

PREMATURE VENTRICULAR CONTRACTION: R ON T PHENOMENON

- The PVCs occur so early that they fall on the T wave of the preceding beat.
- These PVCs occur during the refractory period of the ventricles, a vulnerable period because the cardiac cells have not fully repolarized.

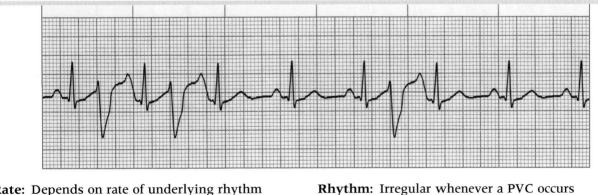

Rate: Depends on rate of underlying rhythm

Rhythm: Irregular whenever a PVC occurs

P Waves: None associated with the PVC

PR Interval: None associated with the PVC

QRS: Wide (>0.10 sec), bizarre appearance

♡ *Clinical Tip:*

In an acute ischemic situation, R on T phenomenon may be especially dangerous because the ventricles may be more vulnerable to VT or VF.

PREMATURE CONTRACTION: INTERPOLATED PVC

* The PVC occurs between two regular complexes; it may appear sandwiched in between two normal beats.
* An interpolated PVC does not interfere with the normal cardiac cycle.

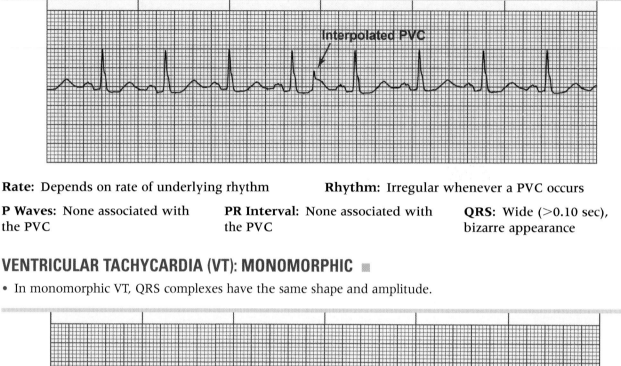

Rate: Depends on rate of underlying rhythm

Rhythm: Irregular whenever a PVC occurs

P Waves: None associated with the PVC

PR Interval: None associated with the PVC

QRS: Wide (>0.10 sec), bizarre appearance

VENTRICULAR TACHYCARDIA (VT): MONOMORPHIC

* In monomorphic VT, QRS complexes have the same shape and amplitude.

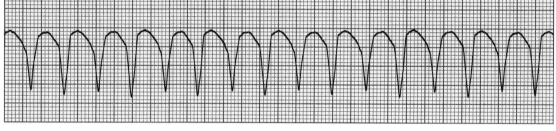

Rate: 100–250 bpm

Rhythm: Regular

P Waves: None or not associated with the QRS

PR Interval: None

QRS: Wide (>0.10 sec), bizarre appearance

 Clinical Tip:

It is important to confirm the presence or absence of pulses because monomorphic VT may be perfusing or nonperfusing.

Clinical Tip:

Monomorphic VT will probably deteriorate into VF or unstable VT if sustained and not treated.

VENTRICULAR TACHYCARDIA (VT): POLYMORPHIC ▪

- In polymorphic VT, QRS complexes vary in shape and amplitude.
- The QT interval is normal or long.

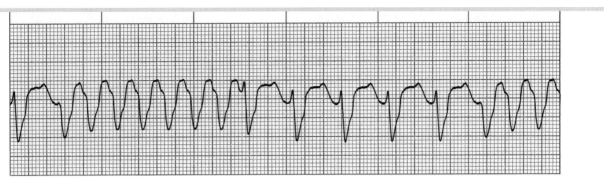

Rate: 100–250 bpm

Rhythm: Regular or irregular

P Waves: None or not associated
with the QRS

PR Interval: None

QRS: Wide (>0.10 sec),
bizarre appearance

 Clinical Tip:

It is important to confirm the presence or absence of pulses because polymorphic VT may be perfusing or
nonperfusing.

Clinical Tip:

Consider electrolyte abnormalities as a possible cause.

TORSADE DE POINTES ▪

- The QRS reverses polarity and the strip shows a spindle effect.
- This rhythm is an unusual variant of polymorphic VT with long QT intervals.
- In French the term means "twisting of points."

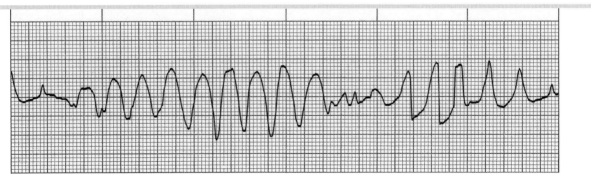

Rate: 200–250 bpm

Rhythm: Irregular

P Waves: None

PR Interval: None

QRS: Wide (>0.10 sec),
bizarre appearance

Clinical Tip:

Torsade de pointes may deteriorate to VF or asystole.

♡ *Clinical Tip:*

Frequent causes are drugs that prolong QT interval, and electrolyte abnormalities such as hypomagnesemia.

VENTRICULAR FIBRILLATION (VF)

• Chaotic electrical activity occurs with no ventricular depolarization or contraction.

The amplitude and frequency of the fibrillatory activity can be used to define the type of fibrillation as coarse, medium, or fine. Small baseline undulations are considered fine; large ones are coarse.

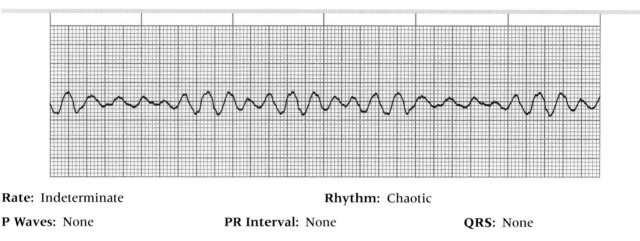

Rate: Indeterminate   **Rhythm:** Chaotic

P Waves: None   **PR Interval:** None   **QRS:** None

♡ *Clinical Tip:*

There is no pulse or cardiac output. Rapid intervention is critical. The longer the delay, the less the chance of conversion.

PULSELESS ELECTRICAL ACTIVITY (PEA)

• The monitor shows an identifiable electrical rhythm, but no pulse is detected.
• The rhythm may be sinus, atrial, junctional, or ventricular.
• PEA is also called electromechanical dissociation (EMD).

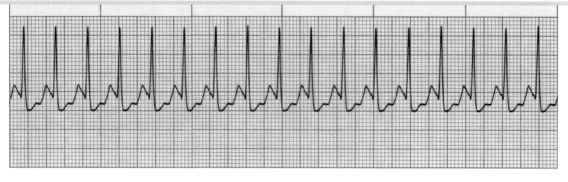

Rate: Reflects underlying rhythm   **Rhythm:** Reflects underlying rhythm

P Waves: Reflect underlying   **PR Interval:** Reflects underlying   **QRS:** Reflects underlying
rhythm   rhythm   rhythm

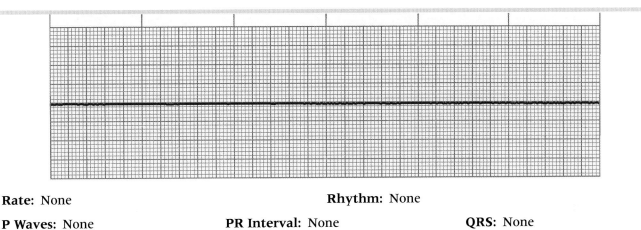

Clinical Tip:

Potential causes of PEA are trauma, tension pneumothorax, thrombosis (pulmonary or coronary), cardiac tamponade, toxins, hypo- or hyperkalemia, hypovolemia, hypoxia, hypoglycemia, hypothermia, and hydrogen ion (acidosis).

ASYSTOLE

• Electrical activity in the ventricles is completely absent.

Rate: None   **Rhythm:** None

P Waves: None   **PR Interval:** None   **QRS:** None

Clinical Tip:

Rule out other causes such as loose leads, no power, or signal gain too low.

Clinical Tip:

Seek to identify the underlying cause as in PEA. Also, search to identify underlying VF.

ECG PRACTICE STRIPS

For instructions on analyzing these practice strips, please see the guidelines given at the end of Chapter 2.

ECG 6•1

Rate: _____   **Rhythm:** _____

P Waves: _____   **PR Interval:** _____   **QRS:** _____

Interpretation: _____

ECG 6•2

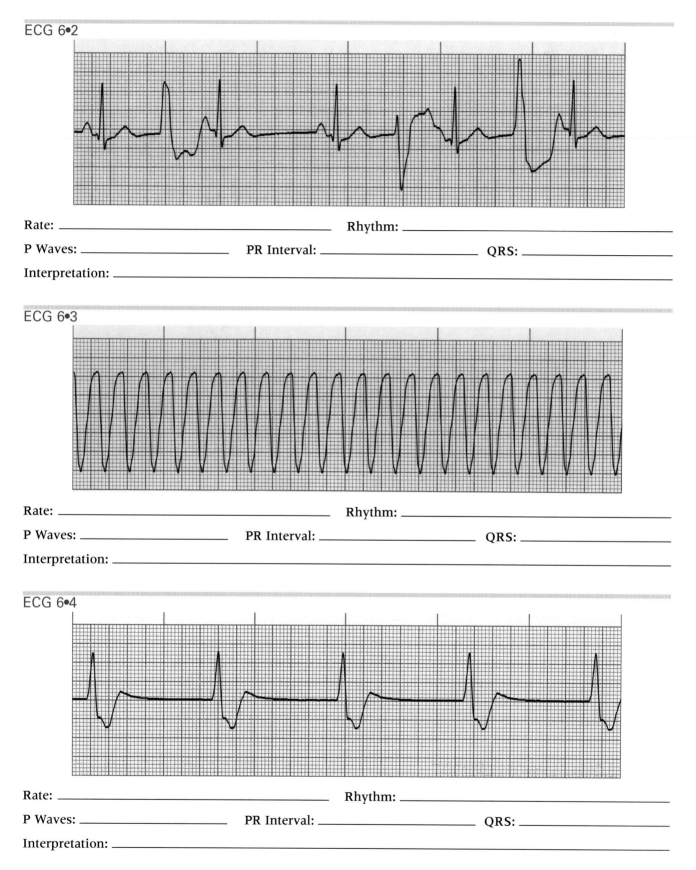

Rate: _____ Rhythm: _____

P Waves: _____ PR Interval: _____ QRS: _____

Interpretation: _____

ECG 6•3

Rate: _____ Rhythm: _____

P Waves: _____ PR Interval: _____ QRS: _____

Interpretation: _____

ECG 6•4

Rate: _____ Rhythm: _____

P Waves: _____ PR Interval: _____ QRS: _____

Interpretation: _____

ECG 6•5

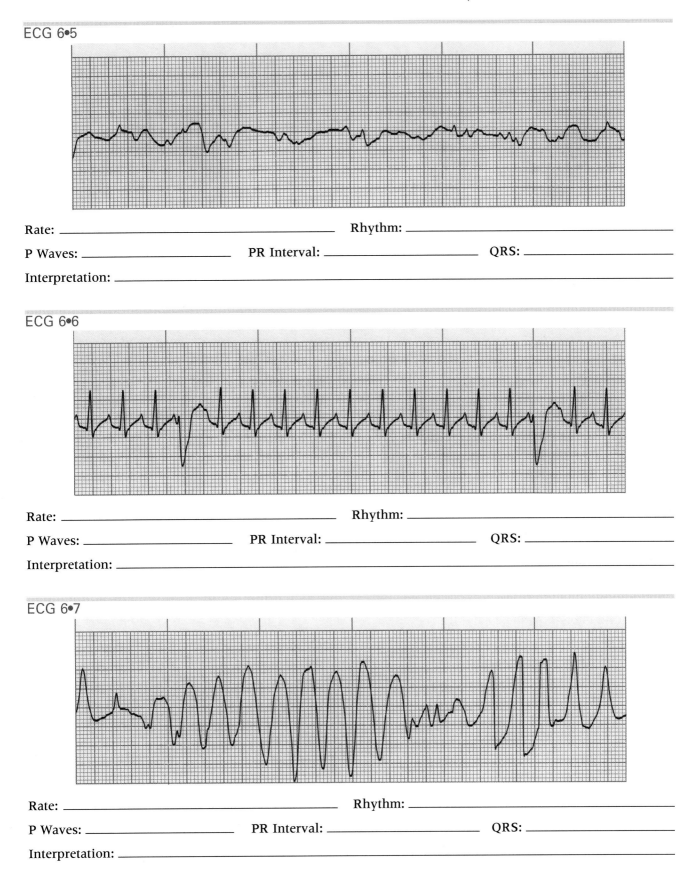

Rate: _____ Rhythm: _____

P Waves: _____ PR Interval: _____ QRS: _____

Interpretation: _____

ECG 6•6

Rate: _____ Rhythm: _____

P Waves: _____ PR Interval: _____ QRS: _____

Interpretation: _____

ECG 6•7

Rate: _____ Rhythm: _____

P Waves: _____ PR Interval: _____ QRS: _____

Interpretation: _____

ECG 6•8

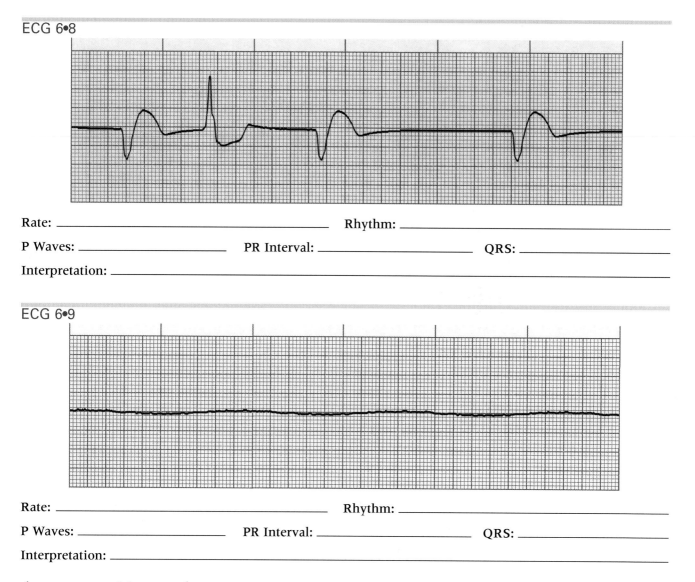

Rate: _____ Rhythm: _____

P Waves: _____ PR Interval: _____ QRS: _____

Interpretation: _____

ECG 6•9

Rate: _____ Rhythm: _____

P Waves: _____ PR Interval: _____ QRS: _____

Interpretation: _____

Answers to Chapter 6

ECG PRACTICE STRIPS

■ ECG 6•1
Rate: 167 bpm
Rhythm: Regular
P Waves: None
PR Interval: None
QRS: Wide—greater than 0.10 sec
Interpretation: Ventricular tachycardia—
    monomorphic

■ ECG 6•2
Rate: 80 bpm (counting PVCs), 41 bpm in under-
    lying rate
Rhythm: Irregular
P Waves: Normal
PR Interval: 0.16 sec
QRS: 0.10 sec
Interpretation: Sinus bradycardia with interpolated
    multiform PVCs

■ ECG 6•3
Rate: 214 bpm
Rhythm: Regular
P Waves: None
PR Interval: None
QRS: Wide—greater than 0.10 sec
Interpretation: Ventricular tachycardia—
    monomorphic

■ ECG 6•4
Rate: 43 bpm
Rhythm: Regular
P Waves: None
PR Interval: None
QRS: Wide—greater than 0.10 sec
Interpretation: Accelerated idioventricular
    rhythm

■ ECG 6•5
Rate: Indeterminate
Rhythm: Chaotic
P Waves: None
PR Interval: None
QRS: None
Interpretation: Ventricular fibrillation

■ ECG 6•6
Rate: 170 bpm (counting PVCs), 150 bpm in under-
  lying rate
Rhythm: Irregular
P Waves: Buried in T wave
PR Interval: Not measurable
QRS: 0.10 sec
Interpretation: Supraventricular tachycardia with
  two uniform PVCs at beats 4 and 15

■ ECG 6•7
Rate: Indeterminate
Rhythm: Irregular
P Waves: None
PR Interval: None
QRS: Wide—greater than 0.10 sec
Interpretation: Torsade de pointes

■ ECG 6•8
Rate: 40 bpm
Rhythm: Irregular
P Waves: None
PR Interval: None
QRS: Wide—greater than 0.10 sec
Interpretation: Idioventricular rhythm with
  one PVC at beat 2

■ ECG 6•9
Rate: None
Rhythm: None
P Waves: None
PR Interval: None
QRS: None
Interpretation: Asystole

Chapter 7

Atrioventricular and Bundle Branch Blocks

Atrioventricular (AV) blocks reflect delay or interruption of impulses through the AV junction due to disease in this region. They are traditionally divided into three categories: first, second, and third degree. This pathological block, caused by such conditions as ischemia, necrosis, degenerative diseases of the conduction system, and drug toxicity, is different from the physiological AV block that occurs in atrial flutter and fibrillation.

Another disorder, involving bundle branch conduction through the ventricles, is bundle branch block (BBB). The problem does not occur until the signal is conducted through the ventricles, although the block originates above them.

All ECG strips, including the practice strips, were recorded in lead II.

FIRST-DEGREE AV BLOCK

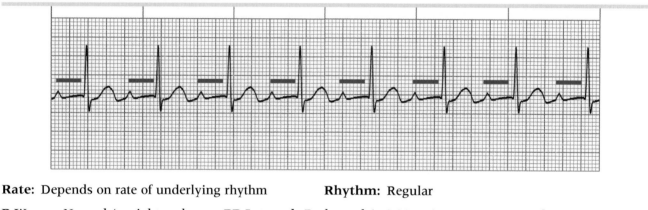

Rate: Depends on rate of underlying rhythm   **Rhythm:** Regular

P Waves: Normal (upright and uniform)   **PR Interval:** Prolonged (>0.20 sec)   **QRS:** Normal (0.06–0.10 sec)

Clinical Tip:

Usually a first-degree AV block is benign, but if associated with an acute MI it may lead to further AV defects.

Clinical Tip:

Often AV block is caused by medications that prolong AV conduction; these include digoxin, calcium channel blockers, and beta blockers.

SECOND-DEGREE AV BLOCK: TYPE I (MOBITZ I OR WENCKEBACH) ▪

- PR intervals become progressively longer until one P wave is totally blocked and produces no QRS complex. After a pause, during which the AV node recovers, this cycle is repeated.

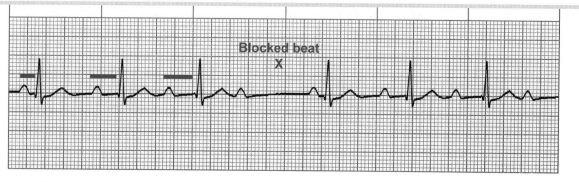

Rate: Depends on rate of underlying rhythm   **Rhythm:** Atrial: regular; ventricular: irregular

P Waves: Normal (upright and uniform), more P waves than QRS   **PR Interval:** Progressively longer until one P wave is blocked and a QRS is dropped   **QRS:** Normal (0.06–0.10 sec)

♡ | *Clinical Tip:*

This rhythm may be caused by medication such as beta blockers, digoxin, and calcium channel blockers. Ischemia involving the right coronary artery is another cause.

SECOND-DEGREE AV BLOCK: TYPE II (MOBITZ II) ▪

- Conduction ratio (P waves to QRS complexes) is commonly 2:1, 3:1, 4:1, or variable.
- QRS complexes are usually wide because this block usually involves both bundle branches.

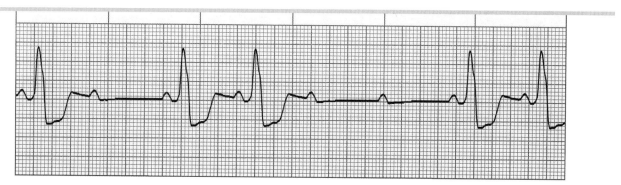

Rate: Atrial: usually 60–100 bpm; ventricular: slower than atrial rate   **Rhythm:** Atrial regular and ventricular may be regular or irregular

P Waves: Normal (upright and uniform); more P waves than QRSs   **PR Interval:** Normal or prolonged but constant   **QRS:** May be normal, but usually wide (>0.10 sec) if the bundle branches are involved

♡ | *Clinical Tip:*

Resulting bradycardia can compromise cardiac output and lead to complete AV block. This rhythm often occurs with cardiac ischemia or an MI.

THIRD-DEGREE AV BLOCK ▧

- Conduction between the atria and the ventricles is totally absent because of complete electrical block at or below the AV node. This is known as AV dissociation.
- "Complete heart block" is another name for this rhythm.

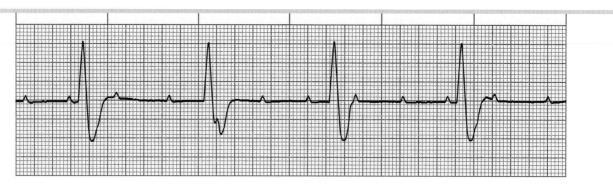

Rate: Atrial: 60–100 bpm; ventricular: 40–60 bpm if escape focus is junctional, <40 bpm if escape focus is ventricular

Rhythm: Usually regular, but atria and ventricles act independently

P Waves: Normal (upright and uniform); may be superimposed on QRS complexes or T waves

PR Interval: Varies greatly

QRS: Normal if ventricles are activated by junctional escape focus; wide if escape focus is ventricular

♡ | *Clinical Tip:*

Third-degree AV block may be associated with ischemia involving the left coronary arteries.

BUNDLE BRANCH BLOCK (BBB) ▧

- Either the left or the right ventricle may depolarize late, creating a "wide" or "notched" QRS complex.

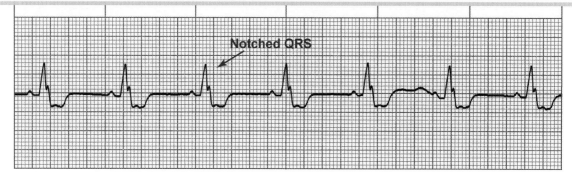

Notched QRS

Rate: Depends on rate of underlying rhythm

Rhythm: Regular

P Waves: Normal (upright and uniform)

PR Interval: Normal (0.12–0.20 sec)

QRS: Wide (>0.10 sec) with or without a notched appearance

♡ | *Clinical Tip:*

Bundle branch block commonly occurs in coronary artery disease.

ECG PRACTICE STRIPS ▪

For instructions on analyzing these practice strips, please see the guidelines given at the end of Chapter 2.

ECG 7•1

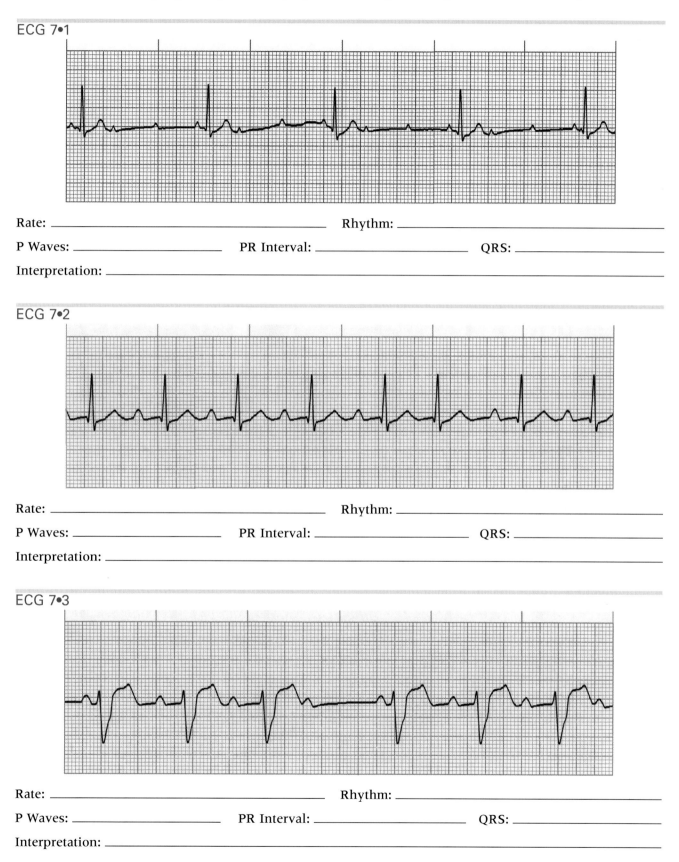

Rate: _____ Rhythm: _____

P Waves: _____ PR Interval: _____ QRS: _____

Interpretation: _____

ECG 7•2

Rate: _____ Rhythm: _____

P Waves: _____ PR Interval: _____ QRS: _____

Interpretation: _____

ECG 7•3

Rate: _____ Rhythm: _____

P Waves: _____ PR Interval: _____ QRS: _____

Interpretation: _____

ECG 7•4

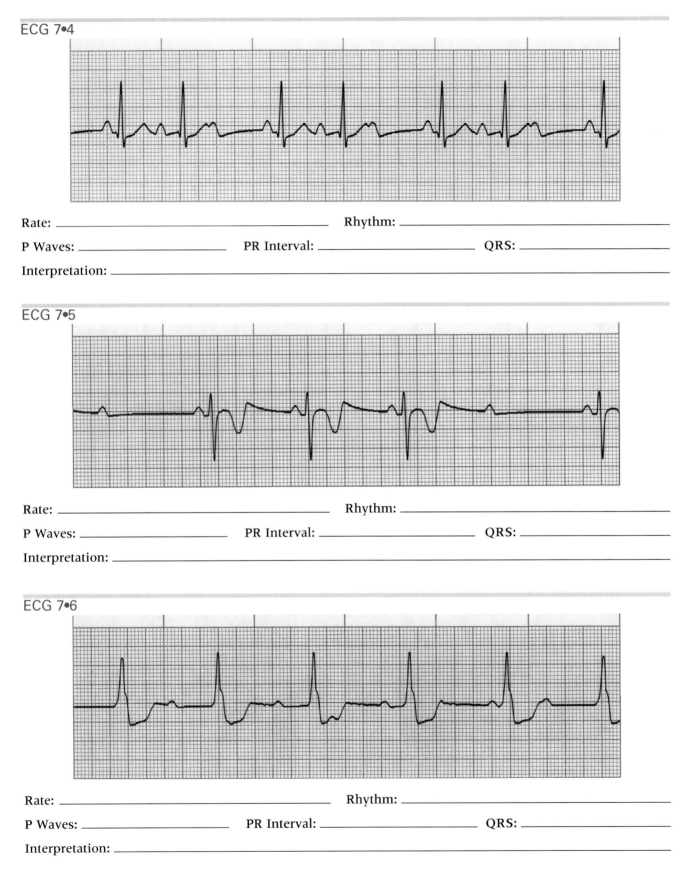

Rate: _____   Rhythm: _____

P Waves: _____   PR Interval: _____   QRS: _____

Interpretation: _____

ECG 7•5

Rate: _____   Rhythm: _____

P Waves: _____   PR Interval: _____   QRS: _____

Interpretation: _____

ECG 7•6

Rate: _____   Rhythm: _____

P Waves: _____   PR Interval: _____   QRS: _____

Interpretation: _____

ECG 7•7

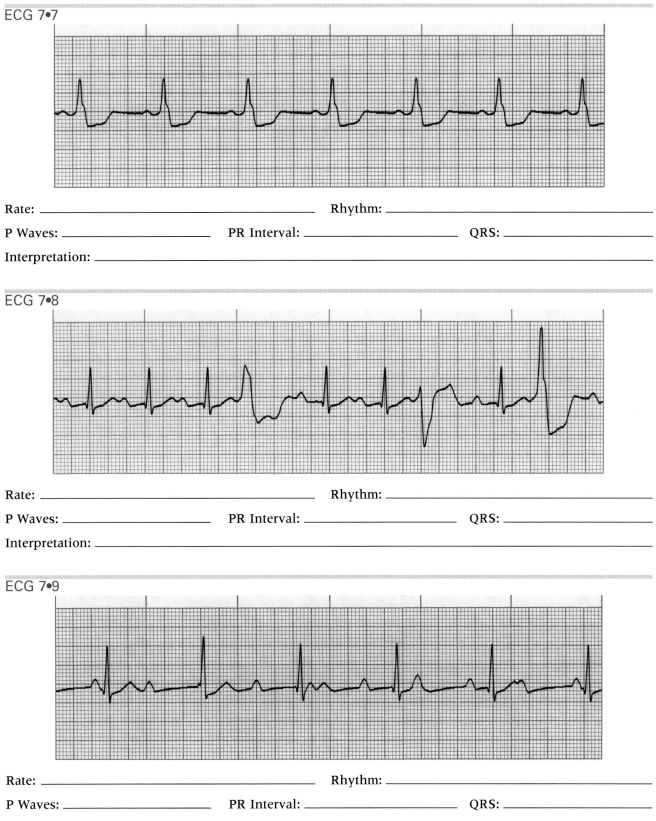

Rate: _____ Rhythm: _____

P Waves: _____ PR Interval: _____ QRS: _____

Interpretation: _____

ECG 7•8

Rate: _____ Rhythm: _____

P Waves: _____ PR Interval: _____ QRS: _____

Interpretation: _____

ECG 7•9

Rate: _____ Rhythm: _____

P Waves: _____ PR Interval: _____ QRS: _____

Interpretation: _____

Answers to Chapter 7

ECG PRACTICE STRIPS ▪

▪ ECG 7•1
Rate: Atrial 125 bpm, ventricular 44 bpm
Rhythm: Atrial regular, ventricular regular
P Waves: Normal
PR Interval: 0.12 sec and constant
QRS: 0.10 sec
Interpretation: Second-degree AV block
    Type II, 3:1 conduction

▪ ECG 7•2
Rate: 80 bpm
Rhythm: Irregular
P Waves: Normal
PR Interval: 0.32 sec
QRS: 0.10 sec
Interpretation: First-degree AV block with a PJC at
    beat 6

▪ ECG 7•3
Rate: 60 bpm
Rhythm: Irregular
P Waves: Normal
PR Interval: Progressive lengthening
QRS: Wide—greater than 0.10 sec
Interpretation: Second-degree AV
    block Type I (Wenckebach) with
    wide QRS

▪ ECG 7•4
Rate: 70 bpm
Rhythm: Irregular
P Waves: Normal
PR Interval: Progressive lengthening
QRS: 0.10 sec
Interpretation: Second-degree AV block
    Type I (Wenckebach)

▪ ECG 7•5
Rate: 40 bpm
Rhythm: Irregular
P Waves: Normal
PR Interval: 0.16 sec and constant
QRS: 0.08 sec
Interpretation: Second-degree AV block Type II with
    inverted T waves

▪ ECG 7•6
Rate: 56 bpm
Rhythm: Regular
P Waves: Normal but not associated with QRS
PR Interval: Variable
QRS: Wide—greater than 0.10 sec with notched
    appearance
Interpretation: Third-degree AV block with a bundle
    branch block

▪ ECG 7•7
Rate: 65 bpm
Rhythm: Regular
P Waves: Normal
PR Interval: 0.20 sec
QRS: 0.16 sec with notched appearance
Interpretation: Normal sinus rhythm with a bundle
    branch block

▪ ECG 7•8
Rate: 90 bpm (counting PVCs), 94 in underlying rate
Rhythm: Irregular
P Waves: Normal
PR Interval: 0.28 sec
QRS: 0.10 sec
Interpretation: Normal sinus rhythm with first-
    degree AV block with multiform PVCs at beats
    4, 7, and 9

▪ ECG 7•9
Rate: 56 bpm
Rhythm: Regular
P Waves: Normal but not associated with QRS
PR Interval: Variable
QRS: 0.10 sec
Interpretation: Third-degree AV block

Chapter 8

Artificial Cardiac Pacemakers

As you found in Chapter 1, myocardial fibers possess highly specialized electrical properties. The components of automaticity, excitability, and conductivity allow a certain number of specialized cardiac cells, called pacemaker cells, to go into action. These cells actually do pace the heart. Each specialized area of the heart has its own intrinsic rate:

- Sinoatrial node: The dominant pacemaker of the heart. Intrinsic rate is 60–100 bpm.
- Atrioventricular node: Intrinsic rate is 40–60 bpm.
- Purkinje system: The bundle branches terminate with this network of fibers. They spread electrical impulses rapidly throughout the ventricular walls. Intrinsic rate is 20–40 bpm.

People with strong, healthy hearts, such as athletes, can sustain an adequate blood flow in their cardiovascular system with heart rates as low as 50 to 60 bpm. But in a person with an unhealthy heart, the natural pacemakers can discharge too slowly or stop altogether. A slow heart rate may be caused by factors such as coronary artery disease or by the side effects of certain medications.

Heart failure can result from an insufficient amount of oxygenated blood being pumped throughout the cardiovascular system. The person begins to suffer from hypotension, bradycardia, diaphoresis, decreased level of consciousness, and possibly an AV block. In this case an artificial pacemaker can save a person's life.

ARTIFICIAL PACEMAKER

An artificial cardiac pacemaker is a device used to electronically stimulate the heart in place of the heart's own natural pacemakers and conduction system. It is composed of one or more electrodes implanted in the heart and connected to a power source that generates regular, timed stimuli. It may be preset to stimulate the heart's activity continuously or intermittently.

Some of the conditions for insertion of a pacemaker are continuous or intermittent third-degree AV block, second-degree AV block Type II, chronic A-fib with bradycardic ventricular response, and sick sinus syndrome (a condition marked by sinus block, severe sinus bradycardia, or alternating periods of bradycardia and tachycardia).

Several types of pacemakers exist, but the most common types used for the conditions just described are the ventricular and dual-chambered pacemakers. Ventricular pacemakers stimulate only the ventricle, while dual-chambered types stimulate both the atrium and ventricle, if needed. The following bullet points explain terms you will find associated with artificial cardiac pacemakers.

Temporary Pacemaker

- A temporary pacemaker is commonly used in an emergency. It paces the heart through epicardial, transvenous, or transcutaneous routes. The pulse generator is located externally. Indications may include symptomatic bradycardia, AV heart block (second- degree Type II or third degree), change in mental status, or pulmonary edema.

Permanent Pacemaker

- A permanent pacemaker may be indicated if there is a chronic or intermittent AV block, sinus arrest, or sick sinus syndrome. It is surgically implanted, usually under local anesthesia. Its circuitry is sealed in an airtight case and the pacemaker is implanted in the body. It uses sensing and pacing device leads.

Single-Chamber Pacemaker

- One lead is placed in the heart and paces a single chamber (either atrium or ventricle).

Table 8.1 ■ PACEMAKER CODES

Chamber Paced	Chamber Sensed	Response to Sensing	Programmable Functions	Response to Tachycardia
A = Atrium V = Ventricle D = Dual (atrium and ventricle) O = None	A = Atrium V = Ventricle D = Dual (atrium and ventricle) O = None	T = Triggers pacing I = Inhibits pacing D = (triggers and inhibits) O = None	P = Basic programs (rate and output) M = Multiple programs C = Communication (i.e., telemetry) R = Rate response O = None	P = Pacing S = Shock D = Dual (pace and shock) O = None

Dual-Chamber Pacemaker

• One lead is placed in the right atrium and the other in the right ventricle. The atrial electrode generates a spike that should be followed by a P wave, and the ventricular electrode generates a spike followed by a wide QRS complex.

PACEMAKER MODES

• Fixed rate (asynchronous): Discharges at a preset rate (usually 70–80 bpm) regardless of the patient's own electrical activity.
• Demand (synchronous): Discharges only when the patient's heart rate drops below the pacemaker's preset (base) rate.

 Clinical Tip:

Patients with pacemakers may receive defibrillation, but avoid placing the defibrillator paddles or pads less than 5 inches from the pacemaker battery pack.

UNDERSTANDING PACEMAKER CODES

An international code was developed in 1974 to identify the preprogrammed pacing, sensing, and response functions of a permanent pacemaker. The code initially consisted of three letters, but in 1980 the system was modified with the addition of two more letters (designating two more functions). The first three letters are the most commonly known because they are used for symptomatic bradycardia.

Understanding the codes used in a permanent pacemaker help to ensure that the pacemaker is set properly. A simple classification of the five-code system is described in TABLE 8-1.

ARTIFICIAL PACEMAKER RHYTHM

• An artificial pacemaker may vary in its rate, rhythm, P waves, P-R interval, and QRS complex.

Rate: Varies according to preset pacemaker rate.

Rhythm: Regular for asynchronous pacemaker; irregular for demand pacemaker unless 100% paced with no intrinsic beats.

P waves: None produced by ventricular pacemaker. Sinus P waves may be seen but are unrelated to QRS. Atrial or dual-chamber pacemaker should have P waves following each atrial spike.

P-R interval: None for ventricular pacer. Atrial or dual-chamber pacemaker produces constant PR intervals.

QRS: Wide (greater than 0.10 sec) following each ventricular spike in a pacemaker rhythm. The patient's own electrical activity may generate a QRS complex that looks different from the paced QRSs. If atrially paced only, the QRS complex may be within normal limits.

 Clinical Tip:

Once an impulse is generated by the pacemaker it appears as a spike, either above or below the baseline (isoelectric line), on the ECG. The spike indicates that the pacemaker has fired.

SINGLE-CHAMBER PACEMAKER RHYTHM—ATRIAL

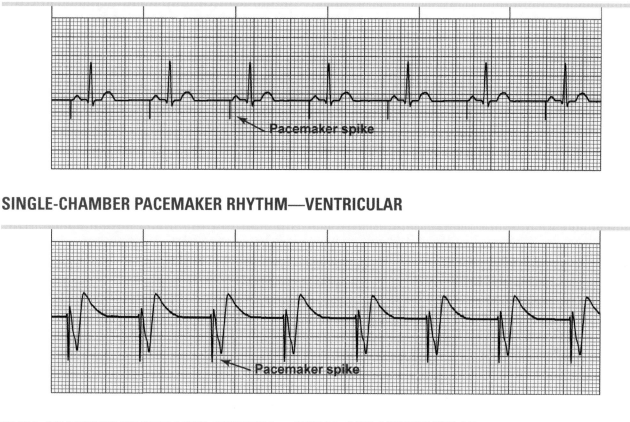

SINGLE-CHAMBER PACEMAKER RHYTHM—VENTRICULAR

DUAL-CHAMBER PACEMAKER RHYTHM—ATRIAL AND VENTRICULAR

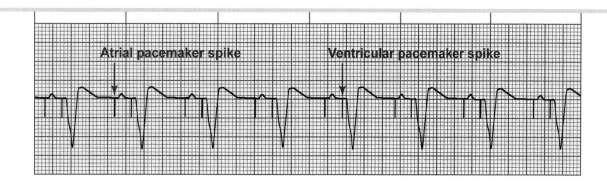

PACEMAKER MALFUNCTIONS

At times a pacemaker may have a malfunction. Common problems are listed in TABLE 8-2.

Clinical Tip:

A pacemaker is said to be in capture when a spike produces an ECG wave or complex.

Table 8.2 ■ PACEMAKER MALFUNCTIONS

Malfunction	Reason
Failure to pace	Pacemaker spikes are absent. The cause may be a dead battery, a disruption in the connecting wires, or improper programming.
Failure to capture	Pacemaker spikes are present, but no P wave or QRS follows the spike. Turning up the pacemaker's voltage often corrects this problem. Lead wires should also be checked—a dislodged or broken lead wire may deliver some, but not all, of the needed energy.
Failure to sense	The pacemaker fires because it fails to detect the heart's intrinsic beats, resulting in abnormal complexes. The cause may be a dead battery, decrease of P wave or QRS voltage, or damage to a pacing lead wire. One serious potential consequence may be an R on T phenomenon.
Oversensing	The pacemaker may be too sensitive and misinterpret muscle movement or other events in the cardiac cycle as depolarization. This error resets the pacemaker inappropriately, increasing the amount of time before the next discharge.

FAILURE TO CAPTURE

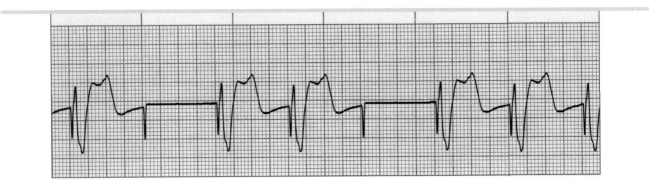

FAILURE TO SENSE

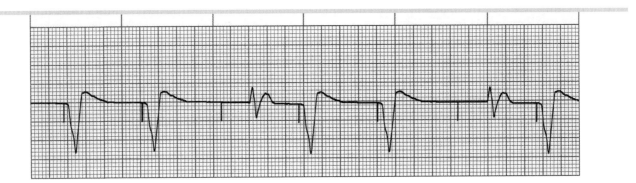

OVERSENSING

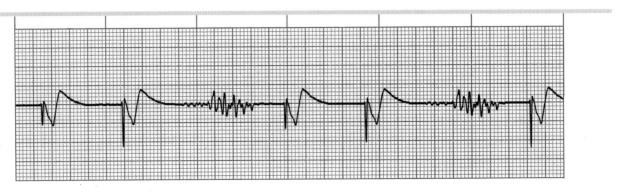

ECG PRACTICE STRIPS ▪

For instructions on analyzing these practice strips, please see the guidelines given at the end of Chapter 2.

ECG 8•1

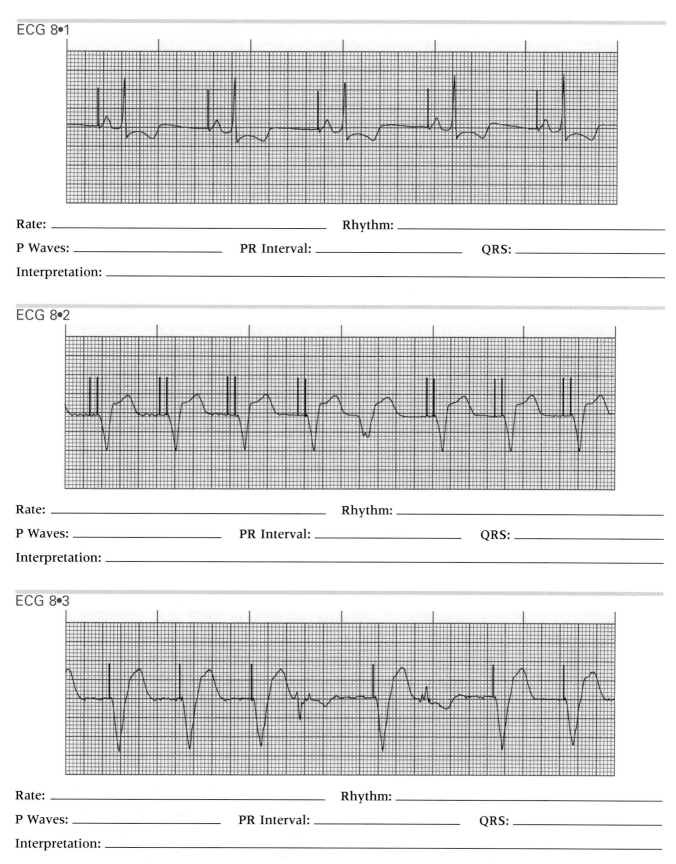

Rate: _____ Rhythm: _____

P Waves: _____ PR Interval: _____ QRS: _____

Interpretation: _____

ECG 8•2

Rate: _____ Rhythm: _____

P Waves: _____ PR Interval: _____ QRS: _____

Interpretation: _____

ECG 8•3

Rate: _____ Rhythm: _____

P Waves: _____ PR Interval: _____ QRS: _____

Interpretation: _____

ECG 8•4

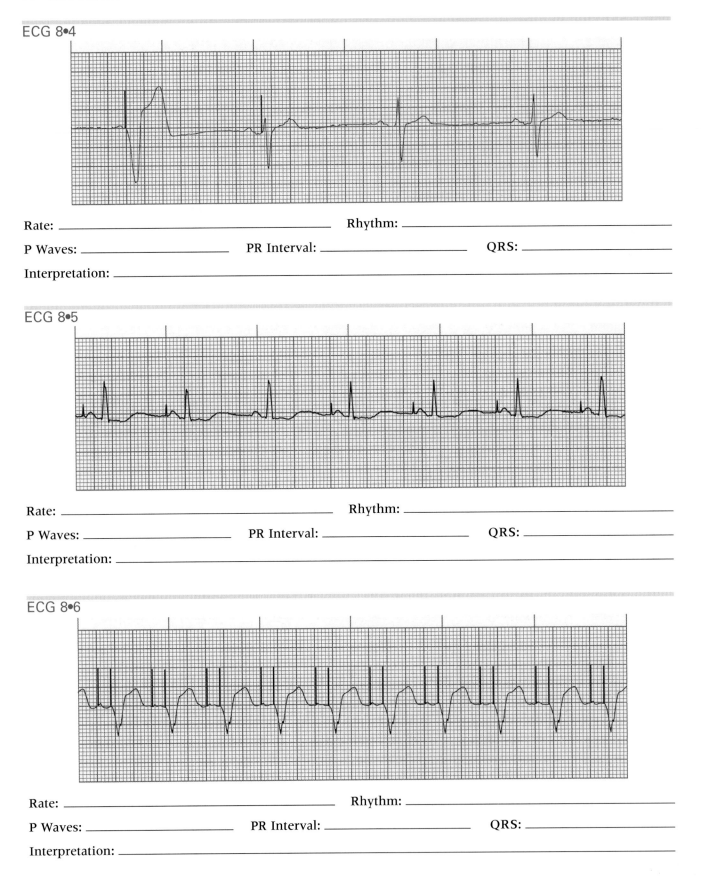

Rate: _____   Rhythm: _____

P Waves: _____   PR Interval: _____   QRS: _____

Interpretation: _____

ECG 8•5

Rate: _____   Rhythm: _____

P Waves: _____   PR Interval: _____   QRS: _____

Interpretation: _____

ECG 8•6

Rate: _____   Rhythm: _____

P Waves: _____   PR Interval: _____   QRS: _____

Interpretation: _____

ECG 8•7

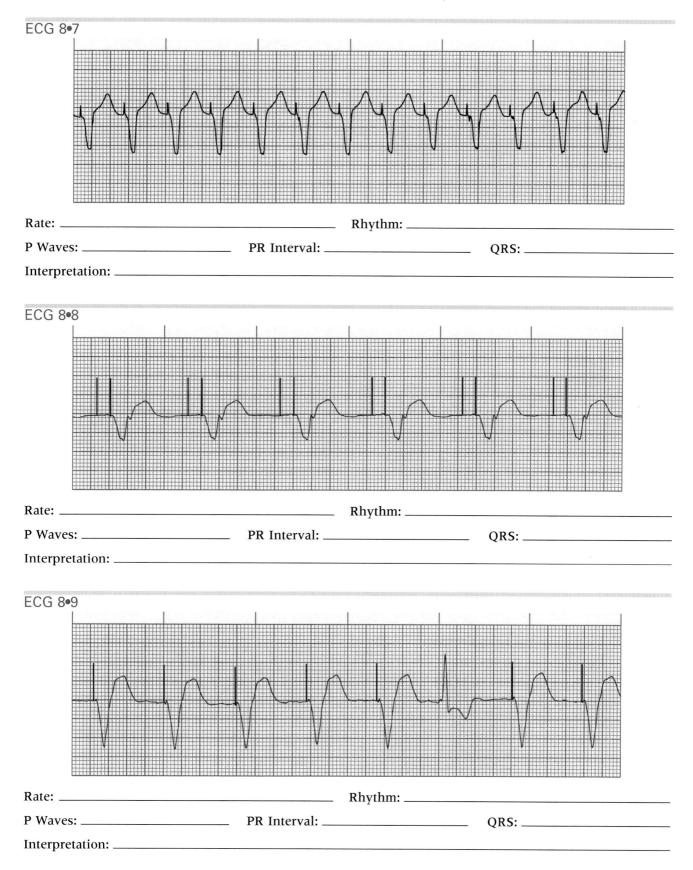

Rate: _____   Rhythm: _____

P Waves: _____   PR Interval: _____   QRS: _____

Interpretation: _____

ECG 8•8

Rate: _____   Rhythm: _____

P Waves: _____   PR Interval: _____   QRS: _____

Interpretation: _____

ECG 8•9

Rate: _____   Rhythm: _____

P Waves: _____   PR Interval: _____   QRS: _____

Interpretation: _____

Answers to Chapter 8

ECG PRACTICE STRIPS ■

■ ECG 8•1
Rate: 50 bpm
Rhythm: Regular
P Waves: Normal following pacemaker
   spike
PR Interval: 0.20 sec
QRS: 0.10 sec
Interpretation: Pacemaker—atrial, with
   ST segment depression and inverted
   T waves

■ ECG 8•2
Rate: 80 bpm
Rhythm: Irregular
P Waves: None following pacemaker spike
PR Interval: None
QRS: Wide—greater than 0.10 sec following
   pacemaker spike
Interpretation: Pacemaker—atrial and ventri-
   cular, with one PVC at beat 5. Notice that
   there is no P wave generated with the atrial
   spike. This would be a failure to capture
   with the atrial spike.

■ ECG 8•3
Rate: 80 bpm
Rhythm: Irregular
P Waves: None
PR Interval: None
QRS: Wide—greater than 0.10 sec following
   pacemaker spike
Interpretation: Pacemaker—ventricular, with
   PVCs at beats 4 and 6

■ ECG 8•4
Rate: 40 bpm
Rhythm: Regular
P Waves: Normal at beats 2 through 4
PR Interval: 0.20 sec at beats 2 through 4
QRS: Wide—greater than 0.10 sec at beat
   1; 0.10 sec at beats 2 through 4
Interpretation: Pacemaker—ventricular
   evolving to sinus complexes, with no
   ventricular pacing, at beats 3 and 4

■ ECG 8•5
Rate: 65 bpm
Rhythm: Regular
P Waves: Normal
PR Interval: 0.16 sec
QRS: 0.10 sec
Interpretation: Pacemaker—atrial, with
   nonpaced P wave at beat 3

■ ECG 8•6
Rate: 100 bpm
Rhythm: Regular
P Waves: Normal with low voltage following
   pacemaker spike
PR Interval: 0.16 sec
QRS: Wide—greater than 0.10 sec with notched
   appearance following pacemaker spike
Interpretation: Pacemaker—atrial and ventricular

■ ECG 8•7
Rate: 125 bpm
Rhythm: Regular
P Waves: None
PR Interval: None
QRS: Wide—greater than 0.10 sec following pace-
   maker spike
Interpretation: Pacemaker—ventricular

■ ECG 8•8
Rate: 60 bpm
Rhythm: Regular
P Waves: None following pacemaker spike
PR Interval: None
QRS: Wide—greater than 0.10 sec following pace-
   maker spike
Interpretation: Pacemaker—atrial and ventricular,
   with no atrial conduction. The atrial spike shows
   failure to capture.

■ ECG 8•9
Rate: 80 bpm
Rhythm: Irregular
P Waves: None
PR Interval: None
QRS: Wide—greater than 0.10 sec following pace-
   maker spike
Interpretation: Pacemaker—ventricular, with one
   junctional complex with ST segment depression
   and inverted T wave at beat 6

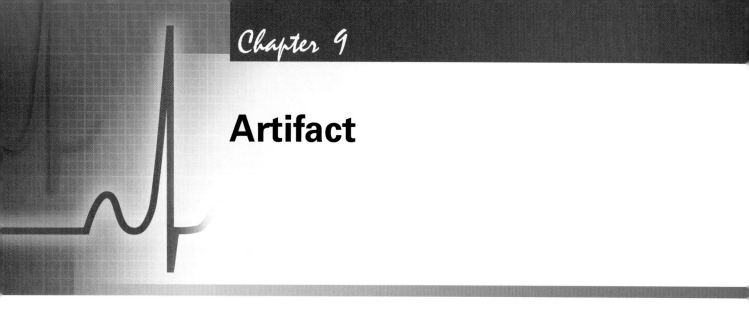

Chapter 9

Artifact

In an ECG tracing, waves, segments, and complexes are produced by the heart's electrical activity. However, deflections are occasionally produced by other influences, known as ECG artifact. Some common causes of artifact are loose electrodes; patient movement and muscle tremors; ECG calibration marks; 60-cycle electrical interference; and malfunction of the ECG machine, patient cable, or lead wires. Artifact can complicate the interpretation of an ECG tracing, so it is important to recognize and eliminate it whenever possible.

LOOSE ELECTRICAL CONNECTION ■

• Bizarre, irregular deflections in the baseline (isoelectric line) of the ECG tracing may be caused by poor electrical contact, a loose electrode, or a broken wire. Make sure all the electrical and patient cable connections are secure.

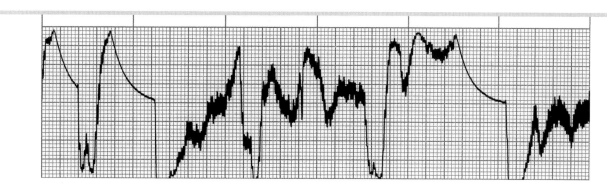

VARIATION WITH RESPIRATION ■

• Patient movement may occur with respiration. The resulting undulations move the entire tracing up and down, reflecting the rhythm of the patient's breathing.

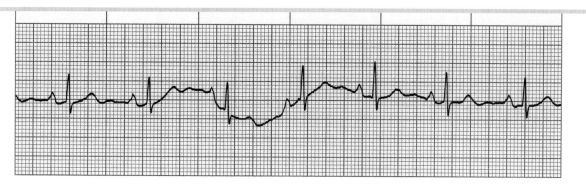

60-CYCLE INTERFERENCE ▪

- Improperly grounded electrical equipment or other electrical interference can cause a phenomenon called 60-cycle interference. If this occurs, check to make sure all electrical equipment is properly grounded and that the patient cable electrical connections are clean.

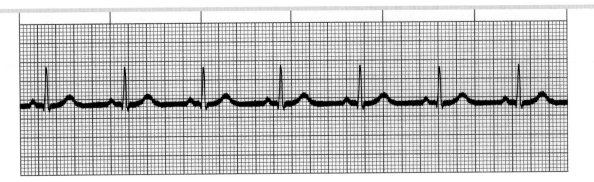

MUSCLE ARTIFACT ▪

- Shivering, tense muscles, seizures, patient movement, and disorders such as Parkinson's disease may cause muscle tremor artifact.

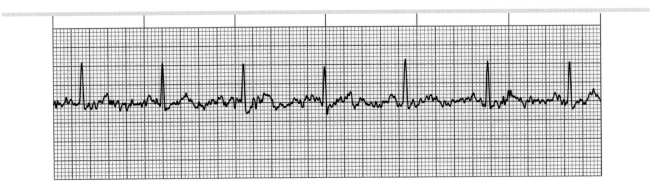

♥ | *Clinical Tip:*
Never confuse muscle artifact with A-fib if the rhythm is regular.

ECG PRACTICE STRIPS ▪

For instructions on analyzing these practice strips, please see the guidelines given at the end of Chapter 2.

ECG 9•1

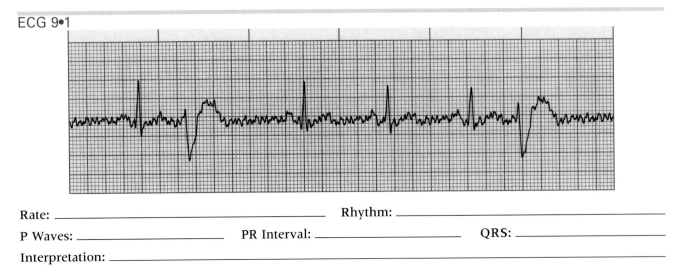

Rate: _____   Rhythm: _____

P Waves: _____   PR Interval: _____   QRS: _____

Interpretation: _____

72

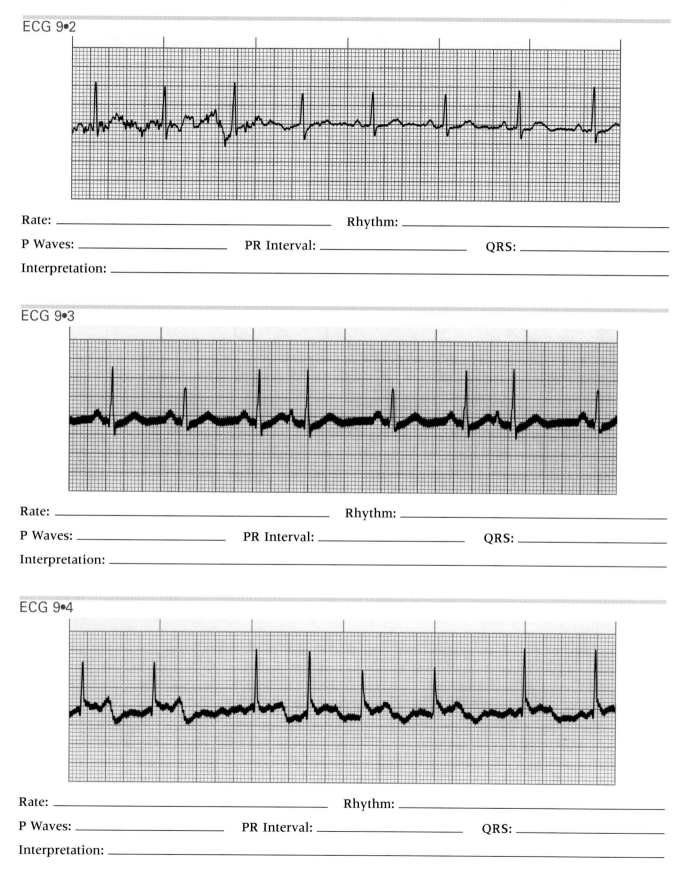

ECG 9•2

Rate: _____ Rhythm: _____

P Waves: _____ PR Interval: _____ QRS: _____

Interpretation: _____

ECG 9•3

Rate: _____ Rhythm: _____

P Waves: _____ PR Interval: _____ QRS: _____

Interpretation: _____

ECG 9•4

Rate: _____ Rhythm: _____

P Waves: _____ PR Interval: _____ QRS: _____

Interpretation: _____

ECG 9•5

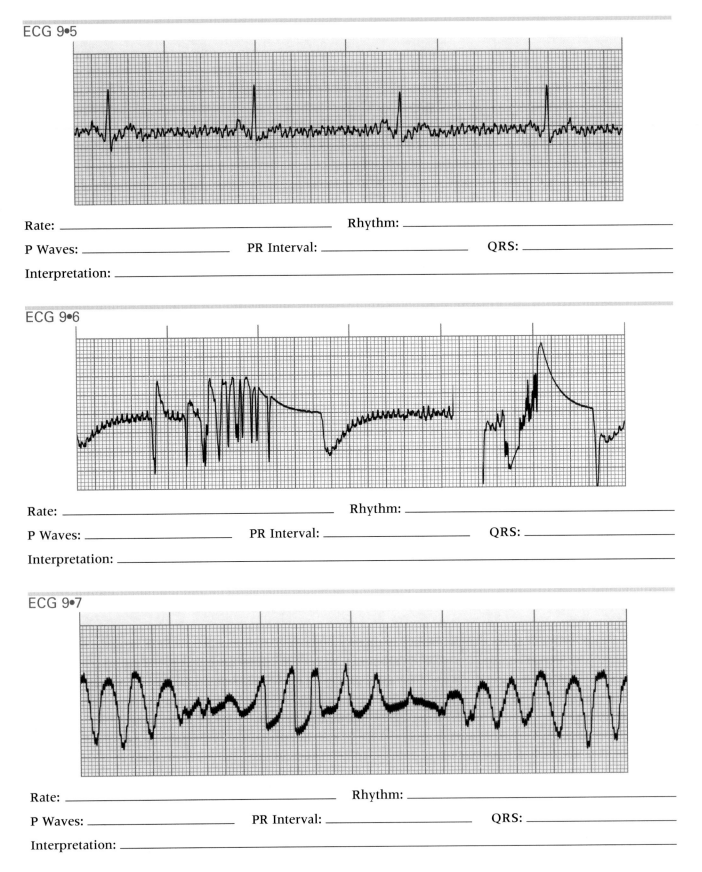

Rate: _____   Rhythm: _____

P Waves: _____   PR Interval: _____   QRS: _____

Interpretation: _____

ECG 9•6

Rate: _____   Rhythm: _____

P Waves: _____   PR Interval: _____   QRS: _____

Interpretation: _____

ECG 9•7

Rate: _____   Rhythm: _____

P Waves: _____   PR Interval: _____   QRS: _____

Interpretation: _____

ECG 9•8

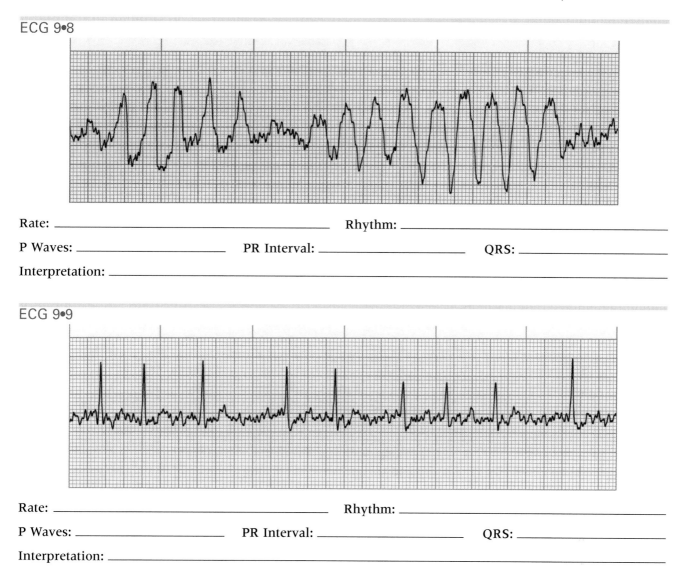

Rate: _____ Rhythm: _____

P Waves: _____ PR Interval: _____ QRS: _____

Interpretation: _____

ECG 9•9

Rate: _____ Rhythm: _____

P Waves: _____ PR Interval: _____ QRS: _____

Interpretation: _____

Answers to Chapter 9

ECG PRACTICE STRIPS ▪

▪ ECG 9•1
Rate: 60 bpm (counting PVCs), 66 bpm in under-lying rate
Rhythm: Irregular
P Waves: Present, but hard to see because of artifact
PR Interval: Not possible to measure
QRS: 0.10 sec
Interpretation: Normal sinus rhythm with uniform PVCs and muscle artifact

▪ ECG 9•2
Rate: 80 bpm
Rhythm: Irregular
P Waves: Normal in beats 5 through 8
PR Interval: 0.16 sec in beats 5 through 8
QRS: 0.10 sec in beats 5 through 8
Interpretation: Normal sinus rhythm beginning with muscle artifact and adjusting to a normal baseline in beats 5 through 8

▪ ECG 9•3
Rate: 80 bpm
Rhythm: Irregular
P Waves: Normal but with artifact
PR Interval: 0.16 sec
QRS: 0.10 sec
Interpretation: Normal sinus rhythm with two PACs at beats 4 and 7 and 60–cycle interference

▪ ECG 9•4
Rate: 80 bpm
Rhythm: Irregular
P Waves: None
PR Interval: None
QRS: 0.10 sec
Interpretation: Atrial fibrillation with 60-cycle interference

■ ECG 9•5

Rate: 38 bpm
Rhythm: Regular
P Waves: Present, but hard to see because of artifact
PR Interval: Not possible to measure
QRS: 0.10 sec
Interpretation: Sinus bradycardia with muscle artifact

■ ECG 9•6

Rate: None
Rhythm: None
P Waves: None
PR Interval: None
QRS: None
Interpretation: Loose electrodes

■ ECG 9•7

Rate: Not possible to measure
Rhythm: Irregular
P Waves: None
PR Interval: None
QRS: Wide—greater than 0.10 sec
Interpretation: Torsade de pointes with 60-cycle
    interference

■ ECG 9•8

Rate: Not possible to measure
Rhythm: Irregular
P Waves: None
PR Interval: None
QRS: Wide—greater than 0.10 sec
Interpretation: Torsade de pointes with
    muscle artifact

■ ECG 9•9

Rate: 90 bpm
Rhythm: Irregular
P Waves: None
PR Interval: None
QRS: 0.10 sec
Interpretation: Atrial fibrillation with muscle
    artifact

Chapter 10

The 12-Lead ECG and Acute Myocardial Infarction

A standard 12-lead ECG provides views of the heart from 12 different angles. This diagnostic test helps to identify pathological conditions, especially bundle branch blocks and T wave changes associated with ischemia, injury, and infarction. The 12-lead ECG also uses ST segment analysis to pinpoint the specific location of a myocardial infarction (MI).

Multiple views give a more comprehensive picture of the heart's electrical activity than a rhythm strip and can be used to assess left ventricular function. Patients with other conditions, such as electrolyte imbalances or adverse conditions caused by certain medications, may also benefit from a 12-lead ECG.

The 12-lead ECG is the type most commonly used in clinical settings. The following list highlights some of its important aspects:

- The 12-lead ECG consists of the six limb leads—I, II, III, aVR, aVL, and aVF—and the six chest leads—V_1, V_2, V_3, V_4, V_5, and V_6.
- The limb leads record electrical activity in the heart's frontal plane. This view shows the middle of the heart from top to bottom. Electrical activity is recorded from the anterior-to-posterior axis.
- The chest leads record electrical activity in the heart's horizontal plane. This transverse view shows the middle of the heart from right to left, dividing it into upper and lower portions. Electrical activity is recorded from either a superior or an inferior approach.
- Measurements are central to 12-lead ECG analysis. The height and depth of waves can offer important diagnostic information in certain conditions, including MI and ventricular hypertrophy.
- The direction of ventricular depolarization is an important factor in determining the axis of the heart.
- In an MI, multiple leads are necessary to recognize its presence and determine its location. If large areas of the heart are affected, the patient can develop cardiogenic shock and fatal arrhythmias.

- ECG signs of an MI are best seen in the reflecting leads—those facing the affected surface of the heart. Reciprocal leads are in the same plane but opposite the area of infarction; they show a "mirror image" of the electrical complex.
- Prehospital EMS systems may use 12-lead ECGs to discover signs of acute MI, such as ST segment elevation, in preparation for in-hospital administration of thrombolytic drugs.
- Once a 12-lead ECG is performed, a 15-lead, or right-sided, ECG may be used for an even more comprehensive view if the right ventricle or the posterior portion of the heart appears to be affected.

Clinical Tip:

Always compare the patient's current 12-lead ECG with the previous one.

Clinical Tip:

Monitor the patient, not just the ECG, for clinical improvement.

TROUBLESHOOTING ECG PROBLEMS

Without proper assessment and treatment, a patient with an abnormal ECG could have a potentially fatal outcome. An accurate and properly monitored patient ECG is extremely important, so remember the following troubleshooting tips:

- Place leads in the correct position. Incorrect placement can give false readings.
- Avoid placing leads over bony areas.
- In patients with large breasts, place the electrodes under the breast. The most accurate tracings are obtained through the smallest amount of fat tissue.

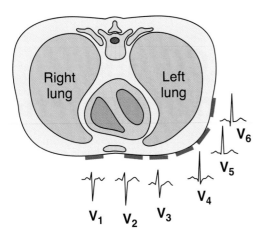

Figure 10.1 ■ Normal R-wave progression in chest leads V₁–V₆.

- Apply tincture of benzoin to the electrode sites if the patient is diaphoretic. The electrodes will adhere to the skin better.
- Shave hair at the electrode site if it interferes with contact between the electrode and skin.
- Discard old electrodes and use new ones if the gel on the back of the electrode dries.

R WAVE PROGRESSION

Normal ventricular depolarization in the heart progresses from right to left and from front to back (FIG. 10-1). In a normal heart, the R wave becomes taller and the S wave smaller as electrical activity crosses the heart from right to left. This phenomenon is called R wave progression and is noted on the chest leads.

Alteration in the normal R wave progression may be seen in left ventricular hypertrophy, COPD, left BBB, or anteroseptal MI.

ELECTRICAL AXIS DEVIATION

The electrical axis is the sum total of all electrical currents generated by the ventricular myocardium during depolarization (FIG. 10-2). Analysis of the axis may help to determine the location and extent of cardiac injury, such as ventricular hypertrophy, BBB, or changes in the position of the heart in the chest (from, e.g., pregnancy or ascites).

The direction of the QRS complex in leads I and aVF determines the axis quadrant in relation to the heart.

♥ | *Clinical Tip:*

Extreme right axis deviation is also called indeterminate, "no man's land," and "northwest."

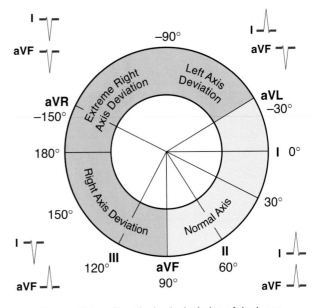

Figure 10.2 ■ Electrical axis deviation of the heart.

ISCHEMIA, INJURY, AND INFARCTION

Ischemia, injury, and infarction are three stages that cardiac tissue goes through when a complete blockage occurs in a coronary artery. The location of the myocardial infarction is a critical factor in determining the most appropriate treatment and predicting probable complications.

Each coronary artery delivers blood to specific areas of the heart. Blockages at different sites can damage various parts of the heart as shown in FIGURES 10-3 and 10-4. Characteristic ECG changes occur in different leads with each type of MI (FIG. 10-5) and can be correlated to the blockages shown in Figures 10-3 and 10-4.

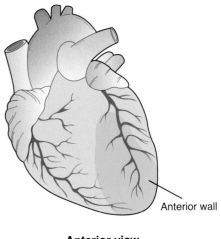

Anterior view

Figure 10.3 ■ Anterior wall of the heart.

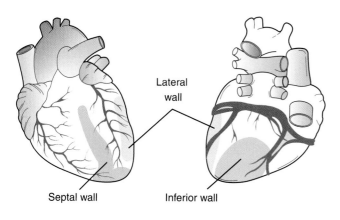

Anterior view · Posterior view

Figure 10.4 ■ Septal, lateral, and inferior walls of the heart.

I lateral	aVR	V₁ septal	V₄ anterior
II inferior	aVL lateral	V₂ septal	V₅ lateral
III inferior	aVF inferior	V₃ anterior	V₆ lateral

Figure 10.5 ■ Location of MI by ECG leads.

 Clinical Tip:

Lead aVR may not show any change in an MI.

 Clinical Tip:

An MI may not be limited to just one region of the heart. For example, if there are changes in leads V₃ and V₄ (anterior) and leads I, aVL, V₅, and V₆ (lateral), the MI is called an anterolateral infarction.

PROGRESSION OF AN ACUTE MYOCARDIAL INFARCTION

An acute MI is a continuum that extends from the normal state to a full infarction (FIG. 10-6):

• Ischemia—Lack of oxygen to the cardiac tissue, represented by ST segment depression, T wave inversion, or both
• Injury—Arterial occlusion with ischemia, represented by ST segment elevation

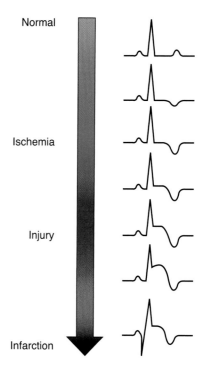

Figure 10.6 ■ Progression of an acute MI.

• Infarction—Death of tissue, represented by a pathological Q wave

 Clinical Tip:

Once the acute MI has ended, the ST segment returns to baseline and the T wave becomes upright, but the Q wave remains abnormal because of scar formation.

ST SEGMENT ELEVATION AND DEPRESSION

A normal ST segment represents early ventricular repolarization. Displacement of the ST segment can be caused by various conditions, shown in FIGURES 10-7 through 10-9.

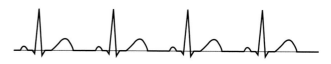

Figure 10.7 ■ ST segment at baseline.

Primary Causes of ST Segment Elevation

• ST segment elevation exceeding 1 mm in the limb leads and 2 mm in the chest leads indicates an evolving acute MI until there is proof to the contrary.

- Early repolarization (normal variant in young adults)
- Pericarditis
- Ventricular aneurysm
- Pulmonary embolism
- Intracranial hemorrhage

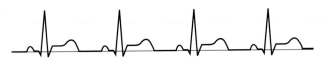

Figure 10.8 ■ Elevated ST segment.

Primary Causes of ST Segment Depression

- Myocardial ischemia
- Left ventricular hypertrophy
- Intraventricular conduction defects
- Medication (e.g., digitalis)
- Reciprocal changes in leads opposite the area of acute injury

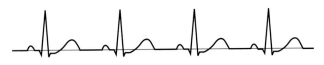

Figure 10.9 ■ Depressed ST segment.

THE NORMAL 12-LEAD ECG

FIGURE 10-10 shows an example of a normal 12-lead ECG.

 Clinical Tip:

A normal ECG does not rule out any acute coronary syndrome.

ANTERIOR MYOCARDIAL INFARCTION

- Occlusion of the left coronary artery—left anterior descending branch
- ECG changes: ST segment elevation with tall T waves and taller-than-normal R waves in leads V_3 and V_4; reciprocal changes in II, III, and aVF

FIGURE 10-11 shows ECG changes typical of an anterior MI.

 Clinical Tip:

Anterior MI frequently involves a large area of the myocardium and can present with cardiogenic shock, second-degree AV block Type II, or third-degree AV block.

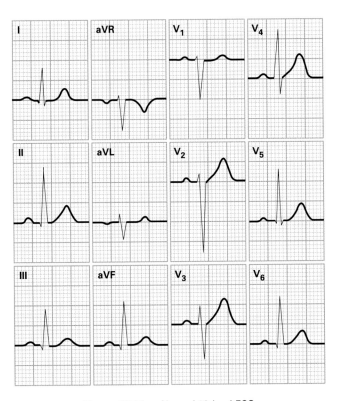

Figure 10.10 ■ Normal 12-lead ECG.

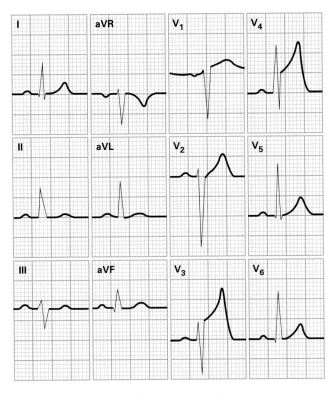

Figure 10.11 ■ Anterior myocardial infarction.

INFERIOR MYOCARDIAL INFARCTION

- Occlusion of the right coronary artery—posterior descending branch

- ECG changes: ST segment elevation in leads II, III, and aVF; reciprocal ST segment depression in I and aVL

FIGURE 10-12 shows a tracing typical of inferior MI.

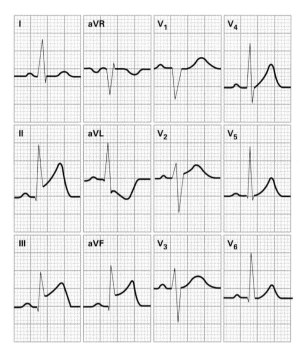

Figure 10.12 ■ Inferior myocardial infarction.

 Clinical Tip:

Be alert for symptomatic sinus bradycardia, AV blocks, hypotension, and hypoperfusion.

LATERAL MYOCARDIAL INFARCTION

- Occlusion of the left coronary artery—circumflex branch
- ECG changes: ST segment elevation in leads I, aVL, V_5, and V_6; reciprocal ST segment depression in V_1, V_2, and V_3

FIGURE 10-13 shows characteristic ECG changes in lateral MI.

Clinical Tip:

Lateral MI is often associated with anterior or inferior wall MI. Be alert for changes that may indicate cardiogenic shock or congestive heart failure.

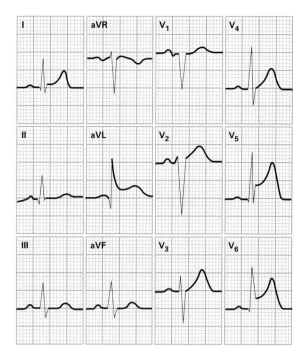

Figure 10.13 ■ Lateral myocardial infarction.

SEPTAL MYOCARDIAL INFARCTION

- Occlusion of the left coronary artery—left anterior descending branch
- ECG changes: pathological Q waves; absence of normal R waves in leads V_1 and V_2

FIGURE 10-14 shows a tracing characteristic of septal MI.

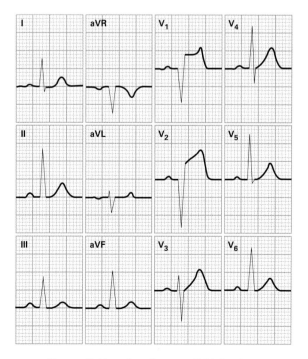

Figure 10.14 ■ Septal myocardial infarction.

💙 *Clinical Tip:*

Septal MI is often associated with an anterior wall MI.

POSTERIOR MYOCARDIAL INFARCTION

- Occlusion of the right coronary artery (posterior descending branch) or the left circumflex artery
- Usually produces tall R waves and ST segment depression in leads V_1, V_2, V_3, and V_4. Complications may include left ventricular dysfunction.
- You may need to view the true posterior leads, V_8 and V_9 (used in the 15-lead ECG) for definite diagnosis of an acute posterior MI. In these leads you will see ST segment elevation.

FIGURE 10-15 shows typical ECG changes in posterior MI.

💙 *Clinical Tip:*

Diagnosis may require a 15-lead ECG because a standard 12-lead does not look directly at the posterior wall.

LEFT BUNDLE BRANCH BLOCK

- QRS complex greater than 0.10 sec
- QRS predominantly negative in leads V_1 and V_2

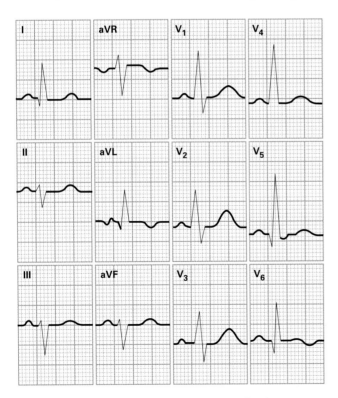

Figure 10.15 ■ Posterior myocardial infarction.

- QRS predominantly positive in V_5 and V_6 and often notched
- Absence of small, normal Q waves in I, aVL, V_5, and V_6
- Wide monophasic R waves in I, aVL, V_1, V_5, and V_6

FIGURE 10-16 shows an example of left BBB.

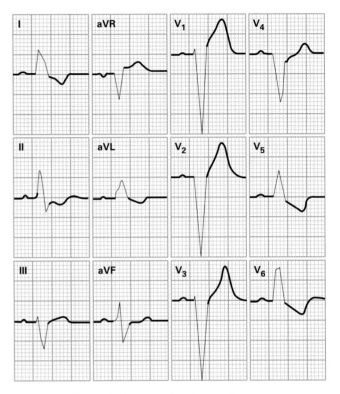

Figure 10.16 ■ Left bundle branch block.

💙 *Clinical Tip:*

Patients may have underlying heart disease, including coronary artery disease, hypertension, cardiomyopathy, and ischemia.

RIGHT BUNDLE BRANCH BLOCK

- QRS complex greater than 0.10 sec
- QRS axis normal or deviated to the right
- Broad S wave in leads I, aVL, V_5, and V_6
- RSR′ pattern in lead V_1 with R′ taller than R
- qRS pattern in V_5 and V_6
- ST-T distorted and in opposite direction to terminal portion of QRS (this is not ST elevation or ST depression).

FIGURE 10-17 shows an example of right BBB.

Clinical Tip:

Patients may have underlying right ventricular hypertrophy, pulmonary edema, cardiomyopathy, congenital heart disease, or rheumatic heart disease.

Clinical Tip:

In bundle branch blocks, the ST segment and T waves are distorted and are in the opposite direction to the terminal portion of the QRS. This is not ST elevation or ST depression.

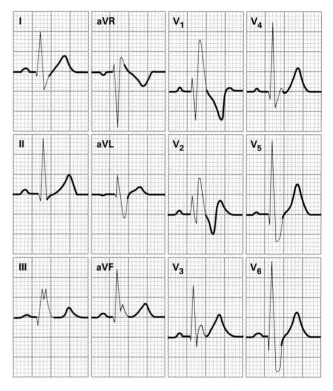

Figure 10.17 ■ Right bundle branch block.

ECG Practice Tests

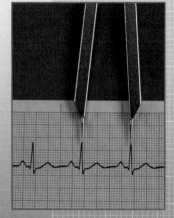

Chapter 11

ECG Practice Test One

For instructions on analyzing these practice test strips, please see the guidelines given at the end of Chapter 2. To help you with your success in ECG interpretation, hints have been provided throughout this chapter. By the time you tackle Chapters 12 through 14, you will have enough experience to proceed without any hints.

TEST STRIP SECTION ONE

ECG 11•1

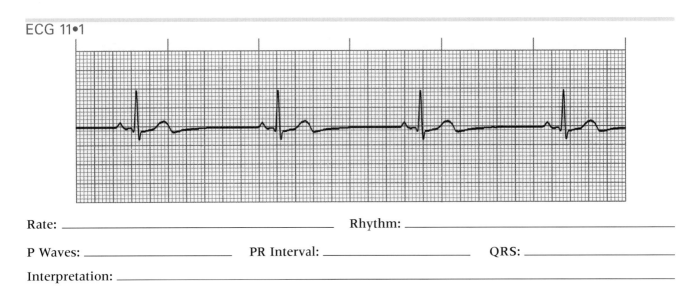

Rate: _____ Rhythm: _____

P Waves: _____ PR Interval: _____ QRS: _____

Interpretation: _____

ECG 11•2

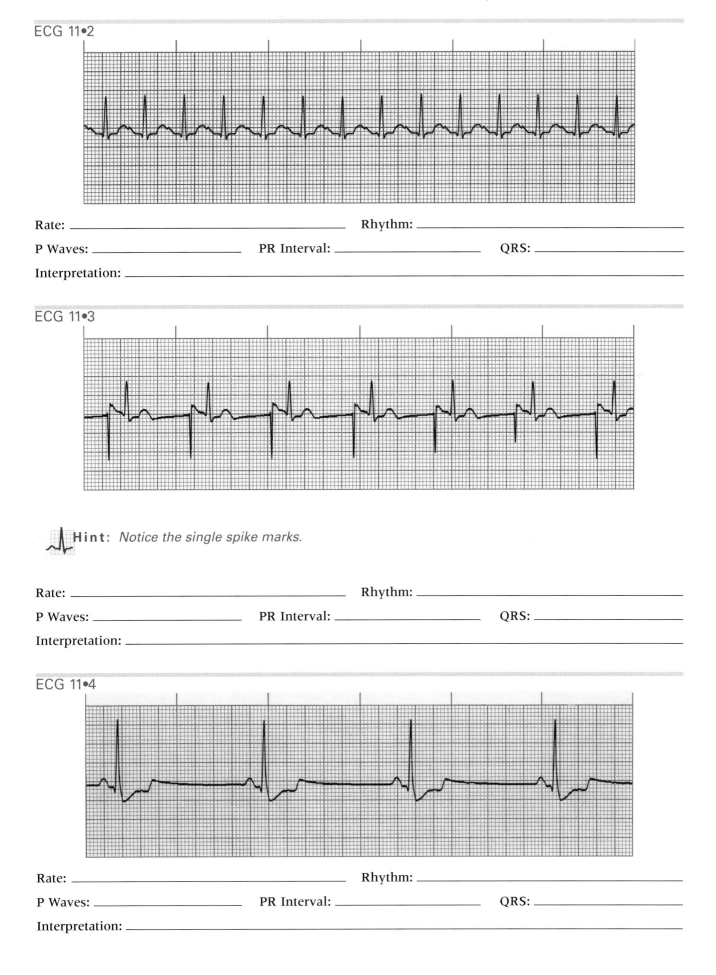

Rate: _____   Rhythm: _____

P Waves: _____   PR Interval: _____   QRS: _____

Interpretation: _____

ECG 11•3

Hint: *Notice the single spike marks.*

Rate: _____   Rhythm: _____

P Waves: _____   PR Interval: _____   QRS: _____

Interpretation: _____

ECG 11•4

Rate: _____   Rhythm: _____

P Waves: _____   PR Interval: _____   QRS: _____

Interpretation: _____

ECG 11•5

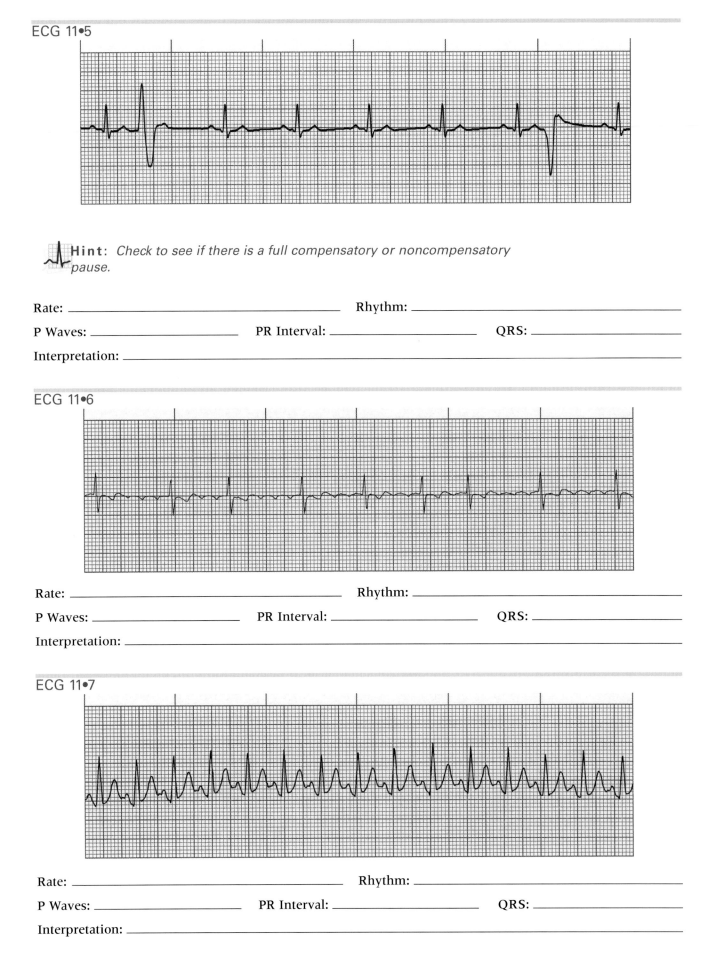

Hint: *Check to see if there is a full compensatory or noncompensatory pause.*

Rate: _____ Rhythm: _____

P Waves: _____ PR Interval: _____ QRS: _____

Interpretation: _____

ECG 11•6

Rate: _____ Rhythm: _____

P Waves: _____ PR Interval: _____ QRS: _____

Interpretation: _____

ECG 11•7

Rate: _____ Rhythm: _____

P Waves: _____ PR Interval: _____ QRS: _____

Interpretation: _____

ECG 11•8

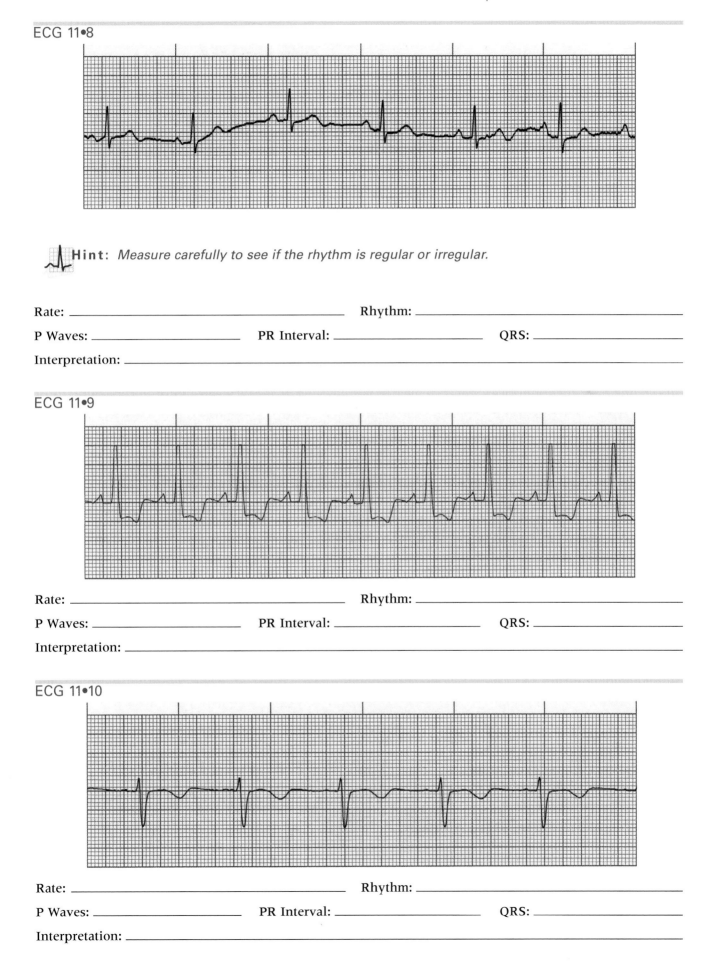

Hint: *Measure carefully to see if the rhythm is regular or irregular.*

Rate: _____ Rhythm: _____

P Waves: _____ PR Interval: _____ QRS: _____

Interpretation: _____

ECG 11•9

Rate: _____ Rhythm: _____

P Waves: _____ PR Interval: _____ QRS: _____

Interpretation: _____

ECG 11•10

Rate: _____ Rhythm: _____

P Waves: _____ PR Interval: _____ QRS: _____

Interpretation: _____

ECG 11•11

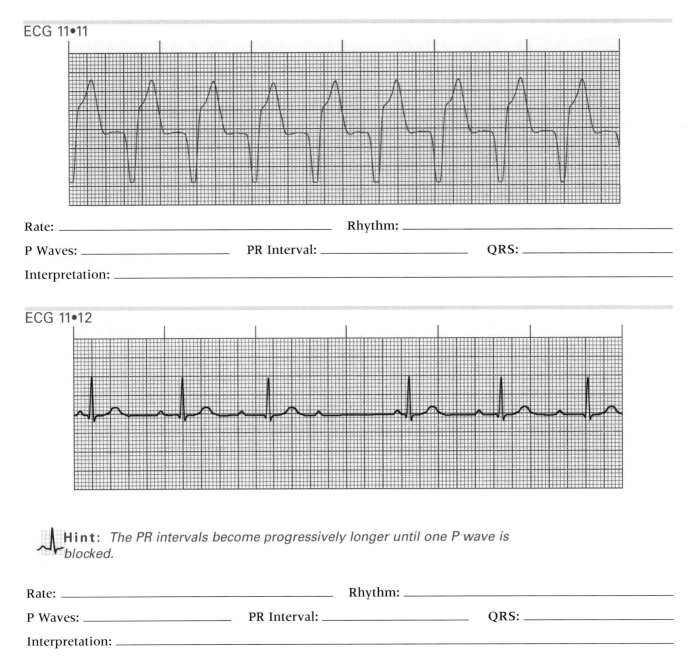

Rate: _____   Rhythm: _____

P Waves: _____   PR Interval: _____   QRS: _____

Interpretation: _____

ECG 11•12

Hint: *The PR intervals become progressively longer until one P wave is blocked.*

Rate: _____   Rhythm: _____

P Waves: _____   PR Interval: _____   QRS: _____

Interpretation: _____

ECG 11•13

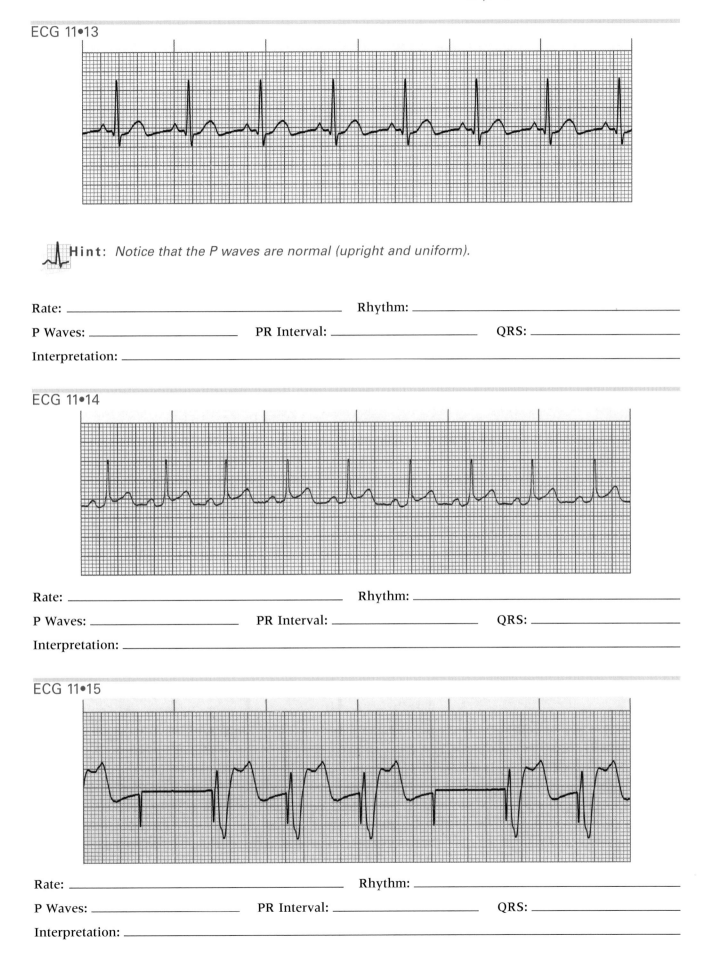

Hint: *Notice that the P waves are normal (upright and uniform).*

Rate: _____ Rhythm: _____

P Waves: _____ PR Interval: _____ QRS: _____

Interpretation: _____

ECG 11•14

Rate: _____ Rhythm: _____

P Waves: _____ PR Interval: _____ QRS: _____

Interpretation: _____

ECG 11•15

Rate: _____ Rhythm: _____

P Waves: _____ PR Interval: _____ QRS: _____

Interpretation: _____

ECG 11•16

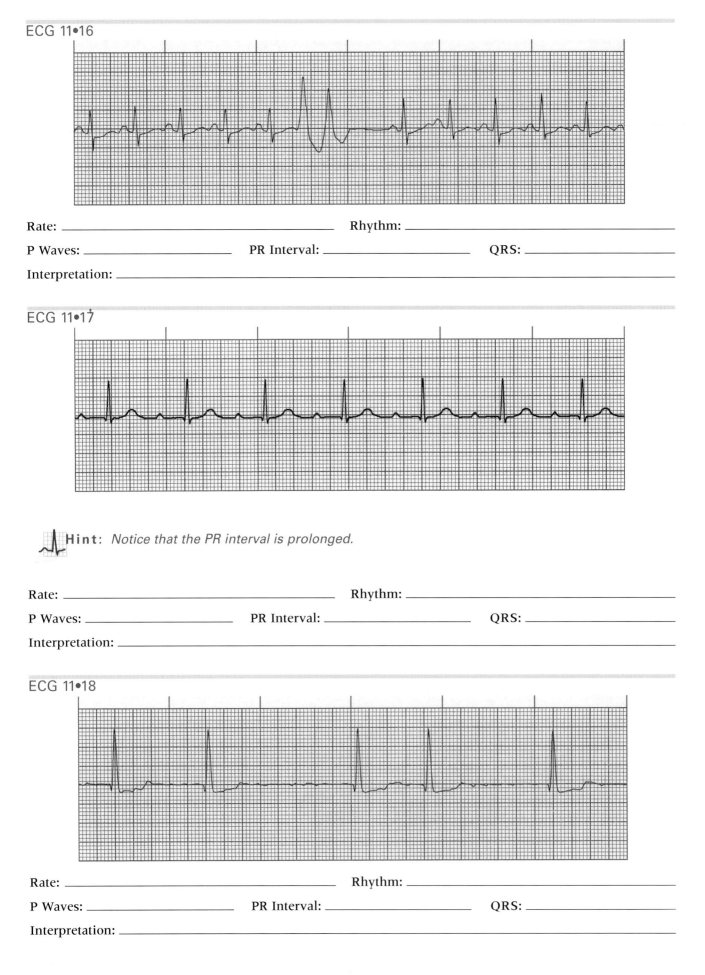

Rate: _____ Rhythm: _____

P Waves: _____ PR Interval: _____ QRS: _____

Interpretation: _____

ECG 11•17

Hint: *Notice that the PR interval is prolonged.*

Rate: _____ Rhythm: _____

P Waves: _____ PR Interval: _____ QRS: _____

Interpretation: _____

ECG 11•18

Rate: _____ Rhythm: _____

P Waves: _____ PR Interval: _____ QRS: _____

Interpretation: _____

ECG 11•19

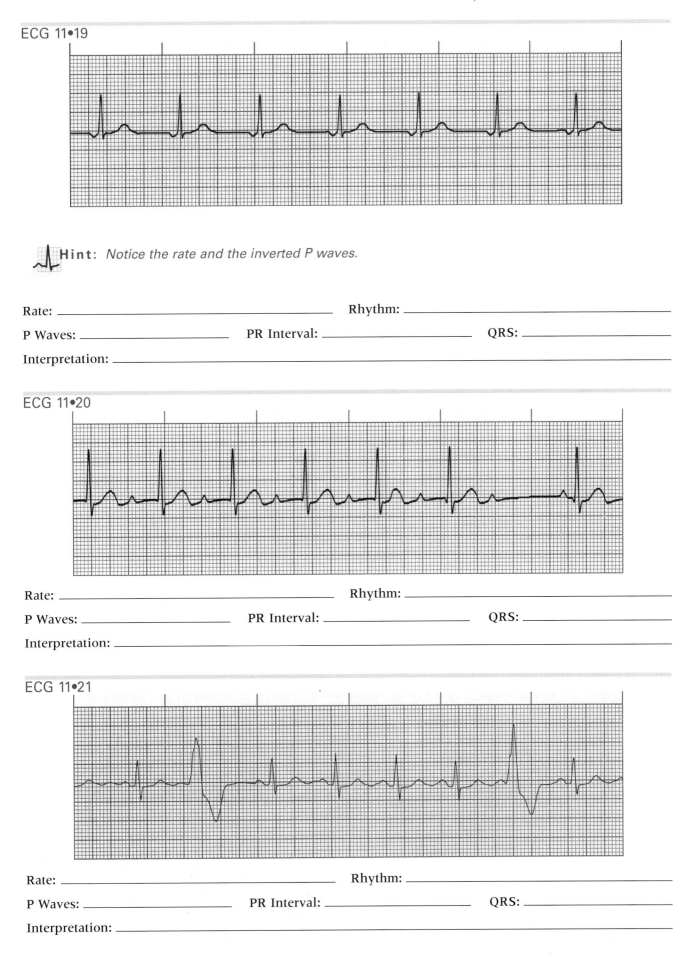

Hint: *Notice the rate and the inverted P waves.*

Rate: _____   Rhythm: _____

P Waves: _____   PR Interval: _____   QRS: _____

Interpretation: _____

ECG 11•20

Rate: _____   Rhythm: _____

P Waves: _____   PR Interval: _____   QRS: _____

Interpretation: _____

ECG 11•21

Rate: _____   Rhythm: _____

P Waves: _____   PR Interval: _____   QRS: _____

Interpretation: _____

ECG 11•22

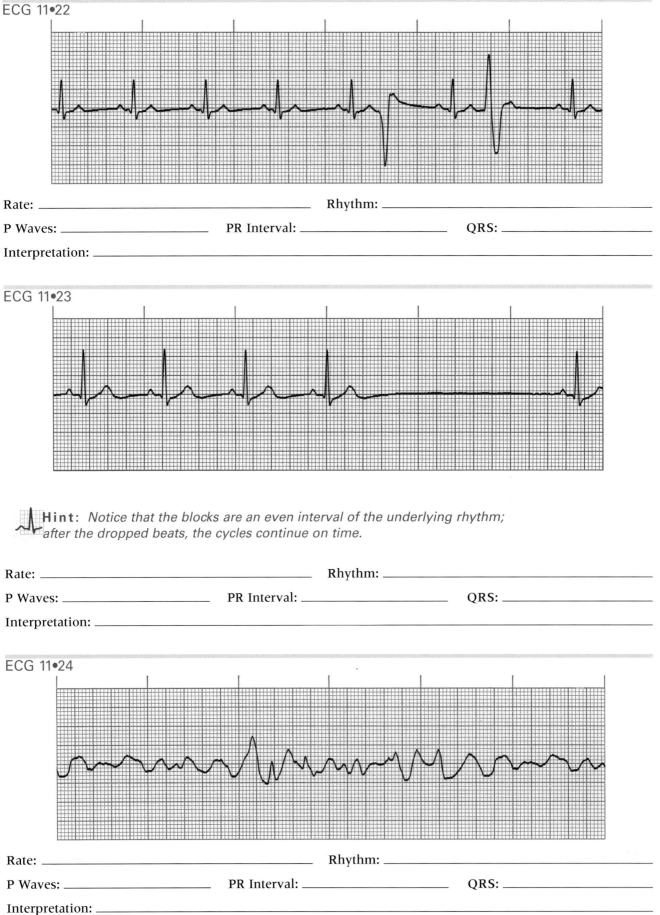

Rate: _____   Rhythm: _____

P Waves: _____   PR Interval: _____   QRS: _____

Interpretation: _____

ECG 11•23

Hint: *Notice that the blocks are an even interval of the underlying rhythm; after the dropped beats, the cycles continue on time.*

Rate: _____   Rhythm: _____

P Waves: _____   PR Interval: _____   QRS: _____

Interpretation: _____

ECG 11•24

Rate: _____   Rhythm: _____

P Waves: _____   PR Interval: _____   QRS: _____

Interpretation: _____

ECG 11•25

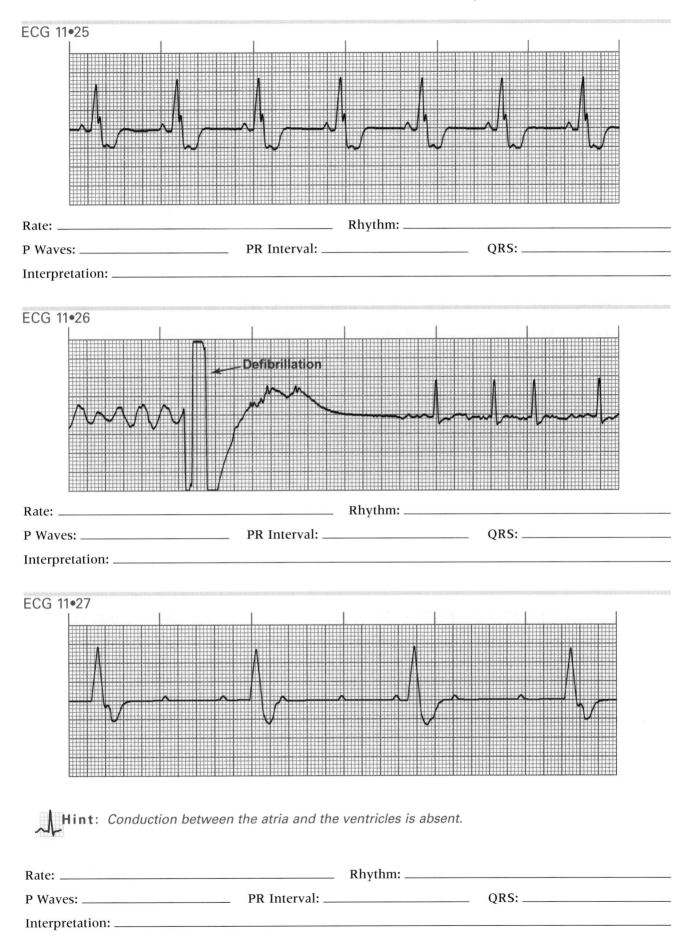

Rate: _____ Rhythm: _____

P Waves: _____ PR Interval: _____ QRS: _____

Interpretation: _____

ECG 11•26

Defibrillation

Rate: _____ Rhythm: _____

P Waves: _____ PR Interval: _____ QRS: _____

Interpretation: _____

ECG 11•27

Hint: *Conduction between the atria and the ventricles is absent.*

Rate: _____ Rhythm: _____

P Waves: _____ PR Interval: _____ QRS: _____

Interpretation: _____

ECG 11•28

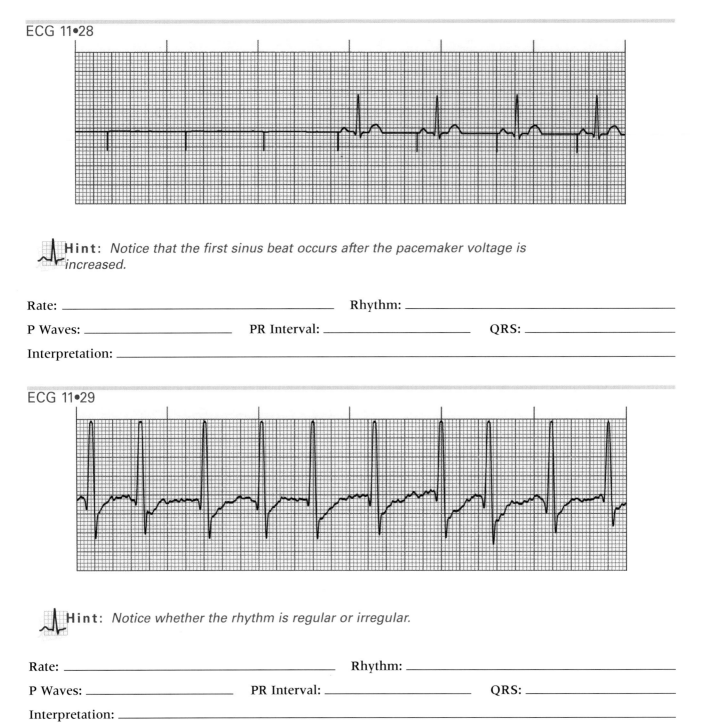

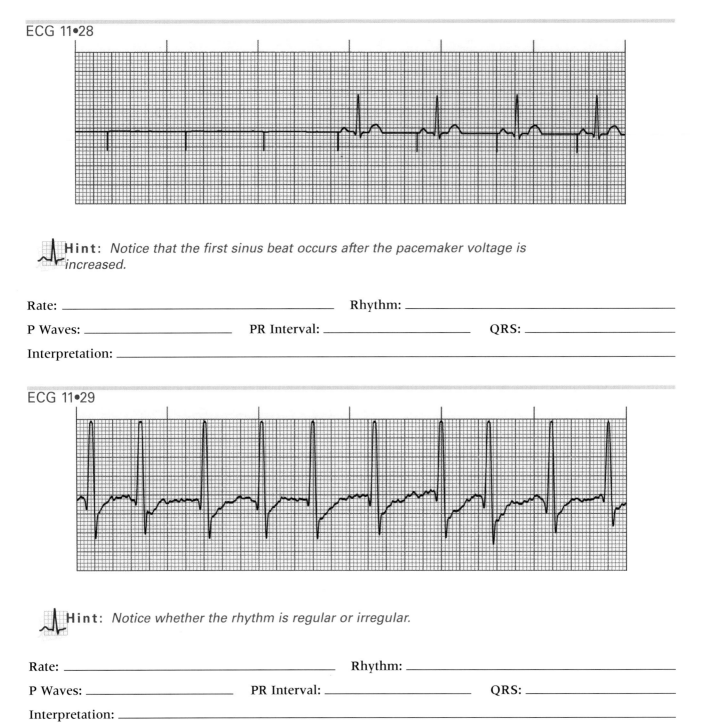Hint: *Notice that the first sinus beat occurs after the pacemaker voltage is increased.*

Rate: _____   Rhythm: _____

P Waves: _____   PR Interval: _____   QRS: _____

Interpretation: _____

ECG 11•29

Hint: *Notice whether the rhythm is regular or irregular.*

Rate: _____   Rhythm: _____

P Waves: _____   PR Interval: _____   QRS: _____

Interpretation: _____

ECG 11•30

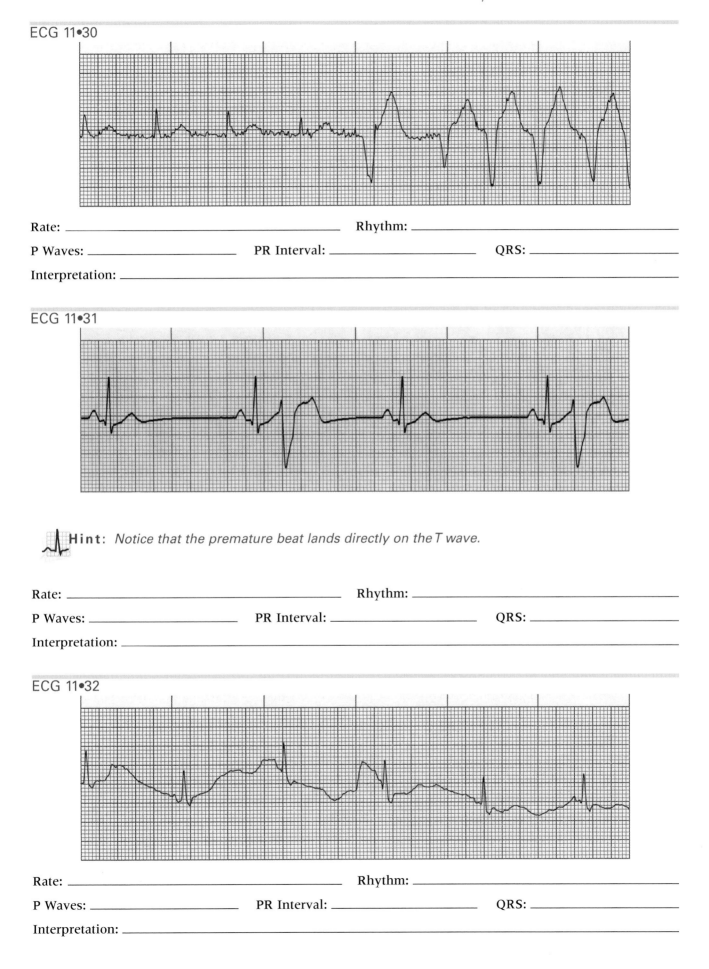

Rate: _____   Rhythm: _____

P Waves: _____   PR Interval: _____   QRS: _____

Interpretation: _____

ECG 11•31

Hint: *Notice that the premature beat lands directly on the T wave.*

Rate: _____   Rhythm: _____

P Waves: _____   PR Interval: _____   QRS: _____

Interpretation: _____

ECG 11•32

Rate: _____   Rhythm: _____

P Waves: _____   PR Interval: _____   QRS: _____

Interpretation: _____

ECG 11•33

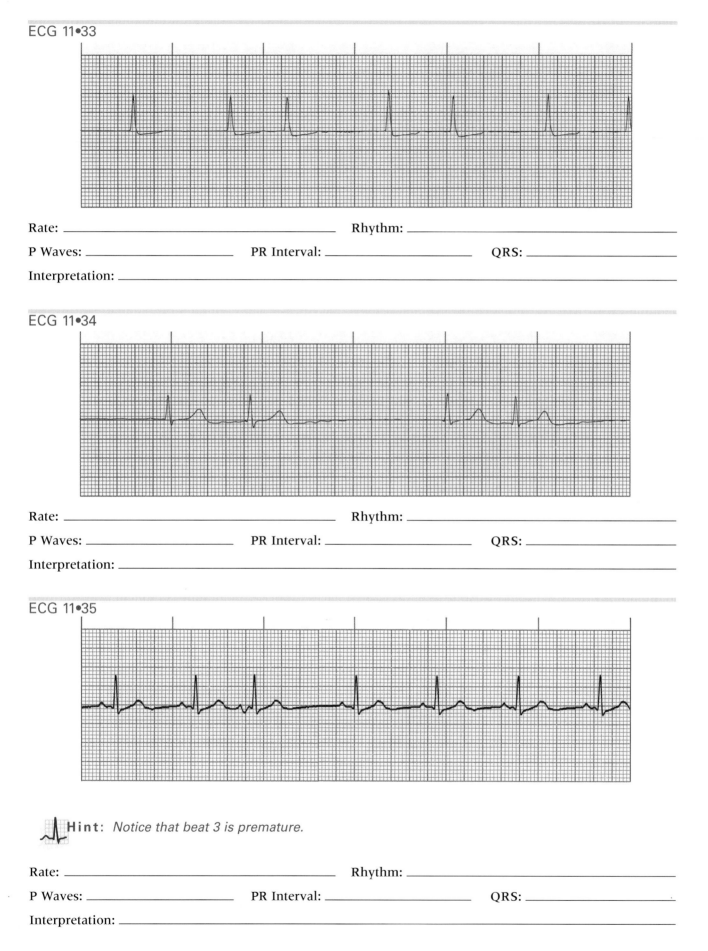

Rate: _____   Rhythm: _____

P Waves: _____   PR Interval: _____   QRS: _____

Interpretation: _____

ECG 11•34

Rate: _____   Rhythm: _____

P Waves: _____   PR Interval: _____   QRS: _____

Interpretation: _____

ECG 11•35

Hint: *Notice that beat 3 is premature.*

Rate: _____   Rhythm: _____

P Waves: _____   PR Interval: _____   QRS: _____

Interpretation: _____

ECG 11•36

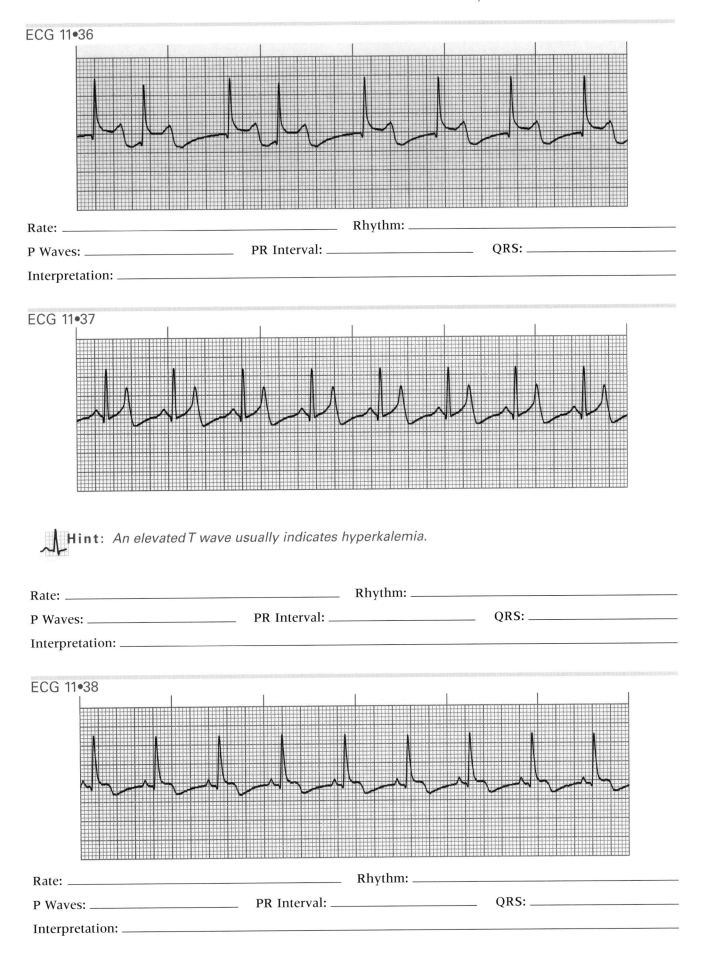

Rate: _____   Rhythm: _____

P Waves: _____   PR Interval: _____   QRS: _____

Interpretation: _____

ECG 11•37

Hint: *An elevated T wave usually indicates hyperkalemia.*

Rate: _____   Rhythm: _____

P Waves: _____   PR Interval: _____   QRS: _____

Interpretation: _____

ECG 11•38

Rate: _____   Rhythm: _____

P Waves: _____   PR Interval: _____   QRS: _____

Interpretation: _____

ECG 11•39

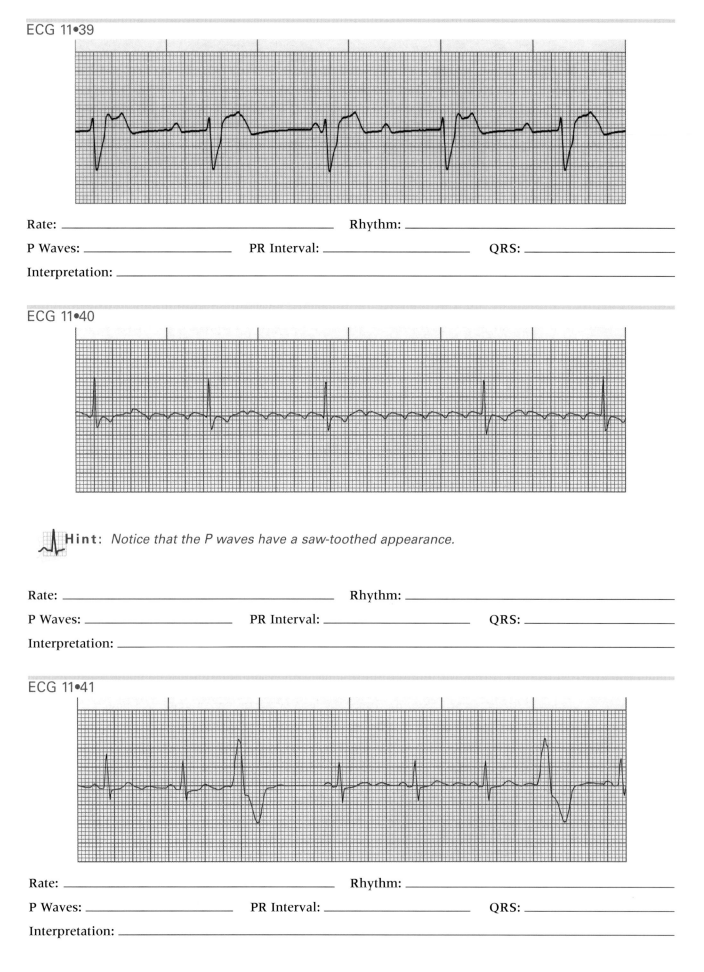

Rate: _____   Rhythm: _____

P Waves: _____   PR Interval: _____   QRS: _____

Interpretation: _____

ECG 11•40

Hint: *Notice that the P waves have a saw-toothed appearance.*

Rate: _____   Rhythm: _____

P Waves: _____   PR Interval: _____   QRS: _____

Interpretation: _____

ECG 11•41

Rate: _____   Rhythm: _____

P Waves: _____   PR Interval: _____   QRS: _____

Interpretation: _____

ECG 11•42

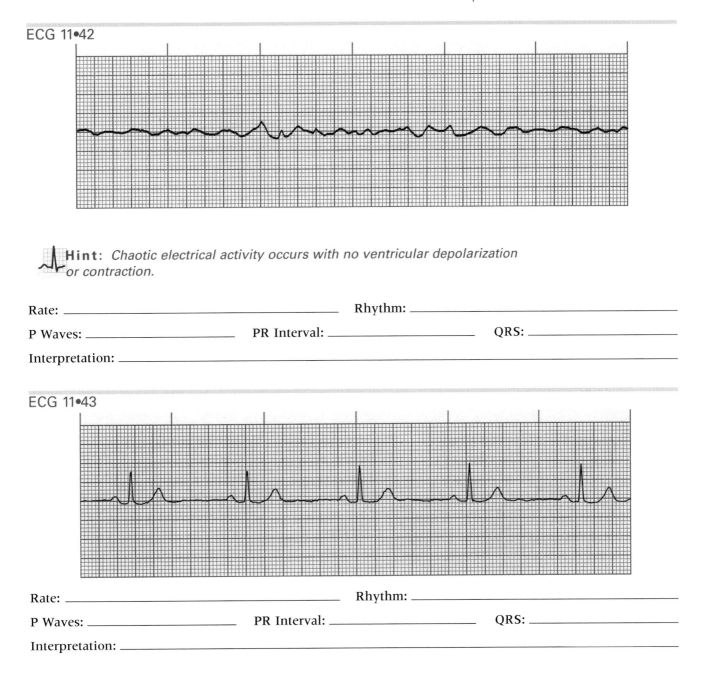

Hint: *Chaotic electrical activity occurs with no ventricular depolarization or contraction.*

Rate: _____ Rhythm: _____

P Waves: _____ PR Interval: _____ QRS: _____

Interpretation: _____

ECG 11•43

Rate: _____ Rhythm: _____

P Waves: _____ PR Interval: _____ QRS: _____

Interpretation: _____

ECG 11•44

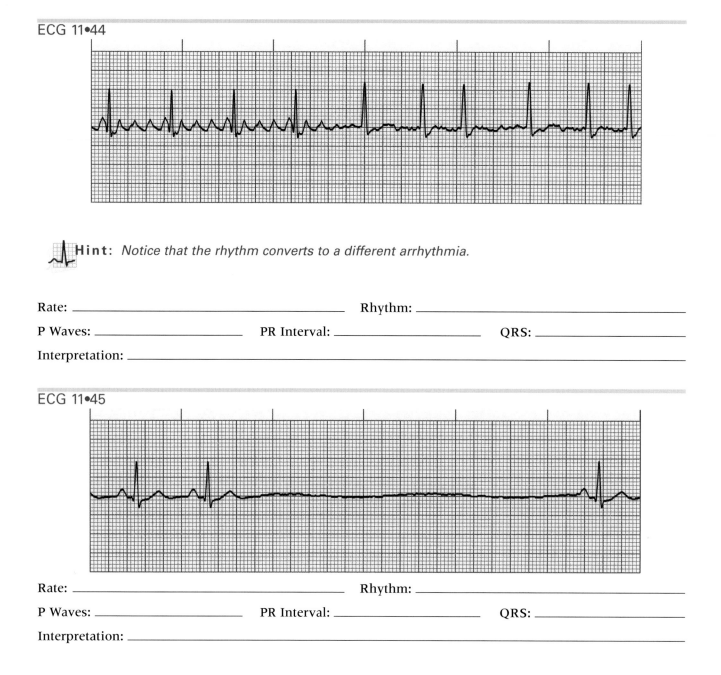

Hint: *Notice that the rhythm converts to a different arrhythmia.*

Rate: _____ Rhythm: _____

P Waves: _____ PR Interval: _____ QRS: _____

Interpretation: _____

ECG 11•45

Rate: _____ Rhythm: _____

P Waves: _____ PR Interval: _____ QRS: _____

Interpretation: _____

ECG 11•46

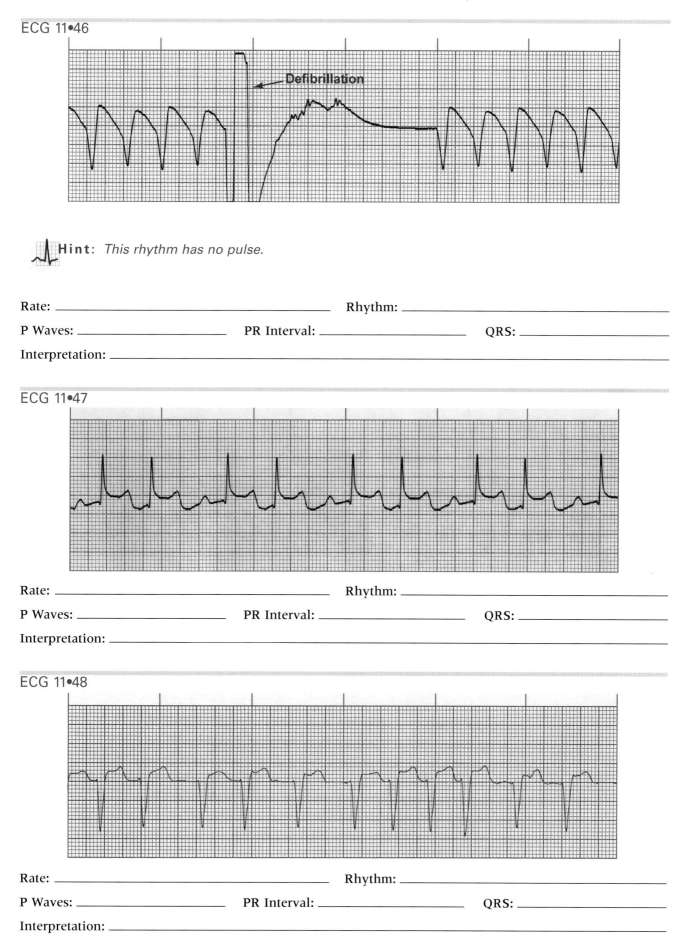

Hint: *This rhythm has no pulse.*

Rate: _____ Rhythm: _____

P Waves: _____ PR Interval: _____ QRS: _____

Interpretation: _____

ECG 11•47

Rate: _____ Rhythm: _____

P Waves: _____ PR Interval: _____ QRS: _____

Interpretation: _____

ECG 11•48

Rate: _____ Rhythm: _____

P Waves: _____ PR Interval: _____ QRS: _____

Interpretation: _____

ECG 11•49

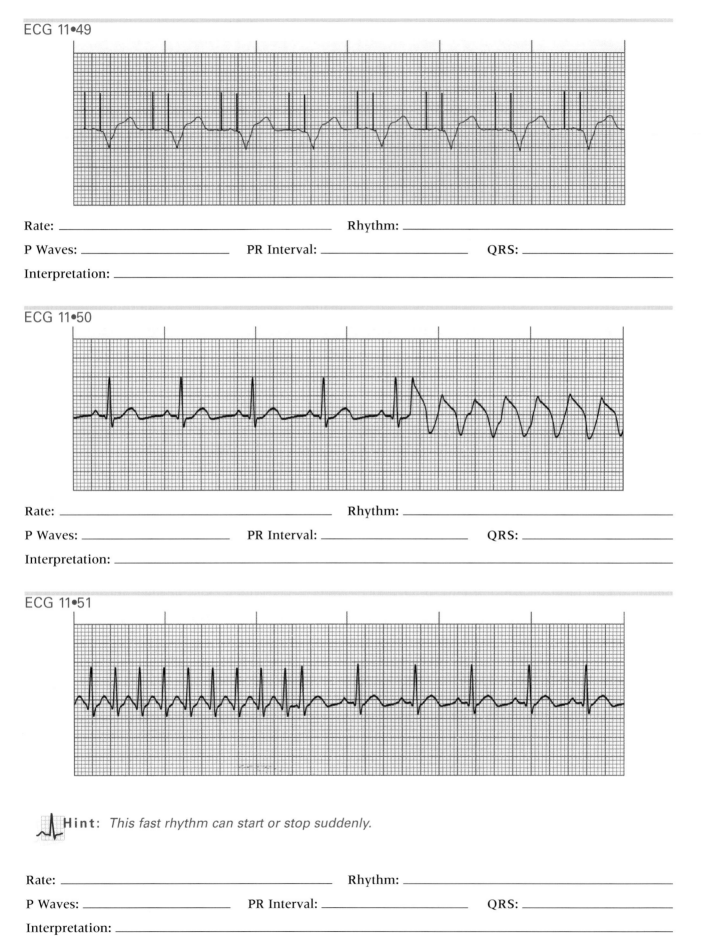

Rate: _____   Rhythm: _____

P Waves: _____   PR Interval: _____   QRS: _____

Interpretation: _____

ECG 11•50

Rate: _____   Rhythm: _____

P Waves: _____   PR Interval: _____   QRS: _____

Interpretation: _____

ECG 11•51

Hint: *This fast rhythm can start or stop suddenly.*

Rate: _____   Rhythm: _____

P Waves: _____   PR Interval: _____   QRS: _____

Interpretation: _____

ECG 11•52

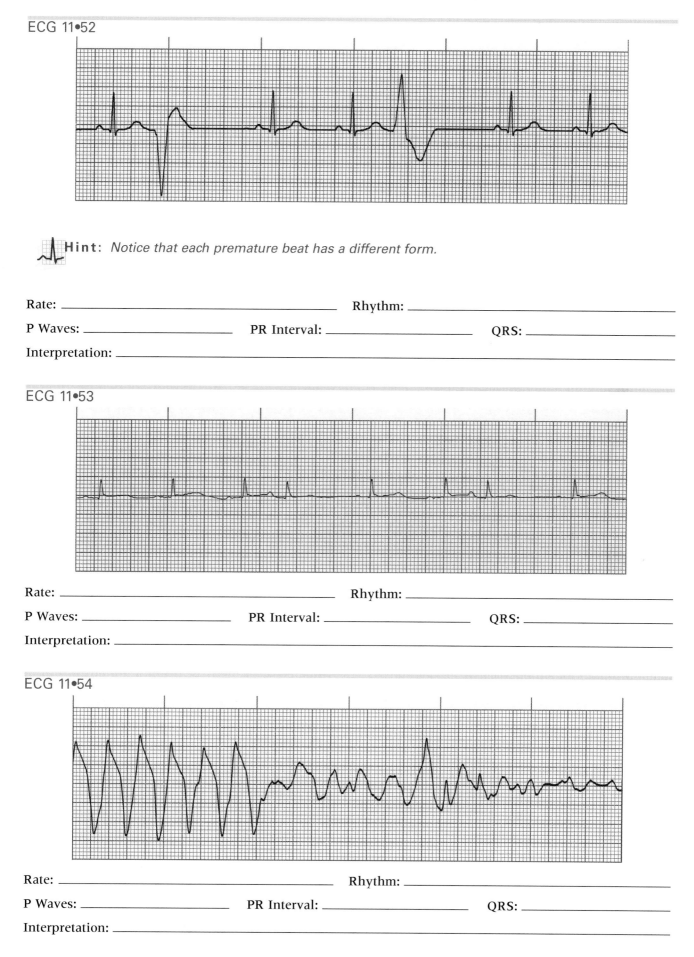

Hint: *Notice that each premature beat has a different form.*

Rate: _____ Rhythm: _____

P Waves: _____ PR Interval: _____ QRS: _____

Interpretation: _____

ECG 11•53

Rate: _____ Rhythm: _____

P Waves: _____ PR Interval: _____ QRS: _____

Interpretation: _____

ECG 11•54

Rate: _____ Rhythm: _____

P Waves: _____ PR Interval: _____ QRS: _____

Interpretation: _____

ECG 11•55

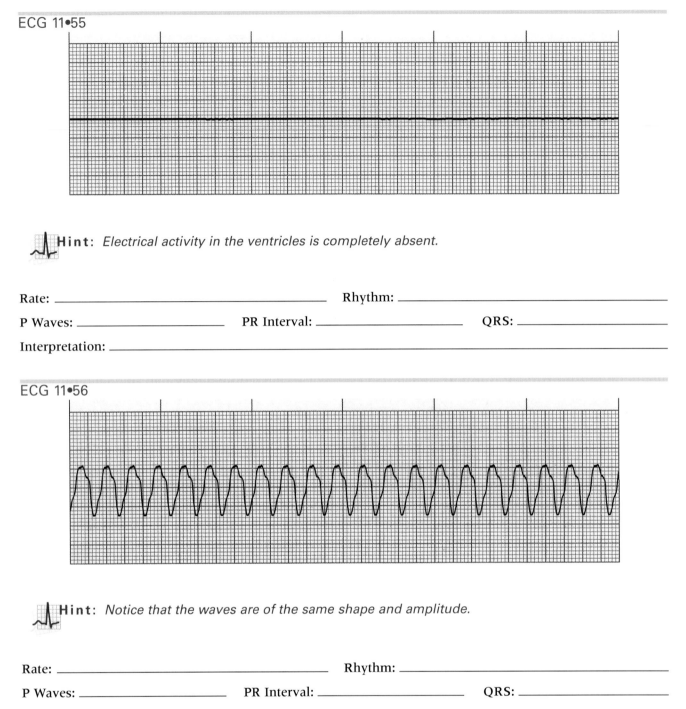

Hint: *Electrical activity in the ventricles is completely absent.*

Rate: _____   Rhythm: _____

P Waves: _____   PR Interval: _____   QRS: _____

Interpretation: _____

ECG 11•56

Hint: *Notice that the waves are of the same shape and amplitude.*

Rate: _____   Rhythm: _____

P Waves: _____   PR Interval: _____   QRS: _____

Interpretation: _____

ECG 11•57

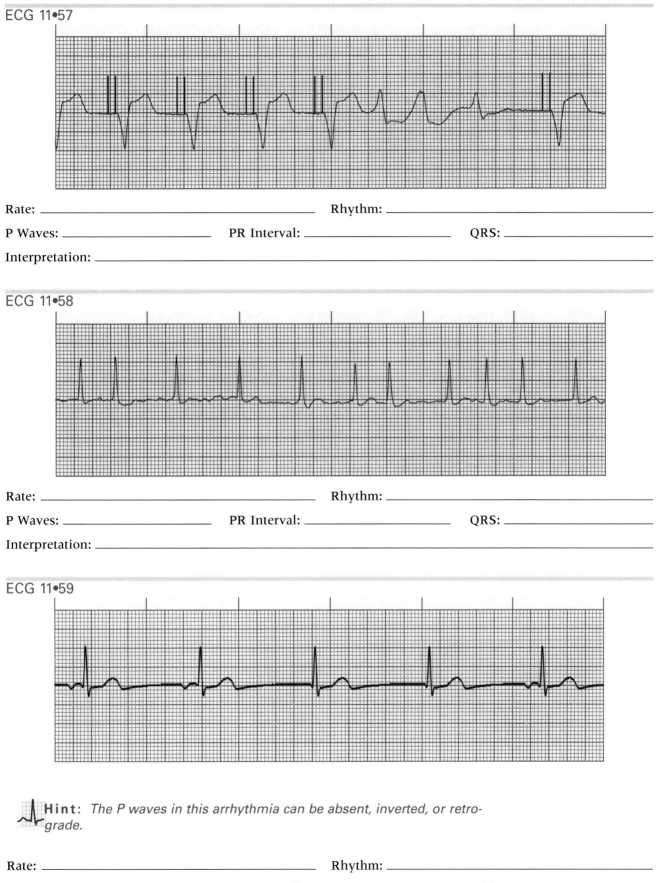

Rate: _____ Rhythm: _____

P Waves: _____ PR Interval: _____ QRS: _____

Interpretation: _____

ECG 11•58

Rate: _____ Rhythm: _____

P Waves: _____ PR Interval: _____ QRS: _____

Interpretation: _____

ECG 11•59

Hint: *The P waves in this arrhythmia can be absent, inverted, or retro-grade.*

Rate: _____ Rhythm: _____

P Waves: _____ PR Interval: _____ QRS: _____

Interpretation: _____

ECG 11•60

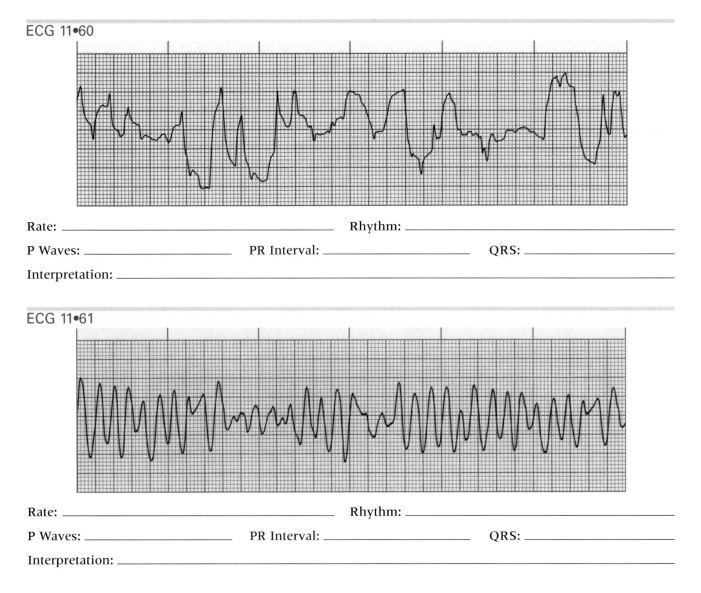

Rate: _____   Rhythm: _____

P Waves: _____   PR Interval: _____   QRS: _____

Interpretation: _____

ECG 11•61

Rate: _____   Rhythm: _____

P Waves: _____   PR Interval: _____   QRS: _____

Interpretation: _____

Hint: *Notice the spindle effect in the rhythm.*

ECG 11•62

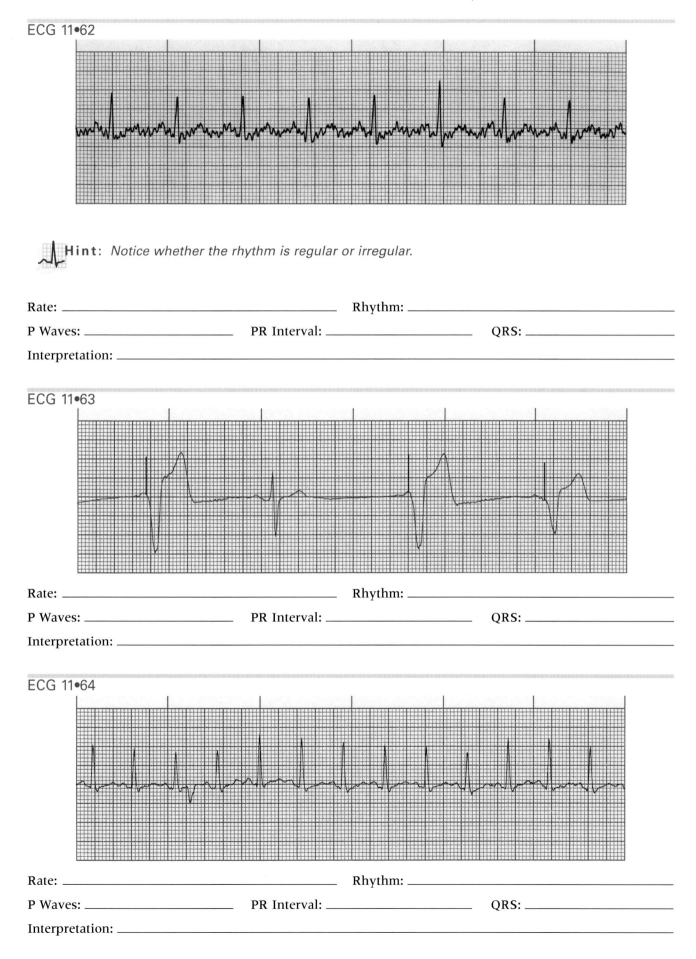

Hint: *Notice whether the rhythm is regular or irregular.*

Rate: _____ Rhythm: _____

P Waves: _____ PR Interval: _____ QRS: _____

Interpretation: _____

ECG 11•63

Rate: _____ Rhythm: _____

P Waves: _____ PR Interval: _____ QRS: _____

Interpretation: _____

ECG 11•64

Rate: _____ Rhythm: _____

P Waves: _____ PR Interval: _____ QRS: _____

Interpretation: _____

ECG 11•65

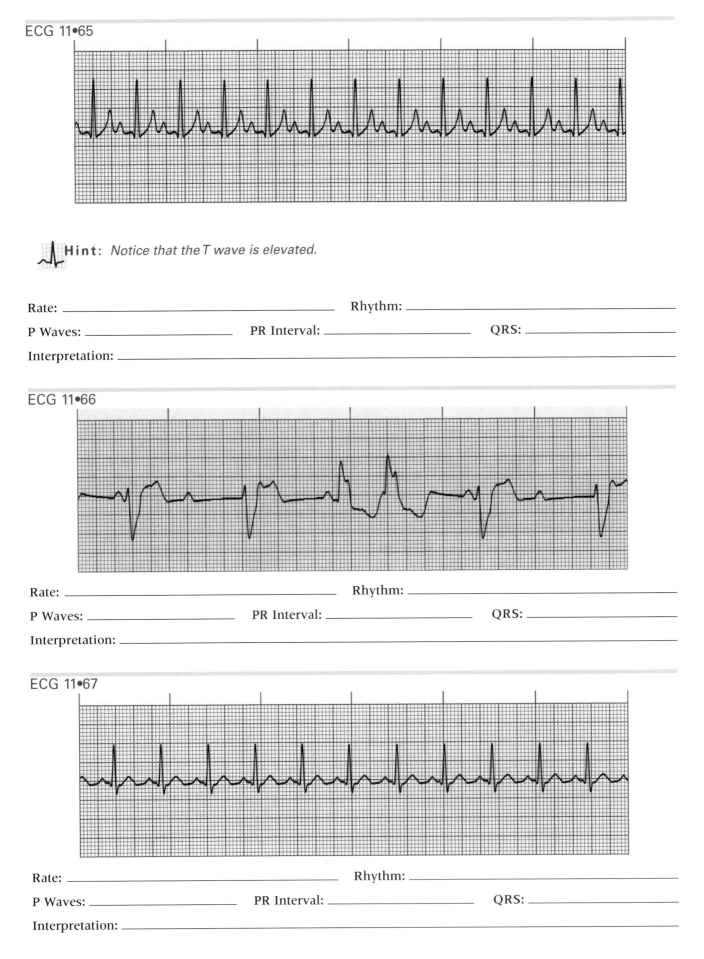

Hint: *Notice that the T wave is elevated.*

Rate: _____ Rhythm: _____

P Waves: _____ PR Interval: _____ QRS: _____

Interpretation: _____

ECG 11•66

Rate: _____ Rhythm: _____

P Waves: _____ PR Interval: _____ QRS: _____

Interpretation: _____

ECG 11•67

Rate: _____ Rhythm: _____

P Waves: _____ PR Interval: _____ QRS: _____

Interpretation: _____

ECG 11•68

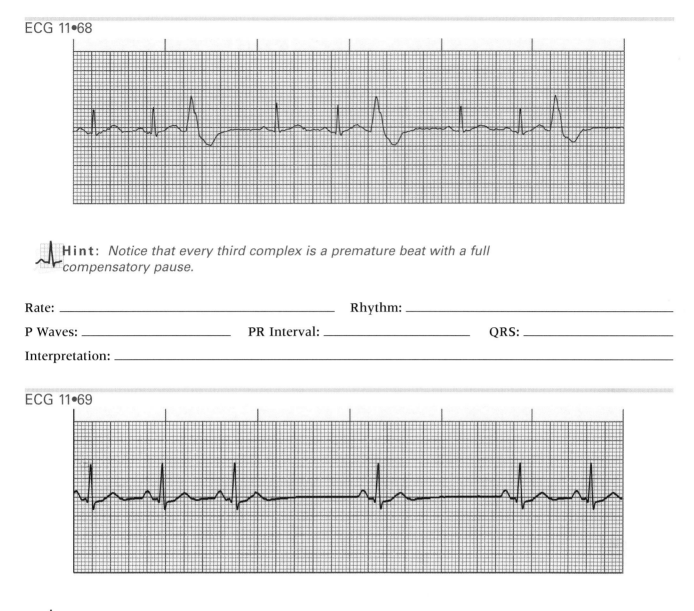

Hint: *Notice that every third complex is a premature beat with a full compensatory pause.*

Rate: _____ Rhythm: _____

P Waves: _____ PR Interval: _____ QRS: _____

Interpretation: _____

ECG 11•69

Hint: *Notice that the dropped beats are at even intervals with the underlying rhythm.*

Rate: _____ Rhythm: _____

P Waves: _____ PR Interval: _____ QRS: _____

Interpretation: _____

ECG 11•70

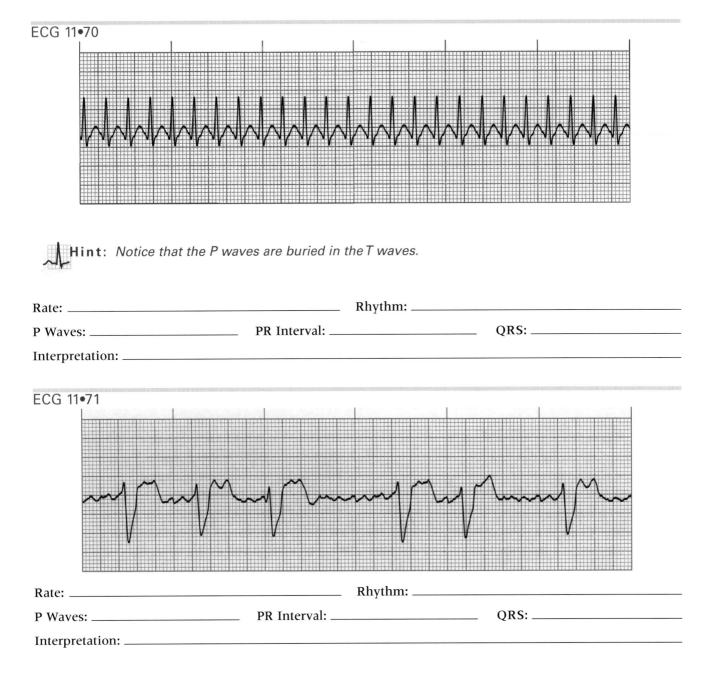

Hint: *Notice that the P waves are buried in the T waves.*

Rate: _____   Rhythm: _____

P Waves: _____   PR Interval: _____   QRS: _____

Interpretation: _____

ECG 11•71

Rate: _____   Rhythm: _____

P Waves: _____   PR Interval: _____   QRS: _____

Interpretation: _____

ECG 11•72

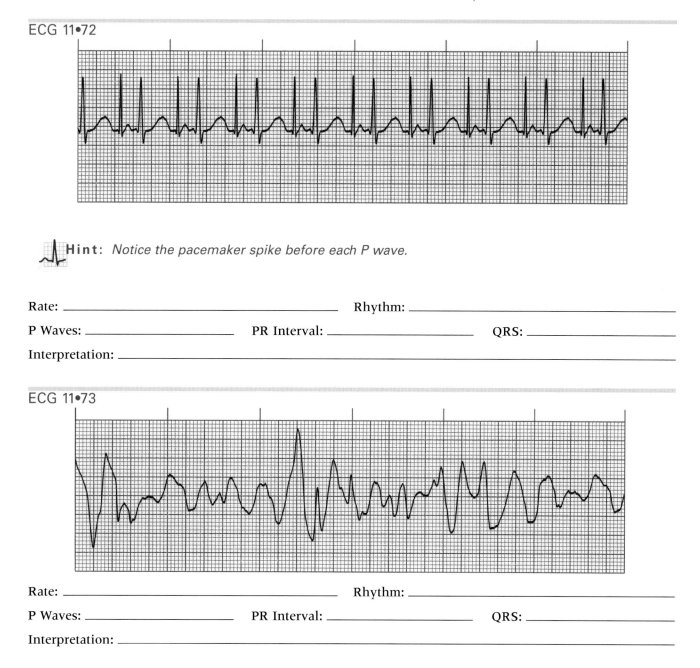

Hint: *Notice the pacemaker spike before each P wave.*

Rate: _____ Rhythm: _____

P Waves: _____ PR Interval: _____ QRS: _____

Interpretation: _____

ECG 11•73

Rate: _____ Rhythm: _____

P Waves: _____ PR Interval: _____ QRS: _____

Interpretation: _____

ECG 11•74

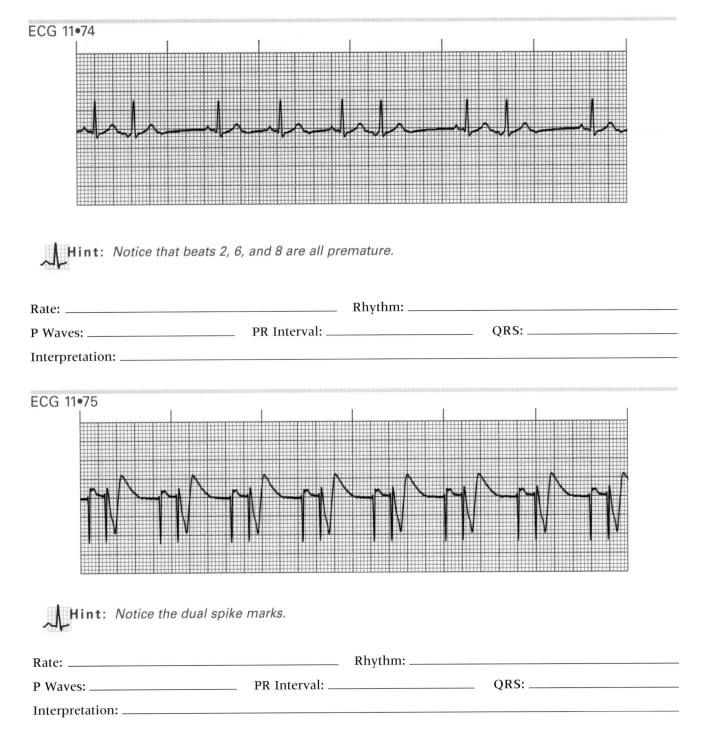

Hint: *Notice that beats 2, 6, and 8 are all premature.*

Rate: _____ Rhythm: _____

P Waves: _____ PR Interval: _____ QRS: _____

Interpretation: _____

ECG 11•75

Hint: *Notice the dual spike marks.*

Rate: _____ Rhythm: _____

P Waves: _____ PR Interval: _____ QRS: _____

Interpretation: _____

Answers to Practice Test One

▧ ECG 11•1
Rate: 38 bpm
Rhythm: Regular
P Waves: Normal
PR Interval: 0.16 sec
QRS: 0.10 sec
Interpretation: Sinus bradycardia

▧ ECG 11•2
Rate: 136 bpm
Rhythm: Regular
P Waves: Normal but encroach on preceding T waves
PR Interval: 0.12 sec
QRS: 0.08 sec
Interpretation: Sinus tachycardia

▧ ECG 11•3
Rate: 68 bpm
Rhythm: Regular
P Waves: Present following pacemaker spike
PR Interval: 0.16 sec
QRS: 0.06 sec
Interpretation: Pacemaker—atrial; ventricular sensed

▧ ECG 11•4
Rate: 38 bpm
Rhythm: Regular
P Waves: Normal
PR Interval: 0.16 sec
QRS: 0.10 sec
Interpretation: Sinus bradycardia with ST segment depression and inverted T waves

▧ ECG 11•5
Rate: 90 bpm (counting PVCs), 75 bpm in now underlying rhythm
Rhythm: Irregular
P Waves: Normal
PR Interval: 0.16 sec
QRS: 0.10 sec
Interpretation: Normal sinus rhythm with two multiform PVCs with noncompensatory pauses

▧ ECG 11•6
Rate: 90 bpm
Rhythm: Irregular
P Waves: Flutter waves
PR Interval: None
QRS: 0.08 sec
Interpretation: Atrial flutter with variable block

▧ ECG 11•7
Rate: 150 bpm
Rhythm: Regular
P Waves: Normal
PR Interval: 0.12 sec
QRS: 0.08 sec
Interpretation: Sinus tachycardia

▧ ECG 11•8
Rate: 60 bpm
Rhythm: Irregular
P Waves: Normal
PR Interval: 0.20 sec
QRS: 0.10 sec
Interpretation: Sinus arrhythmia with respiration artifact

▧ ECG 11•9
Rate: 88 bpm
Rhythm: Regular
P Waves: Normal
PR Interval: 0.20 sec
QRS: 0.10 sec
Interpretation: Normal sinus rhythm with ST segment depression and inverted T waves

▧ ECG 11•10
Rate: 54 bpm
Rhythm: Regular
P Waves: None
PR Interval: None
QRS: 0.12 sec
Interpretation: Junctional rhythm with bundle branch block

▧ ECG 11•11
Rate: 88 bpm
Rhythm: Regular
P Waves: None
PR Interval: None
QRS: 0.16 sec
Interpretation: Accelerated idioventricular rhythm

▧ ECG 11•12
Rate: 60 bpm
Rhythm: Irregular
P Waves: Normal
PR Interval: Progressive prolongation until dropped QRS
QRS: 0.10 sec
Interpretation: Second-degree AV block Type I (Wenckebach)

■ **ECG 11•13**
Rate: 78 bpm
Rhythm: Regular
P Waves: Normal
PR Interval: 0.16 sec
QRS: 0.10 sec
Interpretation: Normal sinus rhythm

■ **ECG 11•14**
Rate: 88 bpm
Rhythm: Regular
P Waves: Normal
PR Interval: 0.20 sec
QRS: 0.08 sec
Interpretation: Normal sinus rhythm with ST
    segment elevation

■ **ECG 11•15**
Rate: 50 bpm
Rhythm: Irregular
P Waves: None
PR Interval: None
QRS: 0.20 sec following pacemaker spike
Interpretation: Pacemaker—ventricular with
    intermittent loss of capture

■ **ECG 11•16**
Rate: 120 bpm (counting PVCs), underlying rhythm
    is 125 bpm
Rhythm: Irregular
P Waves: Normal
PR Interval: 0.16 sec
QRS: 0.08 sec
Interpretation: Sinus tachycardia with ST segment
    depression and couplet PVCs

■ **ECG 11•17**
Rate: 68 bpm
Rhythm: Regular
P Waves: Normal
PR Interval: 0.28 sec
QRS: 0.10 sec
Interpretation: Normal sinus rhythm with first-
    degree AV block

■ **ECG 11•18**
Rate: 50 bpm
Rhythm: Irregular
P Waves: None
PR Interval: None
QRS: 0.10 sec
Interpretation: Atrial fibrillation with ST segment
    depression and slow ventricular response

■ **ECG 11•19**
Rate: 71 bpm
Rhythm: Regular
P Waves: Inverted
PR Interval: 0.08 sec
QRS: 0.08 sec
Interpretation: Accelerated junctional rhythm

■ **ECG 11•20**
Rate: 70 bpm
Rhythm: Irregular
P Waves: Normal
PR Interval: 0.32 sec for beats 2 through 6
QRS: 0.10 sec
Interpretation: Normal sinus rhythm first-degree AV
    block changing to second-degree AV block type I

■ **ECG 11•21**
Rate: 80 bpm (counting PVCs), 88 bpm for underly-
    ing rhythm
Rhythm: Irregular
P Waves: Normal
PR Interval: 0.16 sec
QRS: 0.10 sec
Interpretation: Normal sinus rhythm with PVCs at
    beats 2 and 7

■ **ECG 11•22**
Rate: 90 bpm (counting PVCs), 75 bpm for underly-
    ing rhythm
Rhythm: Irregular
P Waves: Normal
PR Interval: 0.16 sec
QRS: 0.10 sec
Interpretation: Normal sinus rhythm with multiform
    PVCs at beats 6 and 8

■ **ECG 11•23**
Rate: 50 bpm, 68 bpm for underlying rhythm
Rhythm: Irregular
P Waves: Normal
PR Interval: 0.16 sec
QRS: 0.10 sec
Interpretation: Normal sinus rhythm with sinus block
    (two blocked beats)

■ **ECG 11•24**
Rate: Indeterminate
Rhythm: Chaotic
P Waves: None
PR Interval: None
QRS: None
Interpretation: Ventricular fibrillation—coarse
    fibrillatory waves

■ ECG 11•25
Rate: 68 bpm
Rhythm: Regular
P Waves: Normal
PR Interval: 0.12 sec
QRS: 0.12 sec with notched appearance
Interpretation: Normal sinus rhythm with a bundle
    branch block

■ ECG 11•26
Rate: Indeterminate
Rhythm: Irregular
P Waves: None
PR Interval: None
QRS: Variable
Interpretation: Ventricular fibrillation with defibrilla-
    tion converting to atrial fibrillation

■ ECG 11•27
Rate: Atrial 90 bpm, ventricular 35 bpm
Rhythm: Atrial irregular, ventricular regular
P Waves: Normal but not associated with QRS
PR Interval: Variable
QRS: 0.14 sec
Interpretation: Third-degree AV block

■ ECG 11•28
Rate: 70 bpm in second half of strip
Rhythm: Irregular
P Waves: Normal following pacemaker spike
PR Interval: 0.16 sec
QRS: 0.10 sec
Interpretation: Pacemaker—atrial with failure to
    capture at first three pacemaker spikes. When
    the current is increased, there is capture at pace-
    maker spikes 4 through 7.

■ ECG 11•29
Rate: 100 bpm
Rhythm: Irregular
P Waves: None
PR Interval: None
QRS: 0.12 sec
Interpretation: Atrial fibrillation with a bundle
    branch block

■ ECG 11•30
Rate: 90 bpm; 75 bpm in underlying rhythm, over
    100 bpm in VT
Rhythm: Irregular
P Waves: Not seen due to artifact
PR Interval: Indeterminate due to artifact
QRS: 0.08 sec for beats 1 through 4
Interpretation: Probably normal sinus rhythm with
    muscle artifact converting to ventricular tachycar-
    dia at beat 5

■ ECG 11•31
Rate: 60 bpm (counting PVCs), 38 bpm in
    underlying rhythm
Rhythm: Irregular
P Waves: Normal
PR Interval: 0.16 sec
QRS: 0.10 sec
Interpretation: Sinus bradycardia with interpolated
    PVCs (R on T)

■ ECG 11•32
Rate: 56 bpm
Rhythm: Regular
P Waves: Normal
PR Interval: 0.12 sec
QRS: 0.10 sec
Interpretation: Sinus bradycardia with respiration
    artifact

■ ECG 11•33
Rate: 70 bpm
Rhythm: Irregular
P Waves: None
PR Interval: None
QRS: 0.08 sec
Interpretation: Atrial fibrillation with ST segment
    depression

■ ECG 11•34
Rate: 40 bpm
Rhythm: Irregular
P Waves: None
PR Interval: None
QRS: 0.10 sec
Interpretation: Atrial fibrillation with slow ventricu-
    lar response

■ ECG 11•35
Rate: 70 bpm
Rhythm: Irregular
P Waves: Normal
PR Interval: 0.16 sec
QRS: 0.10 sec
Interpretation: Normal sinus rhythm with one
    PAC at beat 3

■ ECG 11•36
Rate: 80 bpm
Rhythm: Irregular
P Waves: None
PR Interval: None
QRS: 0.08 sec
Interpretation: Accelerated junctional rhythm
    with ST segment elevation and PJCs at beats
    2 and 4

■ ECG 11•37
Rate: 79 bpm
Rhythm: Regular
P Waves: Normal
PR Interval: 0.12 sec
QRS: 0.08 sec
Interpretation: Normal sinus rhythm
    with peaked T waves

■ ECG 11•38
Rate: 88 bpm
Rhythm: Regular
P Waves: Normal
PR Interval: 0.12 sec
QRS: 0.10 sec
Interpretation: Normal sinus rhythm with
    ST segment elevation and inverted T waves

■ ECG 11•39
Rate: Atrial 79 bpm, ventricular 47 bpm
Rhythm: Atrial regular, ventricular regular
P Waves: Normal but not associated with QRS
PR Interval: Variable
QRS: 0.16 sec
Interpretation: Third-degree AV block

■ ECG 11•40
Rate: 50 bpm
Rhythm: Irregular
P Waves: Flutter waves
PR Interval: None
QRS: 0.08 sec
Interpretation: Atrial flutter with variable block

■ ECG 11•41
Rate: 80 bpm (counting PVCs), 71 bpm in
    underlying rhythm
Rhythm: Irregular
P Waves: Normal
PR Interval: 0.14 sec
QRS: 0.10 sec
Interpretation: Normal sinus rhythm with
    U waves and two uniform PVCs with
    noncompensatory pauses

■ ECG 11•42
Rate: Indeterminate
Rhythm: Chaotic
P Waves: None
PR Interval: None
QRS: None
Interpretation: Ventricular fibrillation

■ ECG 11•43
Rate: 50 bpm
Rhythm: Regular
P Waves: Normal
PR Interval: 0.20 sec
QRS: 0.08 sec
Interpretation: Sinus bradycardia

■ ECG 11•44
Rate: 100 bpm
Rhythm: Irregular
P Waves: Flutter waves changing to fibrillatory waves
PR Interval: Indeterminate
QRS: 0.08 sec
Interpretation: Atrial flutter converting to atrial
    fibrillation

■ ECG 11•45
Rate: 30 bpm
Rhythm: Irregular
P Waves: Normal
PR Interval: 0.16 sec
QRS: 0.10 sec
Interpretation: Sinus pause (sinus arrest) with
    4.28-sec pause (arrest)

■ ECG 11•46
Rate: 150 bpm before and after defibrillation
Rhythm: Regular in section before and after
    defibrillation
P Waves: None
PR Interval: None
QRS: Wide—greater than 0.10 sec
Interpretation: After checking the patient, there are
    no pulses, ventricular tachycardia defibrillated,
    converting back to ventricular tachycardia with no
    pulses

■ ECG 11•47
Rate: 90 bpm
Rhythm: Irregular
P Waves: Normal
PR Interval: 0.24 sec
QRS: 0.08 sec
Interpretation: Normal sinus rhythm with first-
    degree AV block including ST segment elevation
    and bigeminal PJCs

■ ECG 11•48
Rate: 110 bpm
Rhythm: Irregular
P Waves: None
PR Interval: None
QRS: 0.10 sec
Interpretation: Atrial fibrillation with rapid ventricu-
    lar response

ECG 11•49
Rate: 80 bpm
Rhythm: Regular
P Waves: Present with low amplitude following pacemaker spike
PR Interval: 0.20 sec
QRS: 0.18 sec following pacemaker spike
Interpretation: Pacemaker—atrial and ventricular

ECG 11•50
Rate: 76 bpm in first section; 170–180 bpm in second section
Rhythm: Irregular
P Waves: Normal in first five beats
PR Interval: 0.12 sec in first five beats
QRS: 0.10 sec in the first five beats changing to a wide QRS—greater than 0.10 sec in the last seven ventricular beats
Interpretation: Normal sinus rhythm converting to ventricular tachycardia

ECG 11•51
Rate: 150 bpm; 214 bpm in first section; 100 bpm in second section
Rhythm: Irregular
P Waves: Buried in T wave in beats 1 through 9, none in beat 10, and normal in beats 11 through 15
PR Interval: None in beats 1 through 10, 0.16 sec in beats 11 through 15
QRS: 0.08 sec
Interpretation: Paroxysmal supraventricular tachycardia (supraventricular tachycardia converting to normal sinus rhythm)

ECG 11•52
Rate: 70 bpm (counting PVCs), 68 bpm in underlying rhythm
Rhythm: Irregular
P Waves: Normal
PR Interval: 0.16 sec
QRS: 0.08 sec
Interpretation: Normal sinus rhythm with multiform PVCs at beats 2 and 5 with full compensatory pauses

ECG 11•53
Rate: 80 bpm
Rhythm: Irregular
P Waves: Present with low amplitude
PR Interval: 0.20 sec
QRS: 0.08 sec
Interpretation: Normal sinus rhythm with two PACs at beats 4 and 7

ECG 11•54
Rate: Indeterminate
Rhythm: Chaotic
P Waves: None
PR Interval: None
QRS: First five beats wide—greater than 0.10 sec; for remainder of rhythm—no true QRS complexes
Interpretation: Ventricular tachycardia deteriorating into ventricular fibrillation with coarse fibrillatory waves

ECG 11•55
Rate: None
Rhythm: None
P Waves: None
PR Interval: None
QRS: None
Interpretation: Asystole

ECG 11•56
Rate: 214 bpm
Rhythm: Regular
P Waves: None
PR Interval: None
QRS: Wide—greater than 0.10 sec
Interpretation: Ventricular tachycardia—monomorphic

ECG 11•57
Rate: 80 bpm
Rhythm: Irregular
P Waves: None
PR Interval: None
QRS: 0.12 sec following pacemaker spike
Interpretation: Pacemaker—atrial and ventricular, with no capture of the P waves and with a short run of ventricular tachycardia

ECG 11•58
Rate: 110 bpm
Rhythm: Irregular
P Waves: None
PR Interval: None
QRS: 0.08 sec
Interpretation: Atrial fibrillation with rapid ventricular response

ECG 11•59
Rate: 48 bpm
Rhythm: Regular
P Waves: Absent or inverted
PR Interval: Varies
QRS: 0.10 sec
Interpretation: Junctional rhythm

■ ECG 11•60
Rate: Indeterminate
Rhythm: Irregular
P Waves: None
PR Interval: None
QRS: Wide—greater than 0.10 sec
Interpretation: Ventricular tachycardia—
    polymorphic vs. artifact: assess patient

■ ECG 11•61
Rate: Indeterminate
Rhythm: Irregular
P Waves: None
PR Interval: None
QRS: Wide—greater than 0.10 sec
Interpretation: Torsade de pointes

■ ECG 11•62
Rate: 83 bpm
Rhythm: Regular
P Waves: Normal but distorted due to artifact
PR Interval: Indeterminate
QRS: 0.10 sec
Interpretation: Normal sinus rhythm with muscle
    artifact

■ ECG 11•63
Rate: 40 bpm
Rhythm: Irregular
P Waves: Normal in beat 2
PR Interval: 0.20 sec in beat 2
QRS: 0.10 sec in beat 2; wide—greater than
    0.10 sec—in beats 1, 3, and 4 following
    pacemaker spike
Interpretation: Pacemaker—ventricular with
    intrinsic sinus complex at beat 2

■ ECG 11•64
Rate: 136 bpm
Rhythm: Regular
P Waves: Normal
PR Interval: 0.12 sec
QRS: 0.08 sec
Interpretation: Sinus tachycardia with artifact
    after beat 3

■ ECG 11•65
Rate: 125 bpm
Rhythm: Regular
P Waves: Normal
PR Interval: 0.20 sec
QRS: 0.10 sec
Interpretation: Sinus tachycardia with peaked
    T waves

■ ECG 11•66
Rate: 60 bpm
Rhythm: Irregular
P Waves: Normal but not associated with QRS
PR Interval: Variable
QRS: 0.16 sec
Interpretation: Third-degree AV block with
    couplet PVCs

■ ECG 11•67
Rate: 115 bpm
Rhythm: Regular
P Waves: Normal
PR Interval: 0.12 sec
QRS: 0.10 sec
Interpretation: Sinus tachycardia

■ ECG 11•68
Rate: 90 bpm
Rhythm: Irregular
P Waves: Normal
PR Interval: 0.16 sec
QRS: 0.08 sec
Interpretation: Normal sinus rhythm with ventricular
    trigeminy

■ ECG 11•69
Rate: 60 bpm
Rhythm: Irregular
P Waves: Normal
PR Interval: 0.16 sec
QRS: 0.10 sec
Interpretation: Normal sinus rhythm with sinoatrial
    blocks after beats 3 and 4

■ ECG 11•70
Rate: 250 bpm
Rhythm: Regular
P Waves: Buried in T waves
PR Interval: Not measurable
QRS: 0.08 sec
Interpretation: Supraventricular
    tachycardia

■ ECG 11•71
Rate: 60 bpm
Rhythm: Irregular
P Waves: None
PR Interval: None
QRS: 0.16 sec
Interpretation: Atrial fibrillation with
    bundle branch block

■ ECG 11•72

Rate: 94 bpm
Rhythm: Regular
P Waves: Normal following pacemaker spike
PR Interval: 0.16 sec
QRS: 0.10 sec
Interpretation: Pacemaker—atrial; ventricular

■ ECG 11•73

Rate: Indeterminate
Rhythm: Irregular
P Waves: None
PR Interval: None
QRS: Wide—greater than 0.10 sec
Interpretation: Ventricular tachycardia—
   polymorphic

■ ECG 11•74

Rate: 90 bpm
Rhythm: Irregular
P Waves: Normal
PR Interval: 0.12 sec
QRS: 0.10 sec
Interpretation: Normal sinus rhythm with PJCs
   at beats 2, 6, and 8

■ ECG 11•75

Rate: 75 bpm
Rhythm: Regular
P Waves: Present following pacemaker spike
PR Interval: 0.20 sec
QRS: 0.16 sec following pacemaker spike
Interpretation: Pacemaker—atrial and ventricular

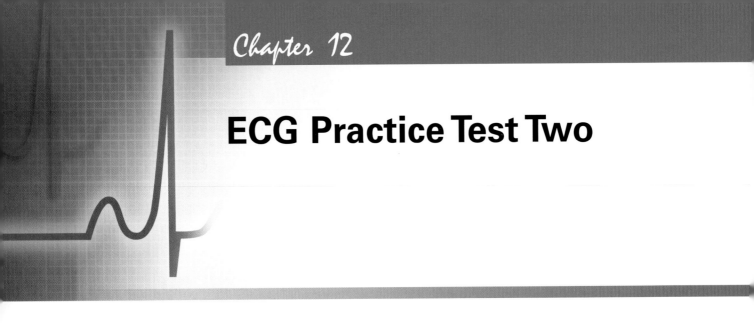

Chapter 12

ECG Practice Test Two

For instructions on analyzing these practice test strips, please see the guidelines given at the end of chapter 2.

TEST STRIP SECTION TWO ■

ECG 12•1

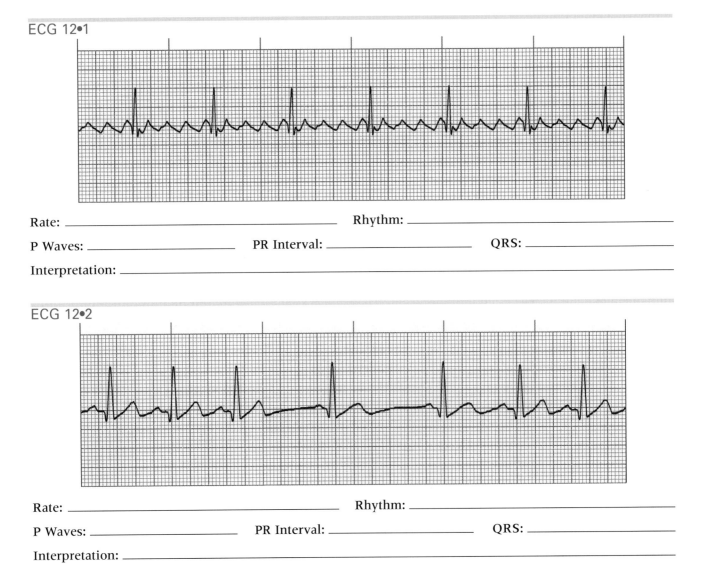

Rate: _____ Rhythm: _____

P Waves: _____ PR Interval: _____ QRS: _____

Interpretation: _____

ECG 12•2

Rate: _____ Rhythm: _____

P Waves: _____ PR Interval: _____ QRS: _____

Interpretation: _____

ECG 12•3

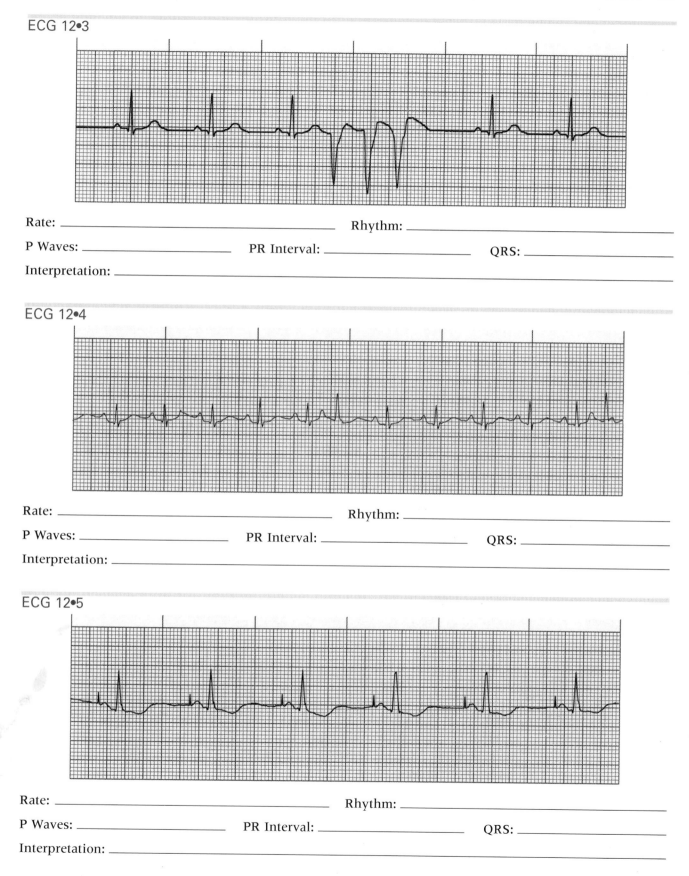

Rate: _____   Rhythm: _____

P Waves: _____   PR Interval: _____   QRS: _____

Interpretation: _____

ECG 12•4

Rate: _____   Rhythm: _____

P Waves: _____   PR Interval: _____   QRS: _____

Interpretation: _____

ECG 12•5

Rate: _____   Rhythm: _____

P Waves: _____   PR Interval: _____   QRS: _____

Interpretation: _____

ECG 12•6

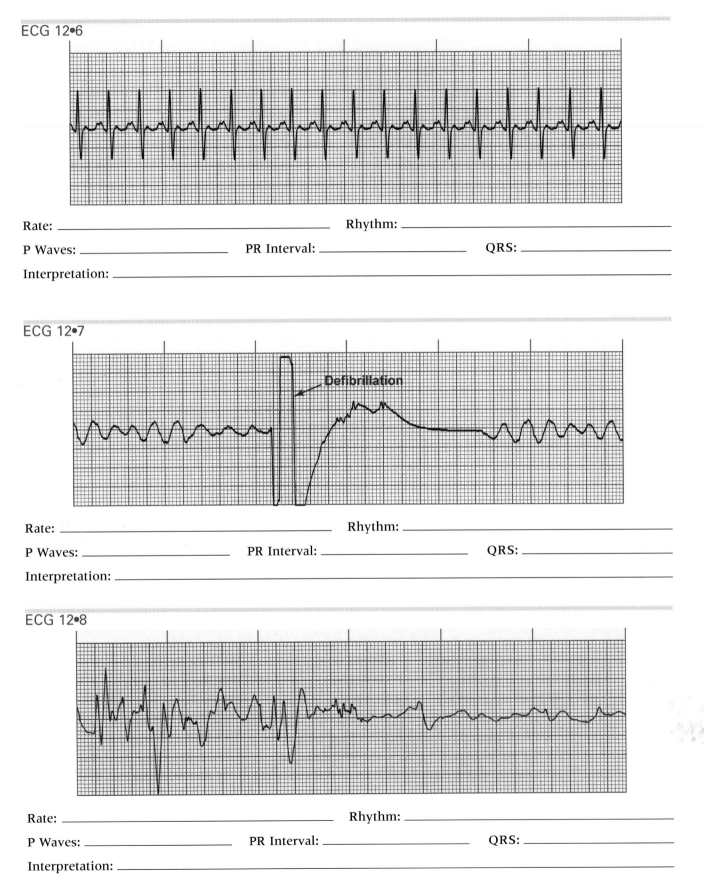

Rate: _____   Rhythm: _____

P Waves: _____   PR Interval: _____   QRS: _____

Interpretation: _____

ECG 12•7

Defibrillation

Rate: _____   Rhythm: _____

P Waves: _____   PR Interval: _____   QRS: _____

Interpretation: _____

ECG 12•8

Rate: _____   Rhythm: _____

P Waves: _____   PR Interval: _____   QRS: _____

Interpretation: _____

ECG 12•9

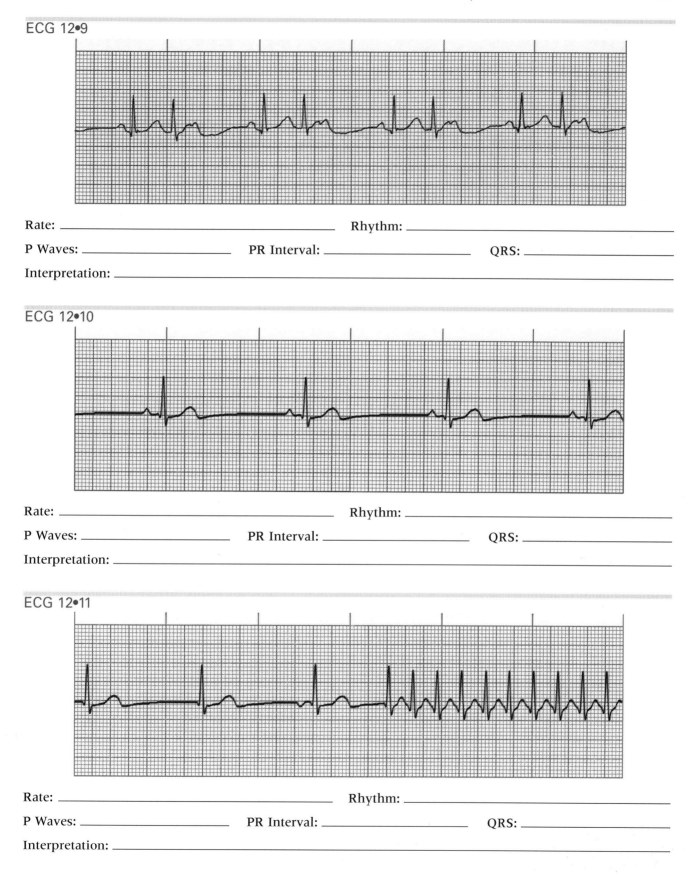

Rate: _____   Rhythm: _____

P Waves: _____   PR Interval: _____   QRS: _____

Interpretation: _____

ECG 12•10

Rate: _____   Rhythm: _____

P Waves: _____   PR Interval: _____   QRS: _____

Interpretation: _____

ECG 12•11

Rate: _____   Rhythm: _____

P Waves: _____   PR Interval: _____   QRS: _____

Interpretation: _____

ECG 12•12

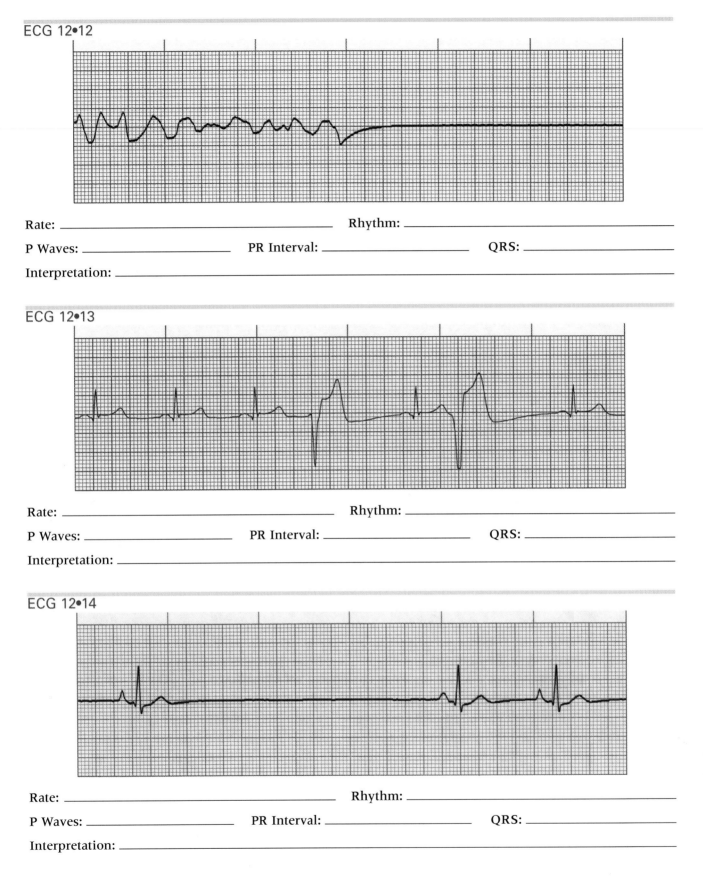

Rate: _____ Rhythm: _____

P Waves: _____ PR Interval: _____ QRS: _____

Interpretation: _____

ECG 12•13

Rate: _____ Rhythm: _____

P Waves: _____ PR Interval: _____ QRS: _____

Interpretation: _____

ECG 12•14

Rate: _____ Rhythm: _____

P Waves: _____ PR Interval: _____ QRS: _____

Interpretation: _____

ECG 12•15

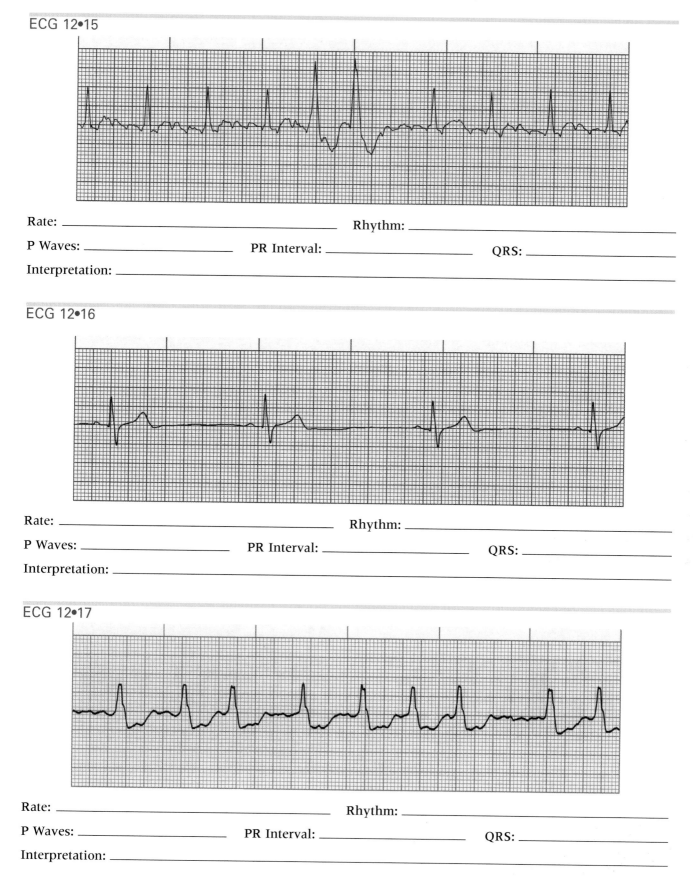

Rate: _____   Rhythm: _____

P Waves: _____   PR Interval: _____   QRS: _____

Interpretation: _____

ECG 12•16

Rate: _____   Rhythm: _____

P Waves: _____   PR Interval: _____   QRS: _____

Interpretation: _____

ECG 12•17

Rate: _____   Rhythm: _____

P Waves: _____   PR Interval: _____   QRS: _____

Interpretation: _____

ECG 12•18

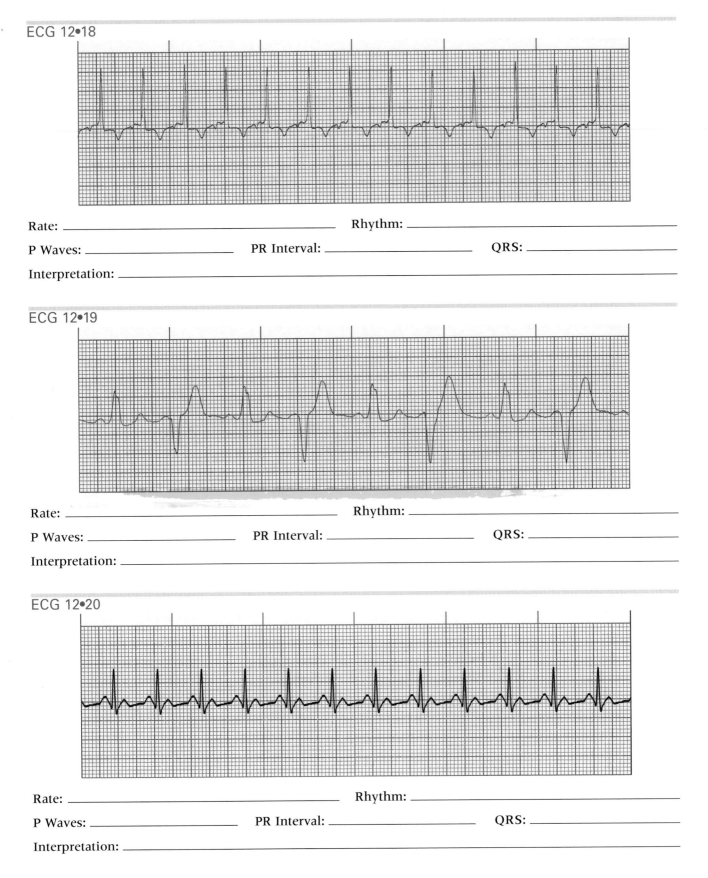

Rate: _____   Rhythm: _____

P Waves: _____   PR Interval: _____   QRS: _____

Interpretation: _____

ECG 12•19

Rate: _____   Rhythm: _____

P Waves: _____   PR Interval: _____   QRS: _____

Interpretation: _____

ECG 12•20

Rate: _____   Rhythm: _____

P Waves: _____   PR Interval: _____   QRS: _____

Interpretation: _____

ECG 12•21

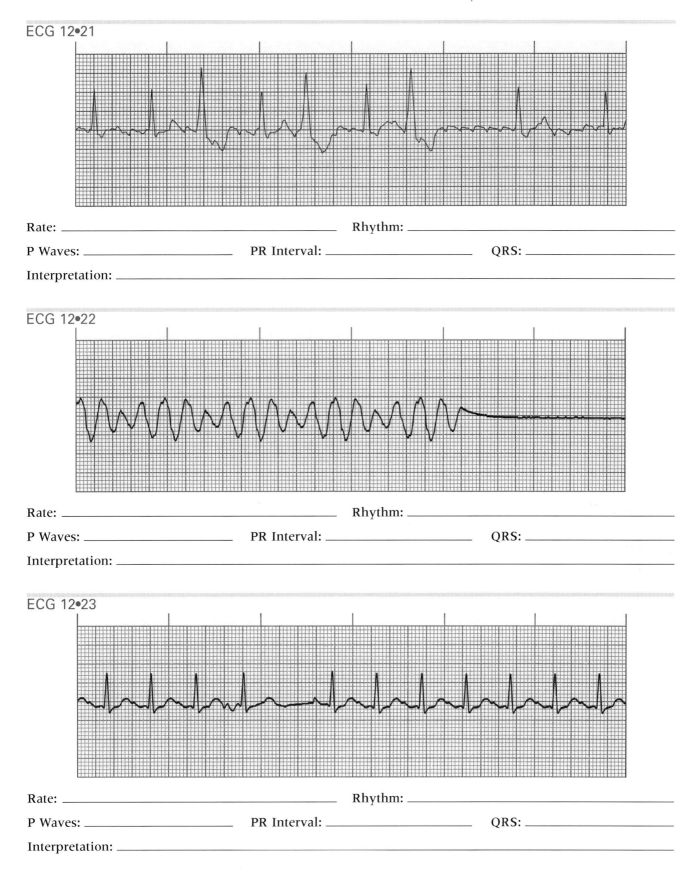

Rate: _____ Rhythm: _____

P Waves: _____ PR Interval: _____ QRS: _____

Interpretation: _____

ECG 12•22

Rate: _____ Rhythm: _____

P Waves: _____ PR Interval: _____ QRS: _____

Interpretation: _____

ECG 12•23

Rate: _____ Rhythm: _____

P Waves: _____ PR Interval: _____ QRS: _____

Interpretation: _____

ECG 12•24

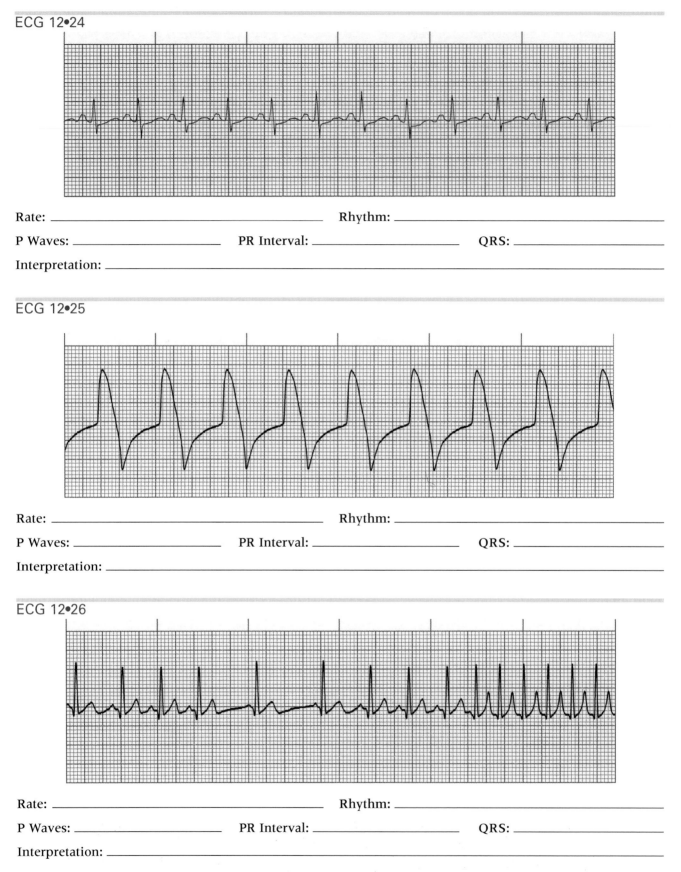

Rate: _____ Rhythm: _____

P Waves: _____ PR Interval: _____ QRS: _____

Interpretation: _____

ECG 12•25

Rate: _____ Rhythm: _____

P Waves: _____ PR Interval: _____ QRS: _____

Interpretation: _____

ECG 12•26

Rate: _____ Rhythm: _____

P Waves: _____ PR Interval: _____ QRS: _____

Interpretation: _____

ECG 12•27

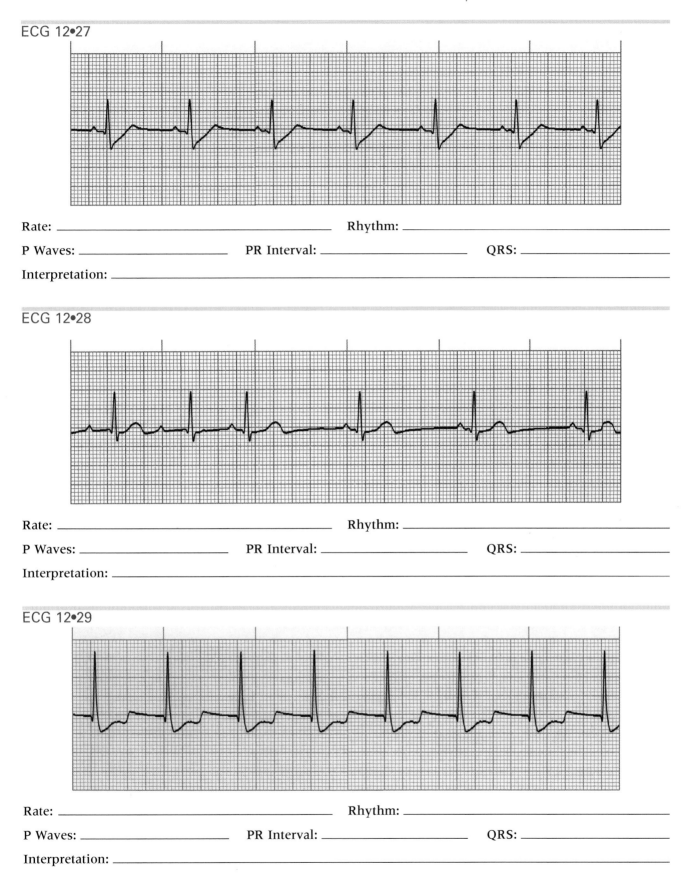

Rate: _____ Rhythm: _____

P Waves: _____ PR Interval: _____ QRS: _____

Interpretation: _____

ECG 12•28

Rate: _____ Rhythm: _____

P Waves: _____ PR Interval: _____ QRS: _____

Interpretation: _____

ECG 12•29

Rate: _____ Rhythm: _____

P Waves: _____ PR Interval: _____ QRS: _____

Interpretation: _____

ECG 12•30

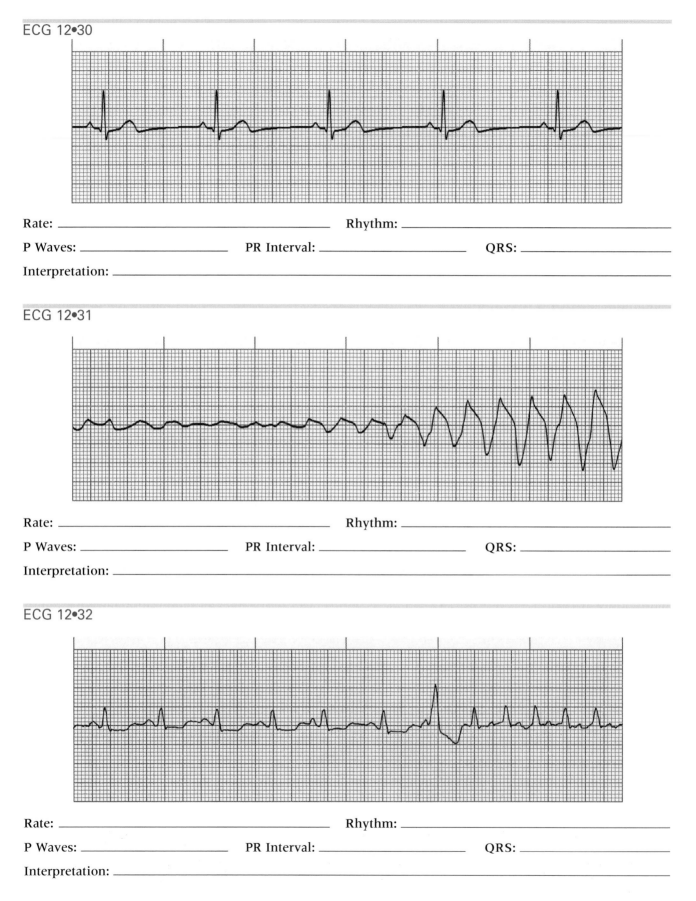

Rate: _____ Rhythm: _____

P Waves: _____ PR Interval: _____ QRS: _____

Interpretation: _____

ECG 12•31

Rate: _____ Rhythm: _____

P Waves: _____ PR Interval: _____ QRS: _____

Interpretation: _____

ECG 12•32

Rate: _____ Rhythm: _____

P Waves: _____ PR Interval: _____ QRS: _____

Interpretation: _____

ECG 12•33

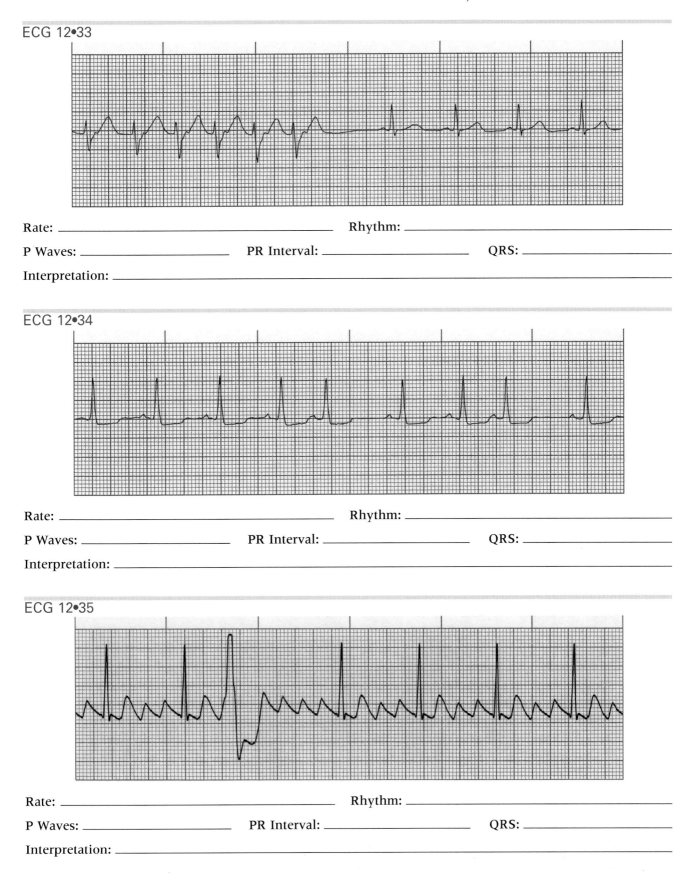

Rate: _____ Rhythm: _____

P Waves: _____ PR Interval: _____ QRS: _____

Interpretation: _____

ECG 12•34

Rate: _____ Rhythm: _____

P Waves: _____ PR Interval: _____ QRS: _____

Interpretation: _____

ECG 12•35

Rate: _____ Rhythm: _____

P Waves: _____ PR Interval: _____ QRS: _____

Interpretation: _____

ECG 12•36

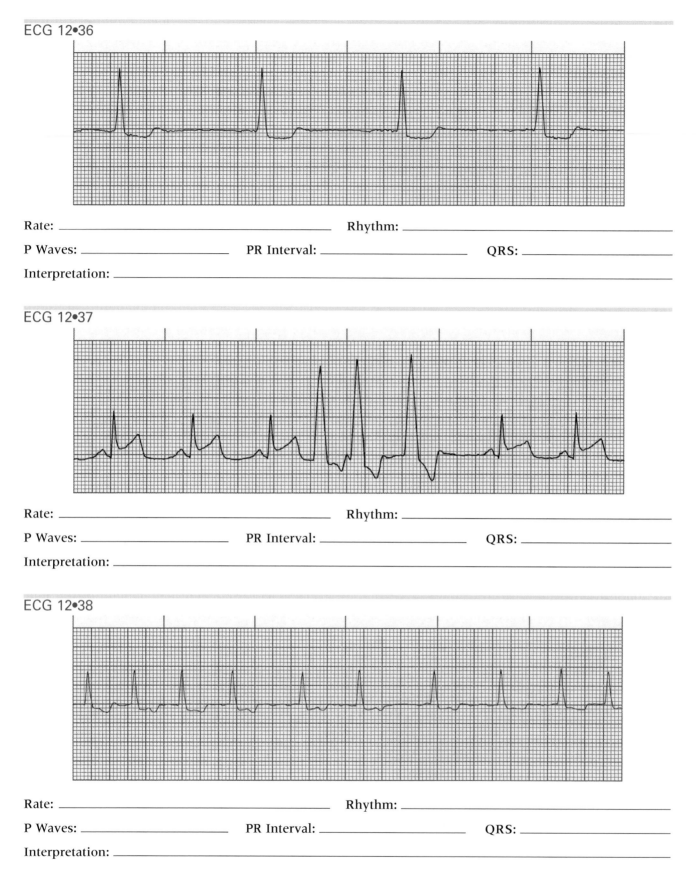

Rate: _____   Rhythm: _____

P Waves: _____   PR Interval: _____   QRS: _____

Interpretation: _____

ECG 12•37

Rate: _____   Rhythm: _____

P Waves: _____   PR Interval: _____   QRS: _____

Interpretation: _____

ECG 12•38

Rate: _____   Rhythm: _____

P Waves: _____   PR Interval: _____   QRS: _____

Interpretation: _____

ECG 12•39

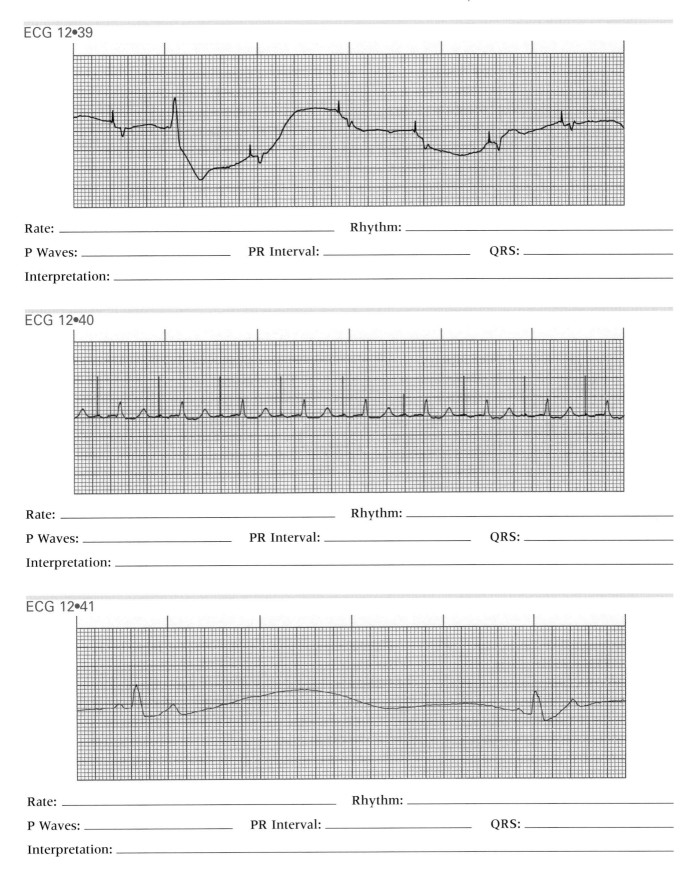

Rate: _____ Rhythm: _____

P Waves: _____ PR Interval: _____ QRS: _____

Interpretation: _____

ECG 12•40

Rate: _____ Rhythm: _____

P Waves: _____ PR Interval: _____ QRS: _____

Interpretation: _____

ECG 12•41

Rate: _____ Rhythm: _____

P Waves: _____ PR Interval: _____ QRS: _____

Interpretation: _____

ECG 12•42

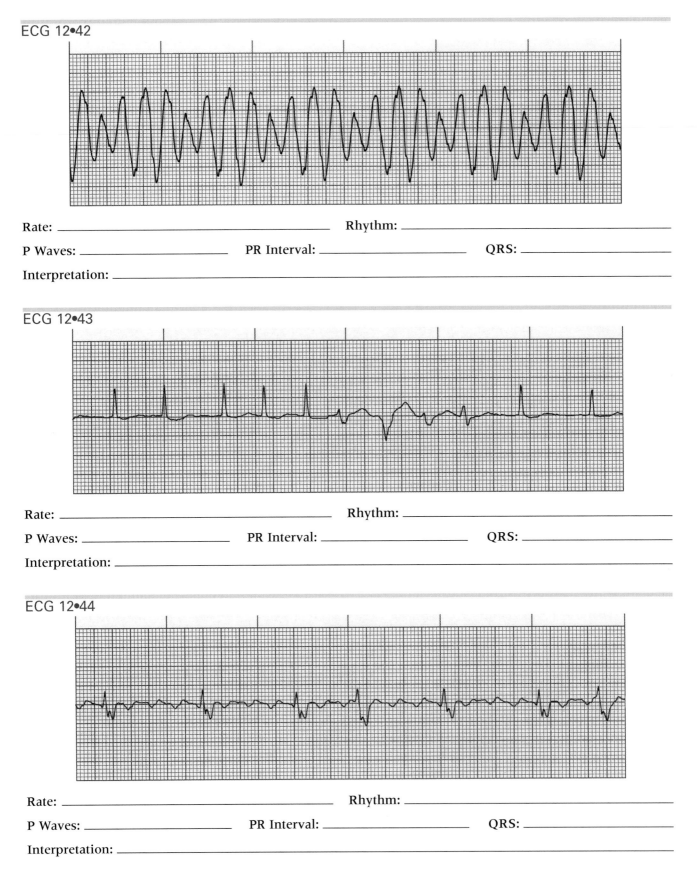

Rate: _____   Rhythm: _____

P Waves: _____   PR Interval: _____   QRS: _____

Interpretation: _____

ECG 12•43

Rate: _____   Rhythm: _____

P Waves: _____   PR Interval: _____   QRS: _____

Interpretation: _____

ECG 12•44

Rate: _____   Rhythm: _____

P Waves: _____   PR Interval: _____   QRS: _____

Interpretation: _____

ECG 12•45

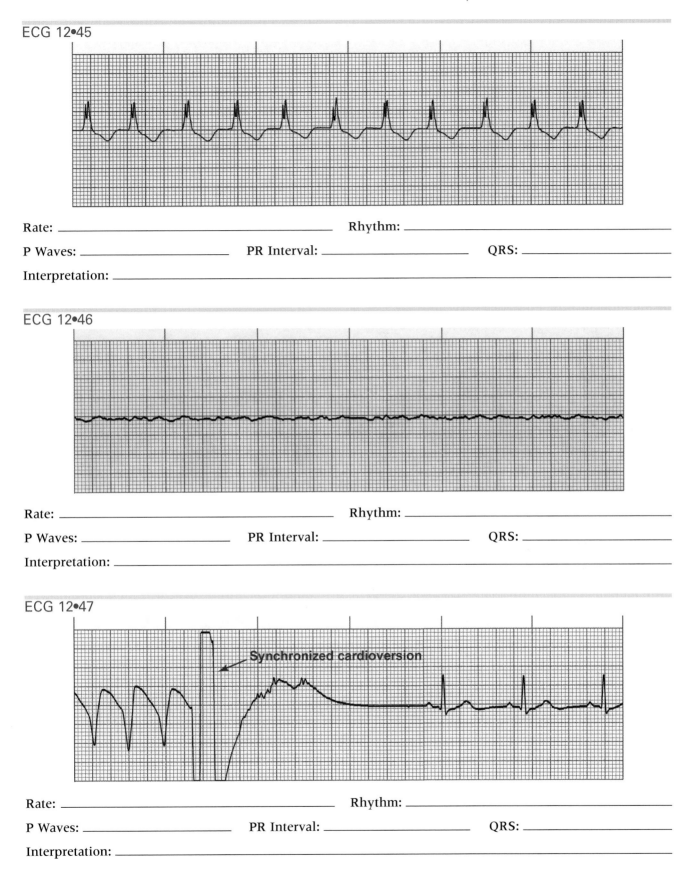

Rate: _____   Rhythm: _____

P Waves: _____   PR Interval: _____   QRS: _____

Interpretation: _____

ECG 12•46

Rate: _____   Rhythm: _____

P Waves: _____   PR Interval: _____   QRS: _____

Interpretation: _____

ECG 12•47

Synchronized cardioversion

Rate: _____   Rhythm: _____

P Waves: _____   PR Interval: _____   QRS: _____

Interpretation: _____

ECG 12•48

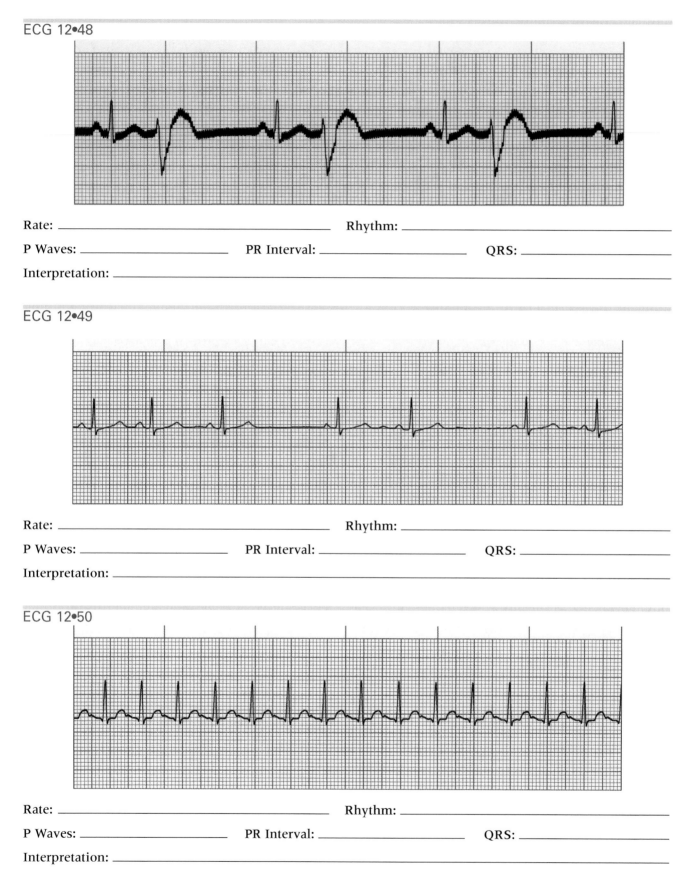

Rate: _____   Rhythm: _____

P Waves: _____   PR Interval: _____   QRS: _____

Interpretation: _____

ECG 12•49

Rate: _____   Rhythm: _____

P Waves: _____   PR Interval: _____   QRS: _____

Interpretation: _____

ECG 12•50

Rate: _____   Rhythm: _____

P Waves: _____   PR Interval: _____   QRS: _____

Interpretation: _____

ECG 12•51

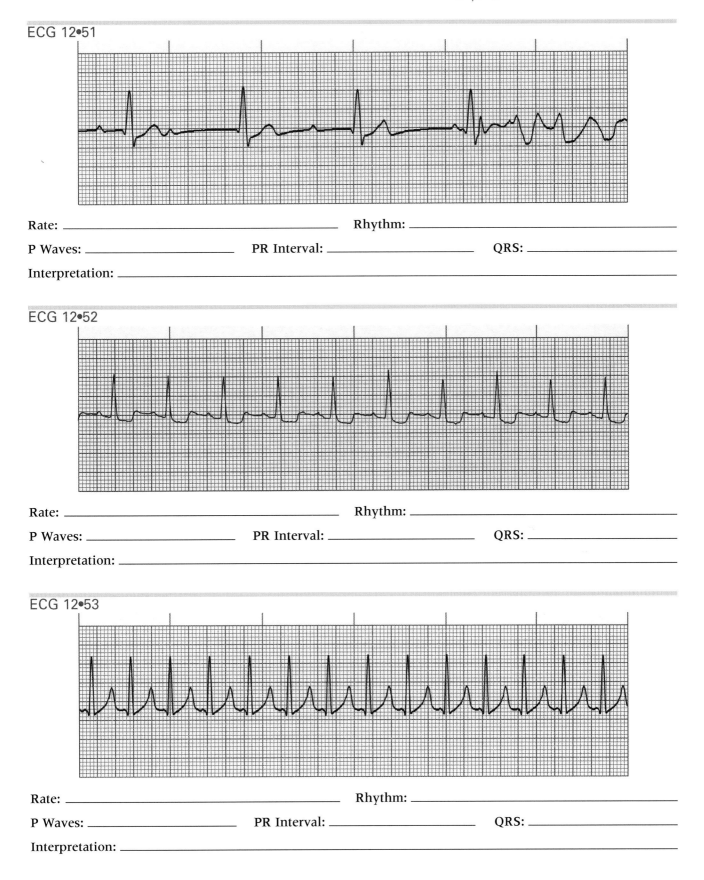

Rate: _____ Rhythm: _____

P Waves: _____ PR Interval: _____ QRS: _____

Interpretation: _____

ECG 12•52

Rate: _____ Rhythm: _____

P Waves: _____ PR Interval: _____ QRS: _____

Interpretation: _____

ECG 12•53

Rate: _____ Rhythm: _____

P Waves: _____ PR Interval: _____ QRS: _____

Interpretation: _____

ECG 12•54

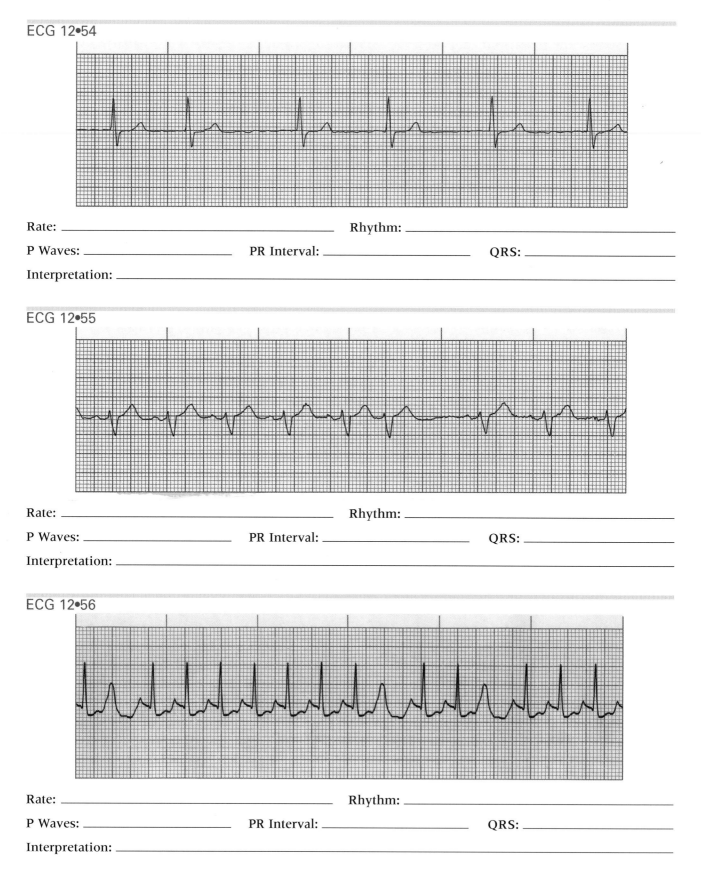

Rate: _____   Rhythm: _____

P Waves: _____   PR Interval: _____   QRS: _____

Interpretation: _____

ECG 12•55

Rate: _____   Rhythm: _____

P Waves: _____   PR Interval: _____   QRS: _____

Interpretation: _____

ECG 12•56

Rate: _____   Rhythm: _____

P Waves: _____   PR Interval: _____   QRS: _____

Interpretation: _____

ECG 12•57

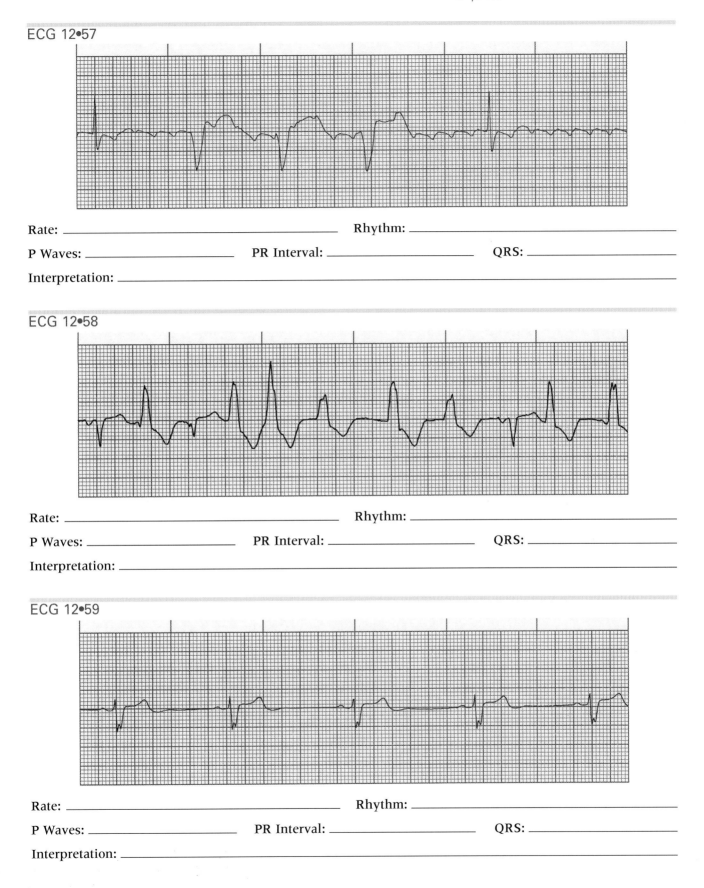

Rate: _____ Rhythm: _____

P Waves: _____ PR Interval: _____ QRS: _____

Interpretation: _____

ECG 12•58

Rate: _____ Rhythm: _____

P Waves: _____ PR Interval: _____ QRS: _____

Interpretation: _____

ECG 12•59

Rate: _____ Rhythm: _____

P Waves: _____ PR Interval: _____ QRS: _____

Interpretation: _____

ECG 12•60

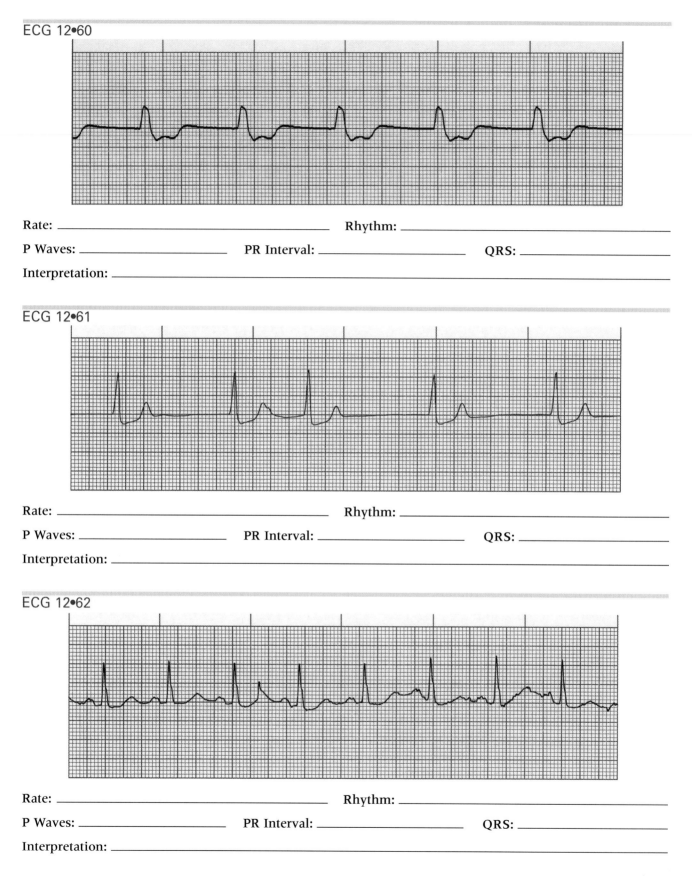

Rate: _____   Rhythm: _____

P Waves: _____   PR Interval: _____   QRS: _____

Interpretation: _____

ECG 12•61

Rate: _____   Rhythm: _____

P Waves: _____   PR Interval: _____   QRS: _____

Interpretation: _____

ECG 12•62

Rate: _____   Rhythm: _____

P Waves: _____   PR Interval: _____   QRS: _____

Interpretation: _____

ECG 12•63

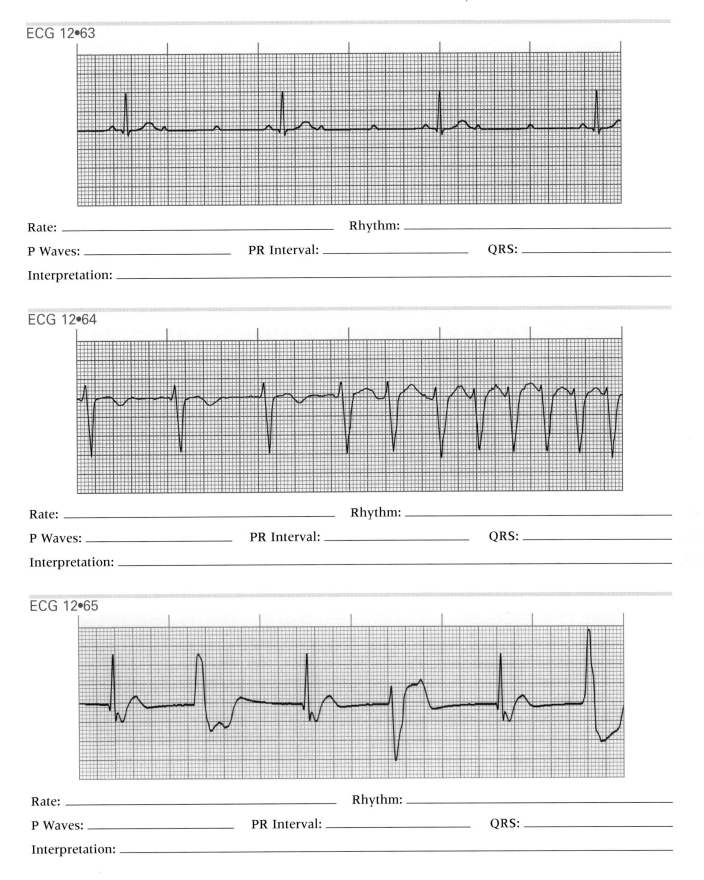

Rate: _____ Rhythm: _____

P Waves: _____ PR Interval: _____ QRS: _____

Interpretation: _____

ECG 12•64

Rate: _____ Rhythm: _____

P Waves: _____ PR Interval: _____ QRS: _____

Interpretation: _____

ECG 12•65

Rate: _____ Rhythm: _____

P Waves: _____ PR Interval: _____ QRS: _____

Interpretation: _____

ECG 12•66

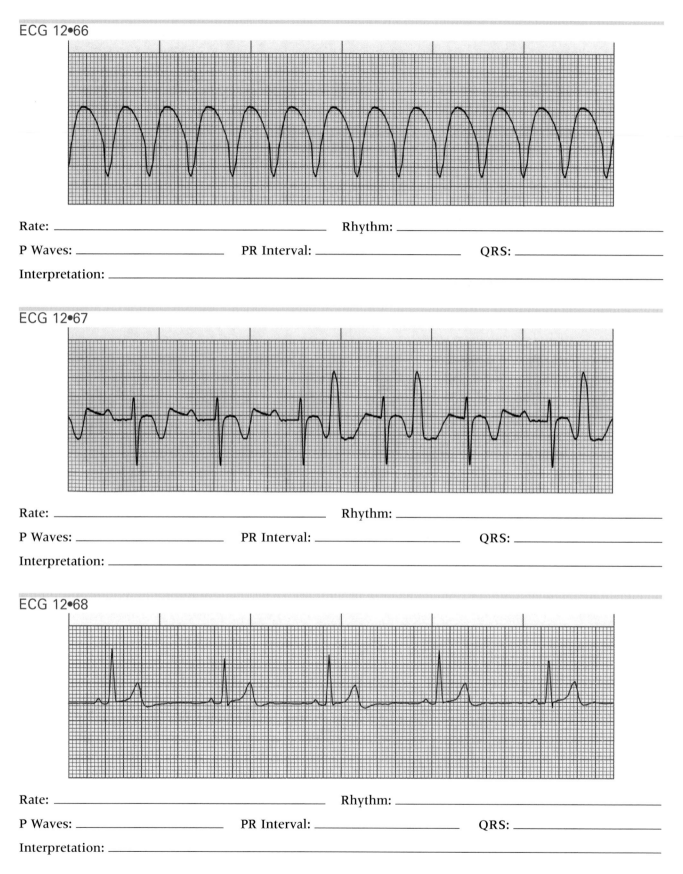

Rate: _____   Rhythm: _____

P Waves: _____   PR Interval: _____   QRS: _____

Interpretation: _____

ECG 12•67

Rate: _____   Rhythm: _____

P Waves: _____   PR Interval: _____   QRS: _____

Interpretation: _____

ECG 12•68

Rate: _____   Rhythm: _____

P Waves: _____   PR Interval: _____   QRS: _____

Interpretation: _____

ECG 12•69

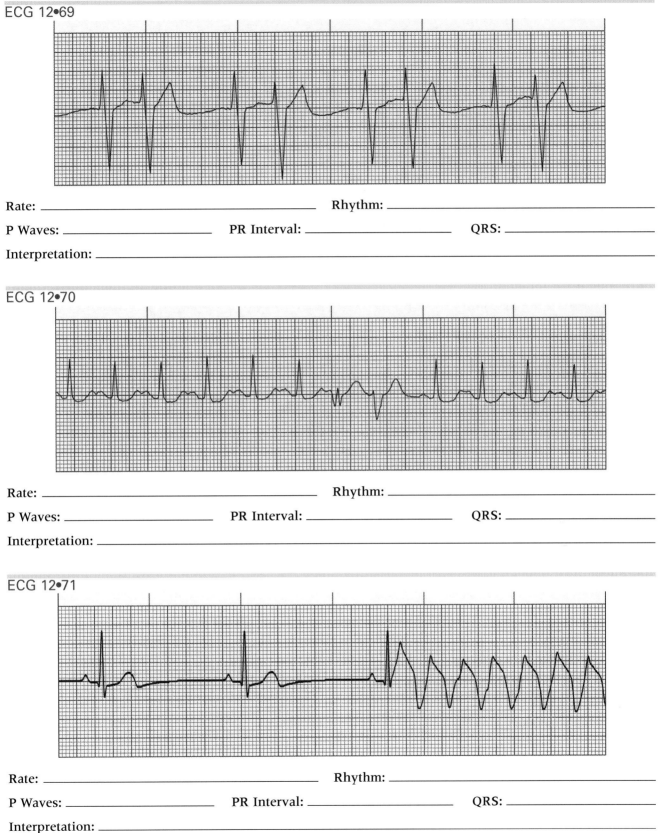

Rate: _____   Rhythm: _____

P Waves: _____   PR Interval: _____   QRS: _____

Interpretation: _____

ECG 12•70

Rate: _____   Rhythm: _____

P Waves: _____   PR Interval: _____   QRS: _____

Interpretation: _____

ECG 12•71

Rate: _____   Rhythm: _____

P Waves: _____   PR Interval: _____   QRS: _____

Interpretation: _____

ECG 12•72

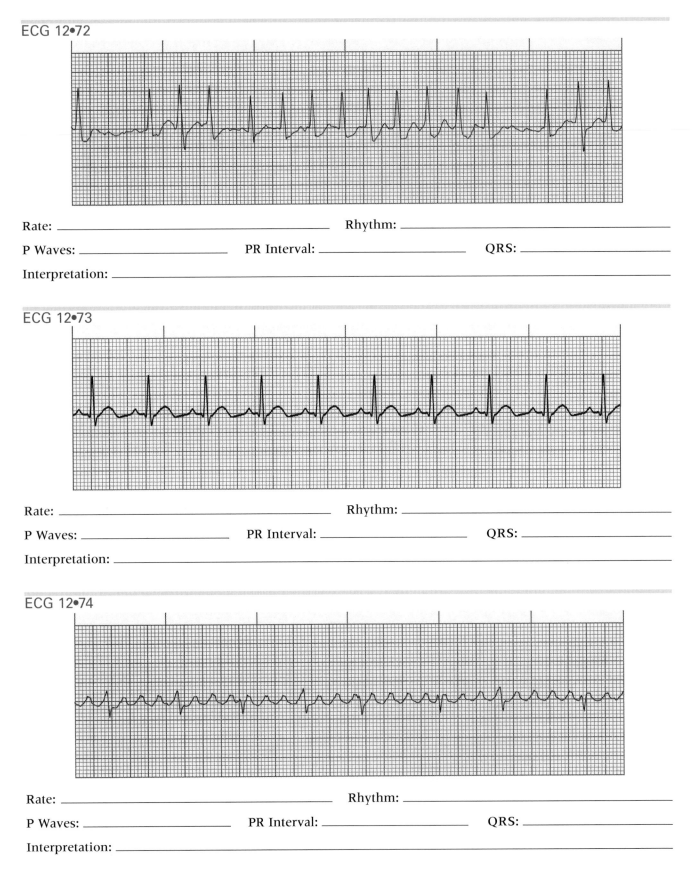

Rate: _____ Rhythm: _____

P Waves: _____ PR Interval: _____ QRS: _____

Interpretation: _____

ECG 12•73

Rate: _____ Rhythm: _____

P Waves: _____ PR Interval: _____ QRS: _____

Interpretation: _____

ECG 12•74

Rate: _____ Rhythm: _____

P Waves: _____ PR Interval: _____ QRS: _____

Interpretation: _____

ECG 12•75

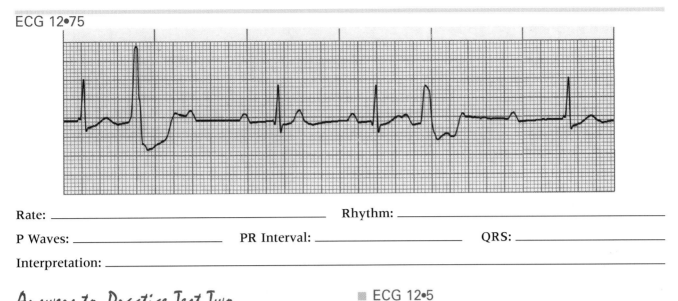

Rate: _____ Rhythm: _____

P Waves: _____ PR Interval: _____ QRS: _____

Interpretation: _____

Answers to Practice Test Two

▦ ECG 12•1

Rate: 68 bpm
Rhythm: Regular
P Waves: Flutter waves
PR Interval: None
QRS: 0.08 sec
Interpretation: Atrial flutter with 4:1 block

▦ ECG 12•2

Rate: 70 bpm
Rhythm: Irregular
P Waves: Vary in form
PR Interval: 0.16 sec
QRS: 0.10 sec
Interpretation: Wandering atrial pacemaker

▦ ECG 12•3

Rate: 80 bpm (counting PVCs), 68 bpm in underlying rhythm
Rhythm: Irregular
P Waves: Normal
PR Interval: 0.16 sec
QRS: 0.10 sec
Interpretation: Normal sinus rhythm with three-beat ventricular tachycardia (triplet PVCs)

▦ ECG 12•4

Rate: 120 bpm, 115 bpm in underlying rhythm
Rhythm: Irregular
P Waves: Normal
PR Interval: 0.16 sec
QRS: 0.08 sec
Interpretation: Sinus tachycardia with PACs at beats 6 and 12

▦ ECG 12•5

Rate: 60 bpm
Rhythm: Regular
P Waves: Normal following pacemaker spike
PR Interval: 0.16 sec
QRS: 0.10 sec
Interpretation: Pacemaker—atrial paced, ventricular sensed with ST segment depression and inverted T waves

▦ ECG 12•6

Rate: 188 bpm
Rhythm: Regular
P Waves: Not clearly visible, probably buried in T waves
PR Interval: 0.06 sec
QRS: 0.10 sec
Interpretation: Atrial tachycardia

▦ ECG 12•7

Rate: Indeterminate
Rhythm: Chaotic
P Waves: None
PR Interval: None
QRS: None
Interpretation: Ventricular fibrillation with defibrillation and return to ventricular fibrillation

▦ ECG 12•8

Rate: Indeterminate
Rhythm: Chaotic
P Waves: None
PR Interval: None
QRS: None
Interpretation: Coarse ventricular fibrillation deteriorating to fine ventricular fibrillation

■ ECG 12•9

Rate: 80 bpm (counting PJCs)
Rhythm: Irregular
P Waves: Normal except none in PJCs
PR Interval: 0.16 sec in sinus beats
QRS: 0.10 sec
Interpretation: Normal sinus rhythm with bigeminal
    PJCs

■ ECG 12•10

Rate: 38 bpm
Rhythm: Regular
P Waves: Normal
PR Interval: 0.16 sec
QRS: 0.08 sec
Interpretation: Sinus bradycardia

■ ECG 12•11

Rate: 130 bpm; 50 bpm in first section, 240 bpm in
    second section
Rhythm: Irregular
P Waves: None in beats 1, 2, and 4; inverted in beat
    3; buried in T waves in beats 5 through 13
PR Interval: None except 0.16 sec in beat 3
QRS: 0.08 sec
Interpretation: Paroxysmal supraventricular tachy-
    cardia (junctional rhythm converting to supraven-
    tricular tachycardia)

■ ECG 12•12

Rate: Indeterminate
Rhythm: Irregular
P Waves: None
PR Interval: None
QRS: None
Interpretation: Ventricular fibrillation deteriorating to
    asystole

■ ECG 12•13

Rate: 70 bpm
Rhythm: Irregular
P Waves: Normal
PR Interval: 0.16 sec
QRS: 0.10 sec
Interpretation: Normal sinus rhythm with PVCs at
    beats 4 and 6

■ ECG 12•14

Rate: 30 bpm
Rhythm: Irregular
P Waves: Normal
PR Interval: 0.16 sec
QRS: 0.10 sec
Interpretation: Sinus bradycardia with a 3.48 sec
    pause (sinus arrest)

■ ECG 12•15

Rate: 100 bpm
Rhythm: Irregular
P Waves: Flutter waves
PR Interval: None
QRS: 0.08 sec
Interpretation: Atrial flutter with 4:1
    conduction and couplet PVCs

■ ECG 12•16

Rate: 40 bpm
Rhythm: Irregular
P Waves: Normal
PR Interval: 0.16 sec
QRS: 0.10 sec
Interpretation: Sinus bradycardia with sinus
    arrhythmia

■ ECG 12•17

Rate: 90 bpm
Rhythm: Irregular
P Waves: None
PR Interval: None
QRS: 0.12 sec
Interpretation: Atrial fibrillation with
    bundle branch block

■ ECG 12•18

Rate: 136 bpm
Rhythm: Regular
P Waves: Inverted
PR Interval: 0.12 sec
QRS: 0.06 sec
Interpretation: Junctional tachycardia
    with inverted T waves

■ ECG 12•19

Rate: 80 bpm
Rhythm: Irregular
P Waves: Normal with beats 1, 3, 5, and 7
PR Interval: 0.16 sec with beats 1, 3, 5,
    and 7
QRS: 0.12 sec
Interpretation: Normal sinus rhythm
    with bundle branch block, and
    bigeminal PVCs

■ ECG 12•20

Rate: 125 bpm
Rhythm: Regular
P Waves: Normal
PR Interval: 0.12 sec
QRS: 0.08 sec
Interpretation: Sinus tachycardia

■ ECG 12•21
Rate: 90 bpm
Rhythm: Irregular
P Waves: Flutter waves
PR Interval: None
QRS: 0.10 sec
Interpretation: Atrial fibrillation with PVCs at beats
3, 5, and 7 changing to atrial flutter

■ ECG 12•22
Rate: Indeterminate
Rhythm: Irregular
P Waves: None
PR Interval: None
QRS: None
Interpretation: Coarse ventricular fibrillation deterio-
rating to asystole

■ ECG 12•23
Rate: 110 bpm
Rhythm: Irregular
P Waves: Present but encroaching on previous T
waves
PR Interval: 0.16 sec
QRS: 0.10 sec
Interpretation: Sinus tachycardia with sinus block

■ ECG 12•24
Rate: 125 bpm
Rhythm: Regular
P Waves: Normal
PR Interval: 0.16 sec
QRS: 0.10 sec
Interpretation: Sinus tachycardia with ST segment
depression

■ ECG 12•25
Rate: 88 bpm
Rhythm: Regular
P Waves: None
PR Interval: None
QRS: Wide—greater than 0.10 sec
Interpretation: Accelerated idioventricular
rhythm

■ ECG 12•26
Rate: 150 bpm
Rhythm: Irregular
P Waves: Normal in first nine beats, then buried in T
waves in last six beats
PR Interval: 0.12 sec for first nine beats, then inde-
terminate for last six beats
QRS: 0.08 sec
Interpretation: Paroxysmal supraventricular tachy-
cardia (sinus arrhythmia converting to supraven-
tricular tachycardia)

■ ECG 12•27
Rate: 68 bpm
Rhythm: Regular
P Waves: Normal
PR Interval: 0.16 sec
QRS: 0.06 sec
Interpretation: Normal sinus rhythm with ST seg-
ment depression

■ ECG 12•28
Rate: 60 bpm
Rhythm: Irregular
P Waves: Normal
PR Interval: 0.28 sec in first two beats, 0.16 sec
in rest of beats
QRS: 0.10 sec
Interpretation: Normal sinus rhythm with first-
degree AV block in beats 1 and 2 changing to sinus
bradycardia

■ ECG 12•29
Rate: 75 bpm
Rhythm: Regular
P Waves: None
PR Interval: None
QRS: 0.10 sec
Interpretation: Accelerated junctional rhythm
with ST segment depression and inverted
T waves

■ ECG 12•30
Rate: 48 bpm
Rhythm: Regular
P Waves: Normal
PR Interval: 0.16 sec
QRS: 0.10 sec
Interpretation: Sinus bradycardia

■ ECG 12•31
Rate: Indeterminate
Rhythm: Chaotic
P Waves: None
PR Interval: None
QRS: Wide—greater than 0.10 sec
Interpretation: Ventricular fibrillation converting
to ventricular tachycardia

■ ECG 12•32
Rate: 120 bpm
Rhythm: Irregular
P Waves: Normal in first 6 beats
PR Interval: 0.16 sec
QRS: 0.10 sec
Interpretation: Normal sinus rhythm with ST segment
depression followed by a PVC at beat 7, with a run
of supraventricular tachycardia following the PVC

■ ECG 12•33
Rate: 100 bpm
Rhythm: Irregular
P Waves: Buried in T waves in first six beats; normal in last four beats
PR Interval: 0.08–0.12 sec
QRS: 0.08–0.12 sec
Interpretation: Paroxysmal supraventricular tachycardia (supraventricular tachycardia with a bundle branch block converting to normal sinus rhythm.)

■ ECG 12•34
Rate: 90 bpm
Rhythm: Irregular
P Waves: Normal
PR Interval: 0.16 sec
QRS: 0.10 sec
Interpretation: Normal sinus rhythm with ST segment depression and PACs at beats 5 and 8

■ ECG 12•35
Rate: 70 bpm
Rhythm: Irregular
P Waves: Flutter waves
PR Interval: None
QRS: 0.10 sec
Interpretation: Atrial flutter with a 4:1 block and one PVC at beat 3 with a full compensatory pause (every fourth flutter wave is buried in the QRS)

■ ECG 12•36
Rate: 40 bpm
Rhythm: Regular
P Waves: None
PR Interval: None
QRS: 0.10 sec
Interpretation: Junctional rhythm with ST segment depression

■ ECG 12•37
Rate: 80 bpm
Rhythm: Irregular
P Waves: Normal
PR Interval: 0.16 sec
QRS: 0.10 sec
Interpretation: Normal sinus rhythm with ST segment elevation and a three-beat run of ventricular tachycardia

■ ECG 12•38
Rate: 100 bpm
Rhythm: Irregular
P Waves: None
PR Interval: None
QRS: 0.10 sec
Interpretation: Atrial fibrillation with ST segment depression and inverted T waves

■ ECG 12•39
Rate: 70 bpm
Rhythm: Irregular
P Waves: None
PR Interval: None
QRS: 0.04 sec following pacemaker spike, 0.12 in second complex
Interpretation: Pacemaker—ventricular, with respiratory artifact and one PVC at beat 2

■ ECG 12•40
Rate: 88 bpm
Rhythm: Regular
P Waves: Pacemaker spike, with small inverted P waves following spike
PR Interval: None
QRS: 0.08 sec
Interpretation: Pacemaker—atrial paced, ventricular sensed

■ ECG 12•41
Rate: 20 bpm
Rhythm: Irregular
P Waves: Normal
PR Interval: 0.20 sec
QRS: 0.16 sec
Interpretation: Sinus arrest with a 4.36 sec pause and respiratory artifact

■ ECG 12•42
Rate: Indeterminate
Rhythm: Irregular
P Waves: None
PR Interval: None
QRS: Wide—greater than 0.10 sec
Interpretation: Ventricular tachycardia—polymorphic

■ ECG 12•43
Rate: 110 bpm
Rhythm: Irregular
P Waves: None
PR Interval: None
QRS: 0.08 sec
Interpretation: Atrial fibrillation with a four-beat multiform ventricular tachycardia

■ ECG 12•44
Rate: 70 bpm
Rhythm: Irregular
P Waves: Flutter waves
PR Interval: None
QRS: 0.16 sec
Interpretation: Atrial flutter with variable block and a bundle branch block

ECG 12•45
Rate: 115 bpm
Rhythm: Regular
P Waves: None
PR Interval: None
QRS: 0.12 sec with notched appearance
Interpretation: Junctional tachycardia with a bundle branch block

ECG 12•46
Rate: Indeterminate
Rhythm: Chaotic
P Waves: None
PR Interval: None
QRS: None
Interpretation: Ventricular fibrillation—fine fibrillatory waves

ECG 12•47
Rate: 155 bpm in the beginning, 68 bpm after cardioversion
Rhythm: Irregular
P Waves: Normal in last three beats
PR Interval: 0.16 sec in last three beats
QRS: Wide—greater than 0.10 sec in first three beats; 0.10 sec in last three beats
Interpretation: Monomorphic ventricular tachycardia with synchronized cardioversion converting to normal sinus rhythm

ECG 12•48
Rate: 70 bpm
Rhythm: Irregular
P Waves: Normal with 60-cycle interference
PR Interval: 0.20 sec
QRS: 0.10 sec
Interpretation: Normal sinus rhythm with bigeminal uniform PVCs and 60-cycle interference

ECG 12•49
Rate: 70 bpm
Rhythm: Irregular
P Waves: Normal
PR Interval: 0.16 sec
QRS: 0.08 sec
Interpretation: Normal sinus rhythm with two 1.28 second pauses (sinus arrest)

ECG 12•50
Rate: 150 bpm
Rhythm: Regular
P Waves: Normal but different in shape from sinus P waves
PR Interval: 0.12 sec
QRS: 0.08 sec
Interpretation: Atrial tachycardia

ECG 12•51
Rate: 40 bpm
Rhythm: Irregular
P Waves: Normal
PR Interval: Variable
QRS: 0.16 sec for first four beats
Interpretation: Third-degree AV block converting to coarse ventricular fibrillation

ECG 12•52
Rate: 100 bpm
Rhythm: Regular
P Waves: Normal
PR Interval: 0.16 sec
QRS: 0.08 sec
Interpretation: Normal sinus rhythm with ST segment depression

ECG 12•53
Rate: 136 bpm
Rhythm: Regular
P Waves: Buried in T waves
PR Interval: Not able to measure
QRS: 0.10 sec
Interpretation: Supraventricular tachycardia

ECG 12•54
Rate: 60 bpm
Rhythm: Irregular
P Waves: None
PR Interval: None
QRS: 0.08 sec
Interpretation: Atrial fibrillation

ECG 12•55
Rate: 90 bpm
Rhythm: Irregular
P Waves: Normal except that the P wave for beat 6 (a PAC) is buried in the preceding T wave
PR Interval: 0.16 sec
QRS: 0.12 sec
Interpretation: Normal sinus rhythm with a bundle branch block and a PAC at beat 6

ECG 12•56
Rate: 160 bpm
Rhythm: Irregular
P Waves: Normal
PR Interval: 0.16 sec
QRS: 0.08 sec
Interpretation: Sinus tachycardia with ST segment depression, inverted T waves, and three uniform PVCs at beats 2, 10, and 13 with full compensatory pauses

■ ECG 12•57
Rate: 50 bpm
Rhythm: Irregular
P Waves: Flutter waves
PR Interval: None
QRS: 0.10 sec for beats 1 and 5
Interpretation: Atrial flutter with a three-beat accel-
    erated ventricular rhythm at beats 2 through 4

■ ECG 12•58
Rate: 110 bpm
Rhythm: Irregular
P Waves: None
PR Interval: None
QRS: Variable
Interpretation: Unknown underlying rhythm with
    multiformed accelerated ventricular rhythm and
    ventricular couplet

■ ECG 12•59
Rate: 46 bpm
Rhythm: Irregular
P Waves: Normal
PR Interval: 0.16 sec
QRS: 0.12 sec
Interpretation: Sinus bradycardia with sinus
    arrhythmia with a bundle branch block

■ ECG 12•60
Rate: 56 bpm
Rhythm: Regular
P Waves: None
PR Interval: None
QRS: 0.18 sec
Interpretation: Accelerated idioventricular rhythm

■ ECG 12•61
Rate: 50 bpm
Rhythm: Irregular
P Waves: None
PR Interval: None
QRS: 0.08 sec
Interpretation: Junctional rhythm with ST
    segment depression and a PJC at beat 3

■ ECG 12•62
Rate: 83 bpm
Rhythm: Regular
P Waves: Normal
PR Interval: 0.20 sec
QRS: 0.08 sec
Interpretation: Normal sinus rhythm with an
    interpolated PVC between beats 3 and 4

■ ECG 12•63
Rate: Atrial 107 bpm, ventricular 35 bpm
Rhythm: Atrial regular, ventricular regular
P Waves: Normal
PR Interval: 0.16 sec
QRS: 0.08 sec
Interpretation: Second-degree AV block Type II with
    3:1 block

■ ECG 12•64
Rate: 110 bpm; 61 bpm in first section, 170 bpm in
    next section
Rhythm: Irregular
P Waves: None
PR Interval: None
QRS: 0.16 sec
Interpretation: Paroxysmal supraventricular tachy-
    cardia (accelerated junctional rhythm with bundle
    branch block followed by supraventricular tachy-
    cardia)

■ ECG 12•65
Rate: 60 bpm
Rhythm: Irregular
P Waves: Retrograde
PR Interval: None
QRS: 0.08 sec
Interpretation: Junctional rhythm with multiform
    bigeminal PVCs

■ ECG 12•66
Rate: 130 bpm
Rhythm: Regular
P Waves: None
PR Interval: None
QRS: Wide—greater than 0.10 sec
Interpretation: Ventricular tachycardia—
    monomorphic

■ ECG 12•67
Rate: 90 bpm (counting PVCs), 65 bpm for underly-
    ing rhythm
Rhythm: Irregular
P Waves: Normal
PR Interval: 0.28 sec
QRS: 0.12 sec
Interpretation: Normal sinus rhythm with first-degree
    AV block, inverted T waves, and interpolated PVCs
    at beats 4, 6, and 9

■ ECG 12•68
Rate: 50 bpm
Rhythm: Regular
P Waves: Normal
PR Interval: 0.16 sec
QRS: 0.08 sec
Interpretation: Sinus bradycardia

■ ECG 12•69
Rate: 80 bpm
Rhythm: Irregular
P Waves: None
PR Interval: None
QRS: 0.16 sec
Interpretation: Accelerated idioventricular rhythm
    with bigeminal PVCs

■ ECG 12•70
Rate: 120 bpm (counting PVCs), 115 bpm in under-
    lying rhythm
Rhythm: Irregular
P Waves: Normal
PR Interval: 0.16 sec
QRS: 0.08 sec
Interpretation: Sinus tachycardia with couplet PVCs
    at beats 7 and 8

■ ECG 12•71
Rate: 39 bpm in first section, 166 bpm in last section
Rhythm: Irregular
P Waves: Normal for first three beats
PR Interval: 0.16 sec for first three beats
QRS: 0.10 sec for first three beats; wide—greater
    than 0.10 sec—for remaining beats
Interpretation: Sinus bradycardia converting to
    monomorphic ventricular tachycardia

■ ECG 12•72
Rate: 160 bpm
Rhythm: Irregular
P Waves: None
PR Interval: None
QRS: 0.08 sec
Interpretation: Atrial fibrillation with rapid ventricu-
    lar response

■ ECG 12•73
Rate: 100 bpm
Rhythm: Regular
P Waves: Normal
PR Interval: 0.16 sec
QRS: 0.10 sec
Interpretation: Normal sinus rhythm

■ ECG 12•74
Rate: 80 bpm
Rhythm: Irregular
P Waves: Flutter waves
PR Interval: None
QRS: Difficult to measure because of flutter waves,
    probably 0.08 sec
Interpretation: Atrial flutter with variable block

■ ECG 12•75
Rate: 60 bpm
Rhythm: Irregular
P Waves: Normal
PR Interval: Variable
QRS: 0.10 sec
Interpretation: Third-degree AV block with multiform
    PVCs at beats 2 and 5

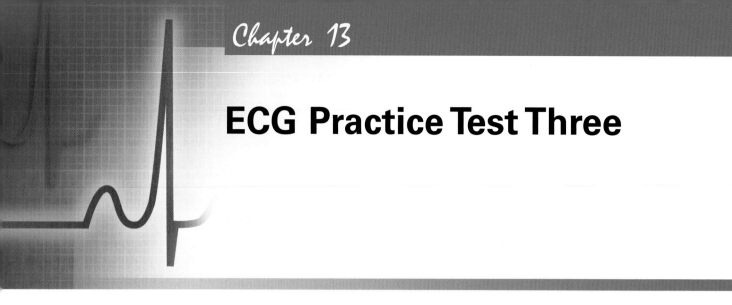

ECG Practice Test Three

For instructions on analyzing these practice test strips, please see the guidelines given at the end of chapter 2.

TEST STRIP SECTION THREE ▪

ECG 13•1

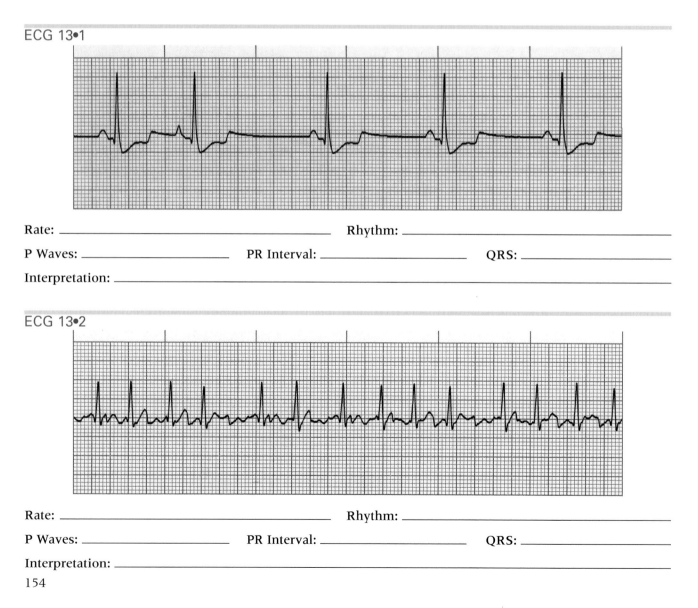

Rate: _____ Rhythm: _____

P Waves: _____ PR Interval: _____ QRS: _____

Interpretation: _____

ECG 13•2

Rate: _____ Rhythm: _____

P Waves: _____ PR Interval: _____ QRS: _____

Interpretation: _____

ECG 13•3

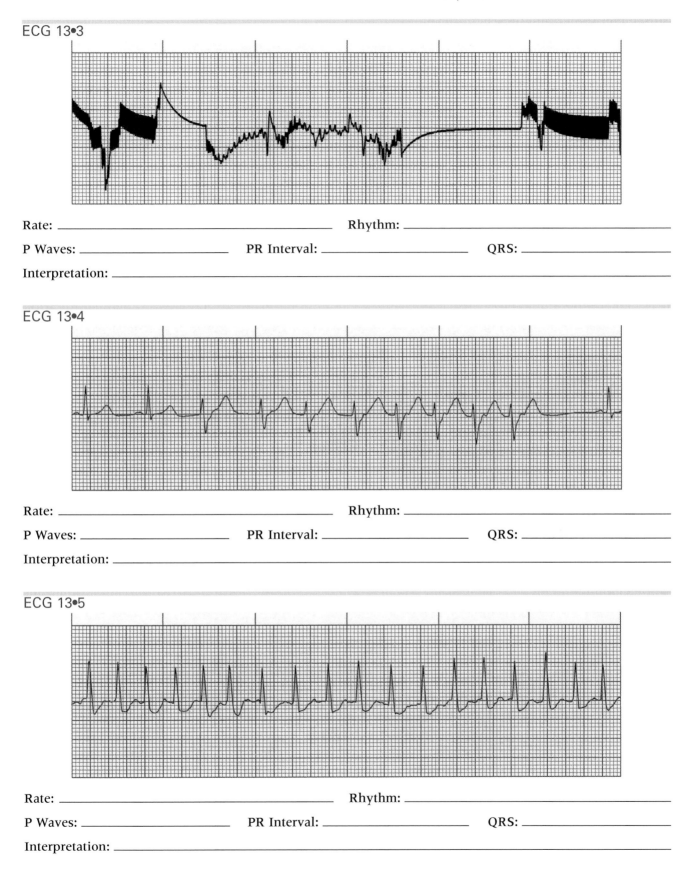

Rate: _____   Rhythm: _____

P Waves: _____   PR Interval: _____   QRS: _____

Interpretation: _____

ECG 13•4

Rate: _____   Rhythm: _____

P Waves: _____   PR Interval: _____   QRS: _____

Interpretation: _____

ECG 13•5

Rate: _____   Rhythm: _____

P Waves: _____   PR Interval: _____   QRS: _____

Interpretation: _____

ECG 13•6

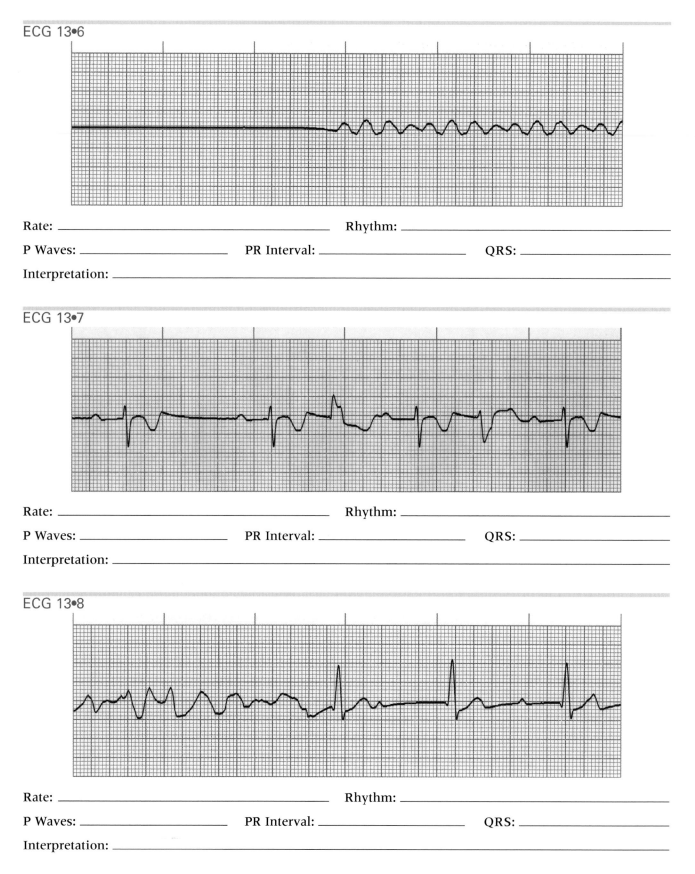

Rate: _____   Rhythm: _____

P Waves: _____   PR Interval: _____   QRS: _____

Interpretation: _____

ECG 13•7

Rate: _____   Rhythm: _____

P Waves: _____   PR Interval: _____   QRS: _____

Interpretation: _____

ECG 13•8

Rate: _____   Rhythm: _____

P Waves: _____   PR Interval: _____   QRS: _____

Interpretation: _____

ECG 13•9

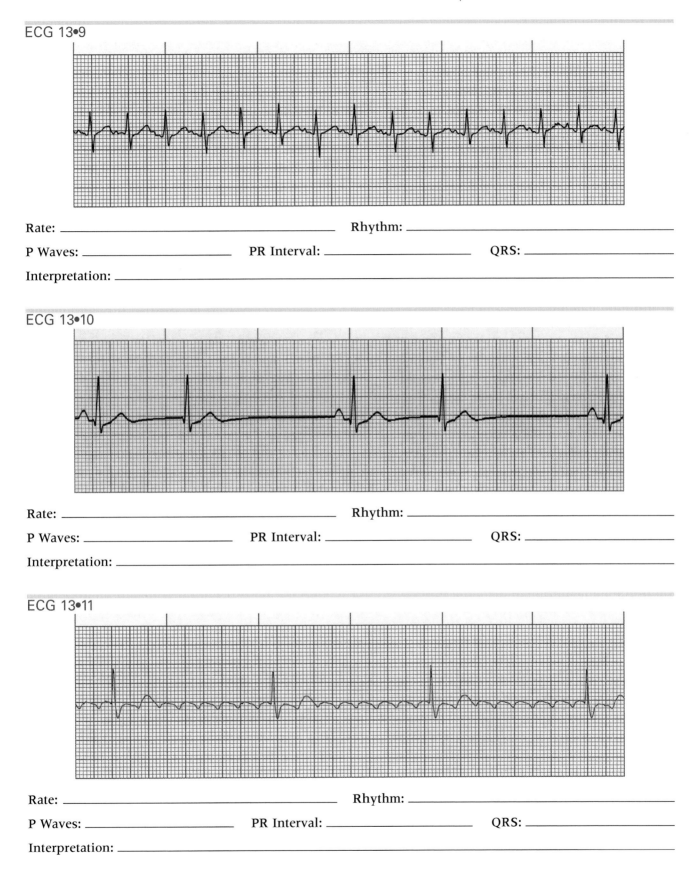

Rate: _____ Rhythm: _____

P Waves: _____ PR Interval: _____ QRS: _____

Interpretation: _____

ECG 13•10

Rate: _____ Rhythm: _____

P Waves: _____ PR Interval: _____ QRS: _____

Interpretation: _____

ECG 13•11

Rate: _____ Rhythm: _____

P Waves: _____ PR Interval: _____ QRS: _____

Interpretation: _____

ECG 13•12

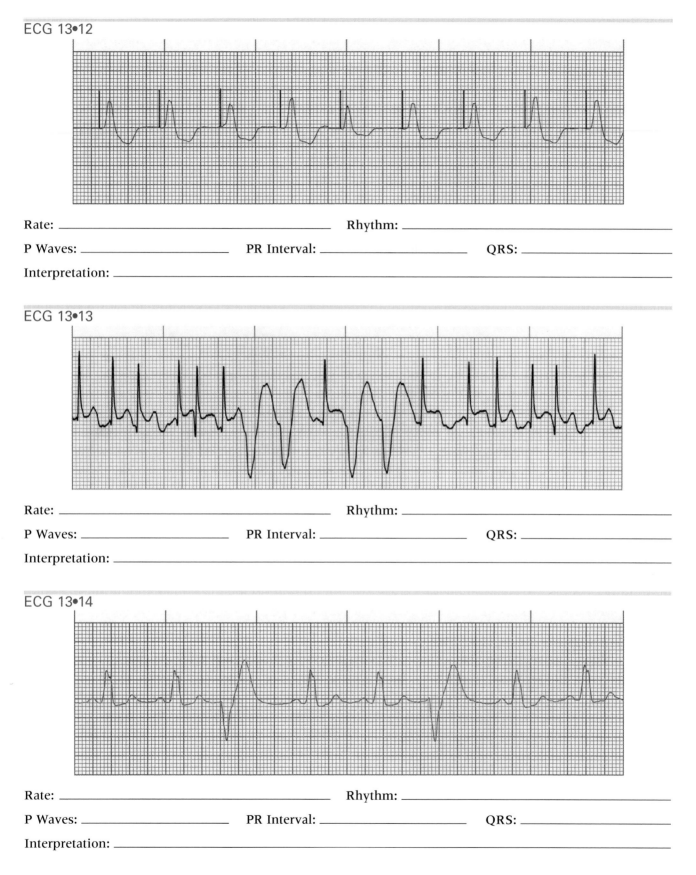

Rate: _____   Rhythm: _____

P Waves: _____   PR Interval: _____   QRS: _____

Interpretation: _____

ECG 13•13

Rate: _____   Rhythm: _____

P Waves: _____   PR Interval: _____   QRS: _____

Interpretation: _____

ECG 13•14

Rate: _____   Rhythm: _____

P Waves: _____   PR Interval: _____   QRS: _____

Interpretation: _____

ECG 13•15

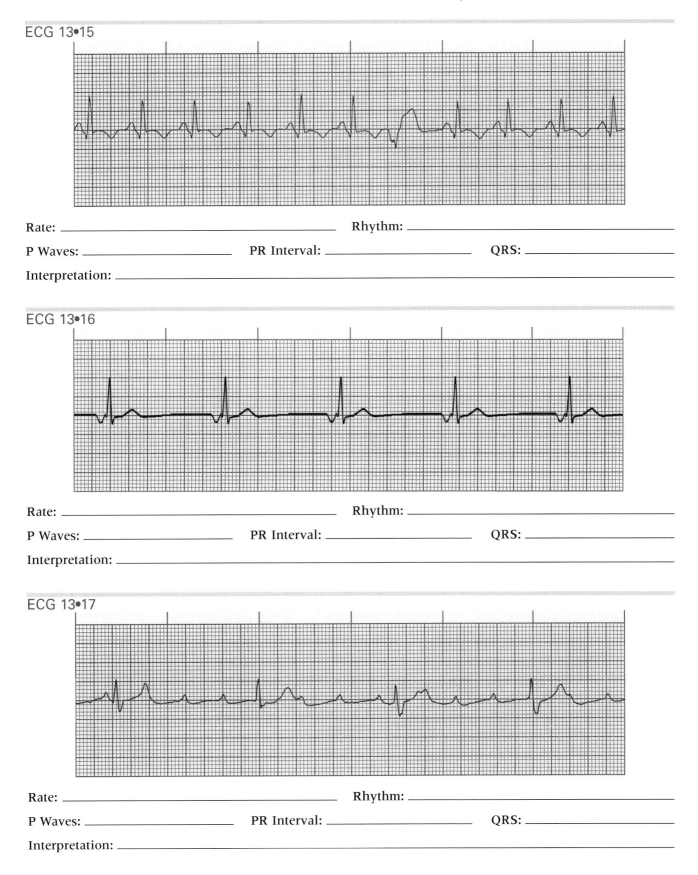

Rate: _____ Rhythm: _____

P Waves: _____ PR Interval: _____ QRS: _____

Interpretation: _____

ECG 13•16

Rate: _____ Rhythm: _____

P Waves: _____ PR Interval: _____ QRS: _____

Interpretation: _____

ECG 13•17

Rate: _____ Rhythm: _____

P Waves: _____ PR Interval: _____ QRS: _____

Interpretation: _____

ECG 13•18

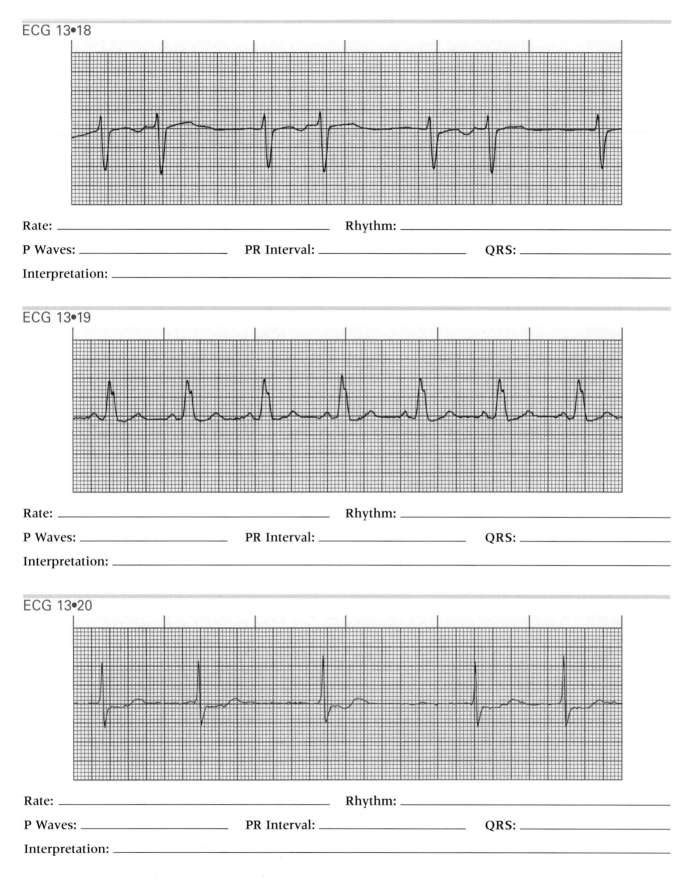

Rate: _____ Rhythm: _____

P Waves: _____ PR Interval: _____ QRS: _____

Interpretation: _____

ECG 13•19

Rate: _____ Rhythm: _____

P Waves: _____ PR Interval: _____ QRS: _____

Interpretation: _____

ECG 13•20

Rate: _____ Rhythm: _____

P Waves: _____ PR Interval: _____ QRS: _____

Interpretation: _____

ECG 13•21

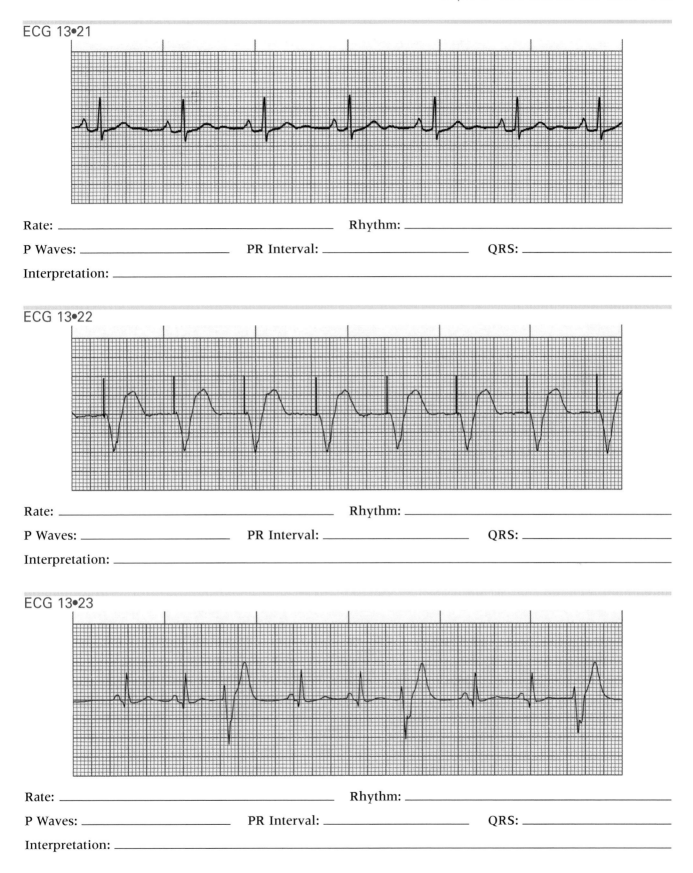

Rate: _____ Rhythm: _____

P Waves: _____ PR Interval: _____ QRS: _____

Interpretation: _____

ECG 13•22

Rate: _____ Rhythm: _____

P Waves: _____ PR Interval: _____ QRS: _____

Interpretation: _____

ECG 13•23

Rate: _____ Rhythm: _____

P Waves: _____ PR Interval: _____ QRS: _____

Interpretation: _____

ECG 13•24

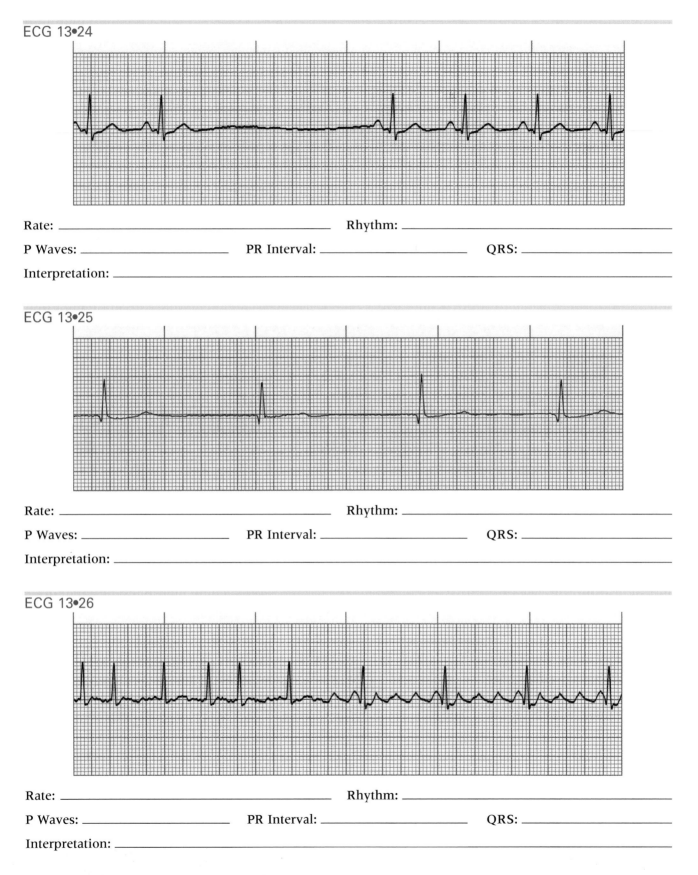

Rate: _____   Rhythm: _____

P Waves: _____   PR Interval: _____   QRS: _____

Interpretation: _____

ECG 13•25

Rate: _____   Rhythm: _____

P Waves: _____   PR Interval: _____   QRS: _____

Interpretation: _____

ECG 13•26

Rate: _____   Rhythm: _____

P Waves: _____   PR Interval: _____   QRS: _____

Interpretation: _____

ECG 13•27

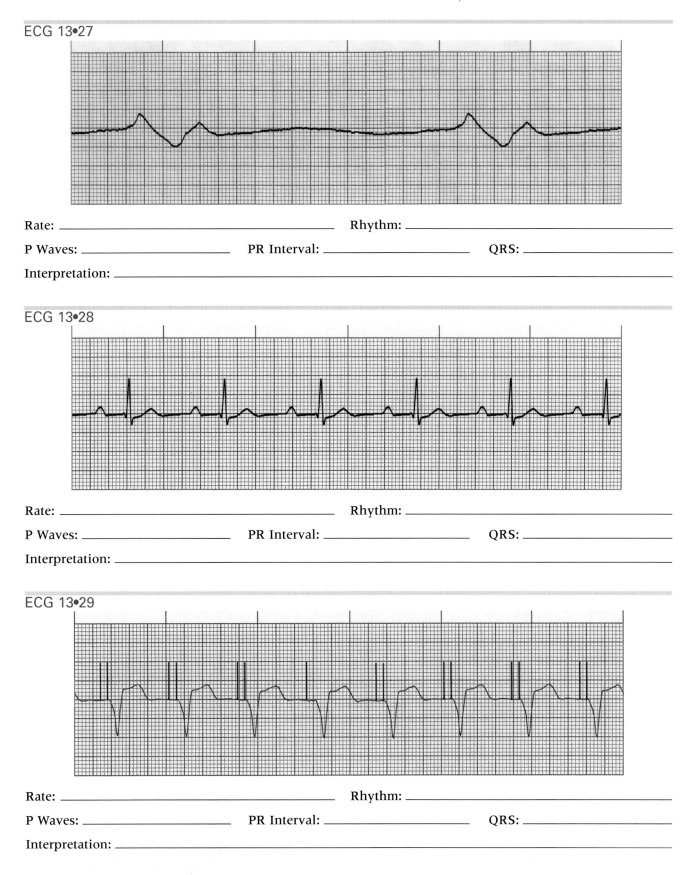

Rate: _____ Rhythm: _____

P Waves: _____ PR Interval: _____ QRS: _____

Interpretation: _____

ECG 13•28

Rate: _____ Rhythm: _____

P Waves: _____ PR Interval: _____ QRS: _____

Interpretation: _____

ECG 13•29

Rate: _____ Rhythm: _____

P Waves: _____ PR Interval: _____ QRS: _____

Interpretation: _____

ECG 13•30

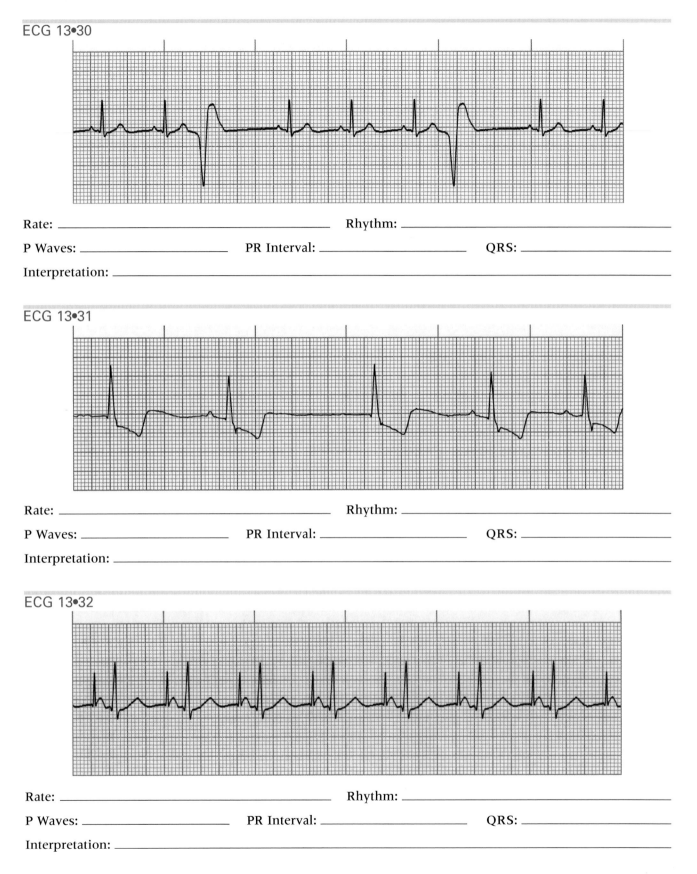

Rate: _____   Rhythm: _____

P Waves: _____   PR Interval: _____   QRS: _____

Interpretation: _____

ECG 13•31

Rate: _____   Rhythm: _____

P Waves: _____   PR Interval: _____   QRS: _____

Interpretation: _____

ECG 13•32

Rate: _____   Rhythm: _____

P Waves: _____   PR Interval: _____   QRS: _____

Interpretation: _____

ECG 13•33

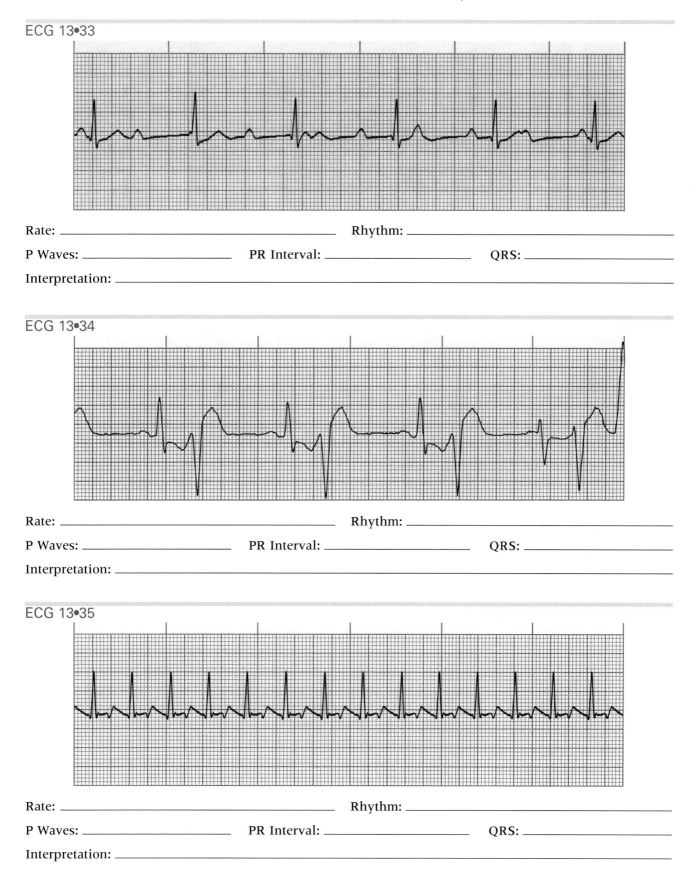

Rate: _____ Rhythm: _____

P Waves: _____ PR Interval: _____ QRS: _____

Interpretation: _____

ECG 13•34

Rate: _____ Rhythm: _____

P Waves: _____ PR Interval: _____ QRS: _____

Interpretation: _____

ECG 13•35

Rate: _____ Rhythm: _____

P Waves: _____ PR Interval: _____ QRS: _____

Interpretation: _____

ECG 13•36

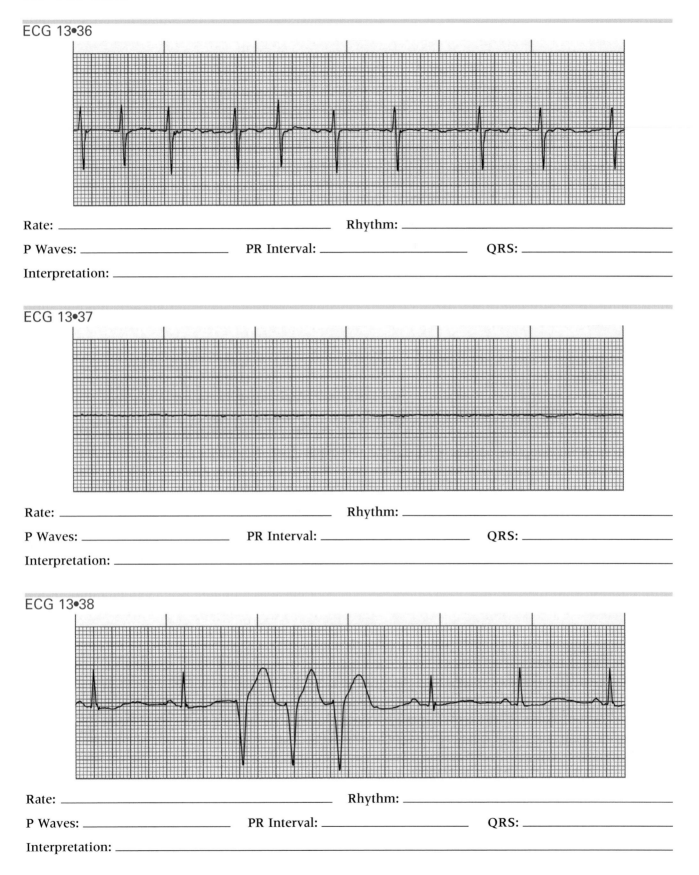

Rate: _____ Rhythm: _____

P Waves: _____ PR Interval: _____ QRS: _____

Interpretation: _____

ECG 13•37

Rate: _____ Rhythm: _____

P Waves: _____ PR Interval: _____ QRS: _____

Interpretation: _____

ECG 13•38

Rate: _____ Rhythm: _____

P Waves: _____ PR Interval: _____ QRS: _____

Interpretation: _____

ECG 13•39

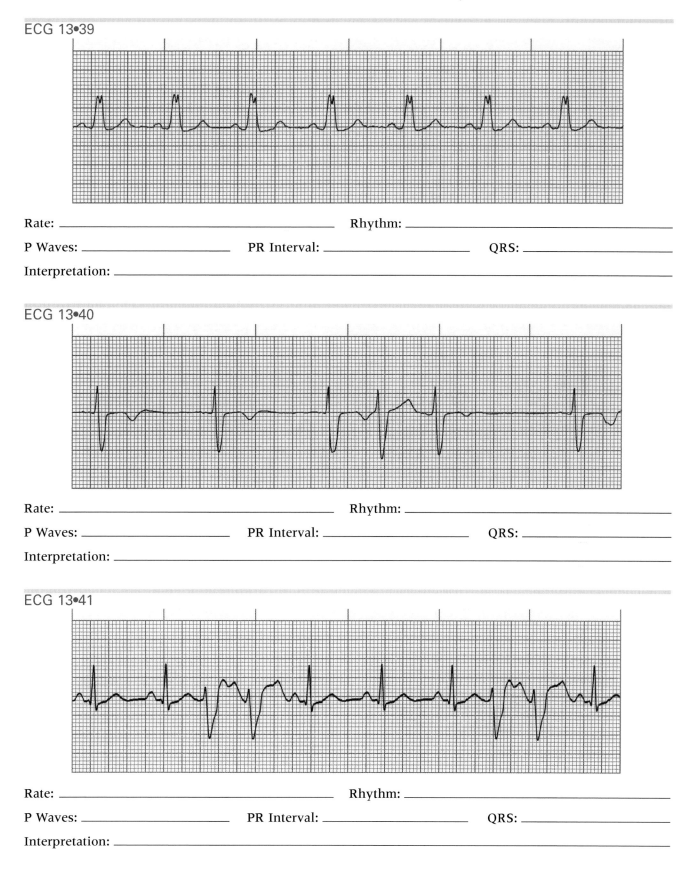

Rate: _____ Rhythm: _____

P Waves: _____ PR Interval: _____ QRS: _____

Interpretation: _____

ECG 13•40

Rate: _____ Rhythm: _____

P Waves: _____ PR Interval: _____ QRS: _____

Interpretation: _____

ECG 13•41

Rate: _____ Rhythm: _____

P Waves: _____ PR Interval: _____ QRS: _____

Interpretation: _____

ECG 13•42

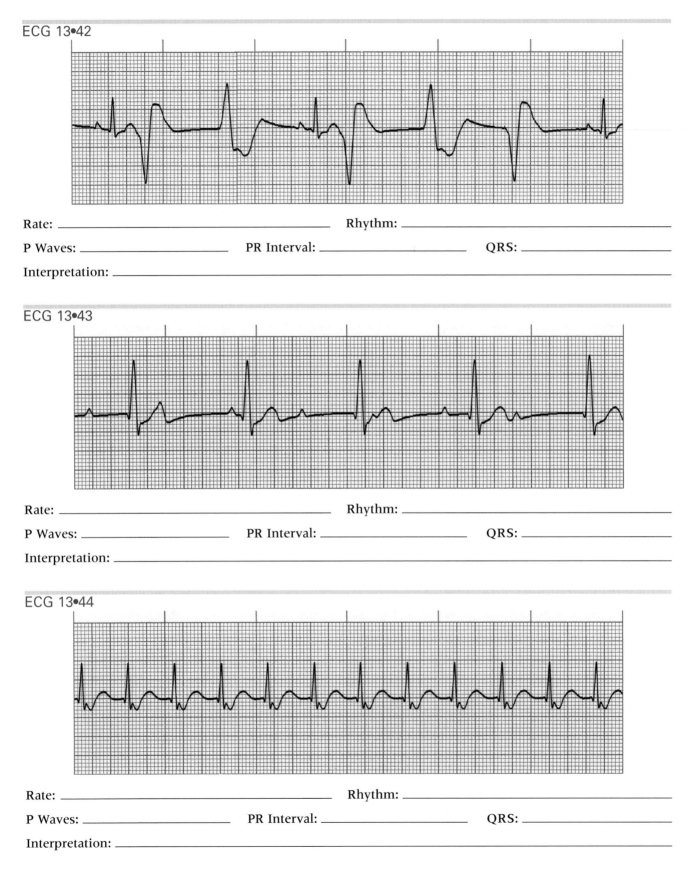

Rate: _____   Rhythm: _____

P Waves: _____   PR Interval: _____   QRS: _____

Interpretation: _____

ECG 13•43

Rate: _____   Rhythm: _____

P Waves: _____   PR Interval: _____   QRS: _____

Interpretation: _____

ECG 13•44

Rate: _____   Rhythm: _____

P Waves: _____   PR Interval: _____   QRS: _____

Interpretation: _____

ECG 13•45

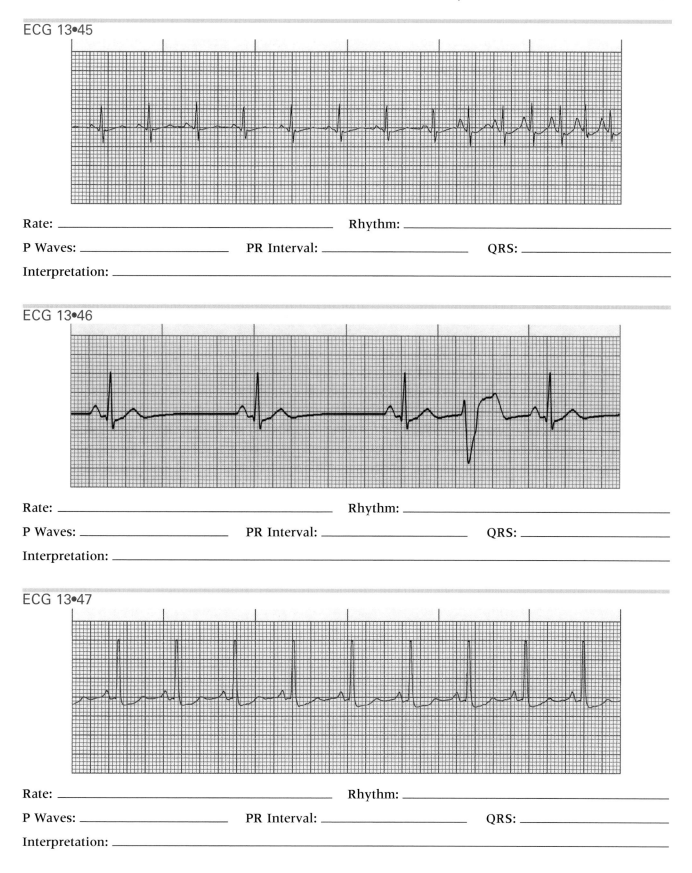

Rate: _____ Rhythm: _____

P Waves: _____ PR Interval: _____ QRS: _____

Interpretation: _____

ECG 13•46

Rate: _____ Rhythm: _____

P Waves: _____ PR Interval: _____ QRS: _____

Interpretation: _____

ECG 13•47

Rate: _____ Rhythm: _____

P Waves: _____ PR Interval: _____ QRS: _____

Interpretation: _____

ECG 13•48

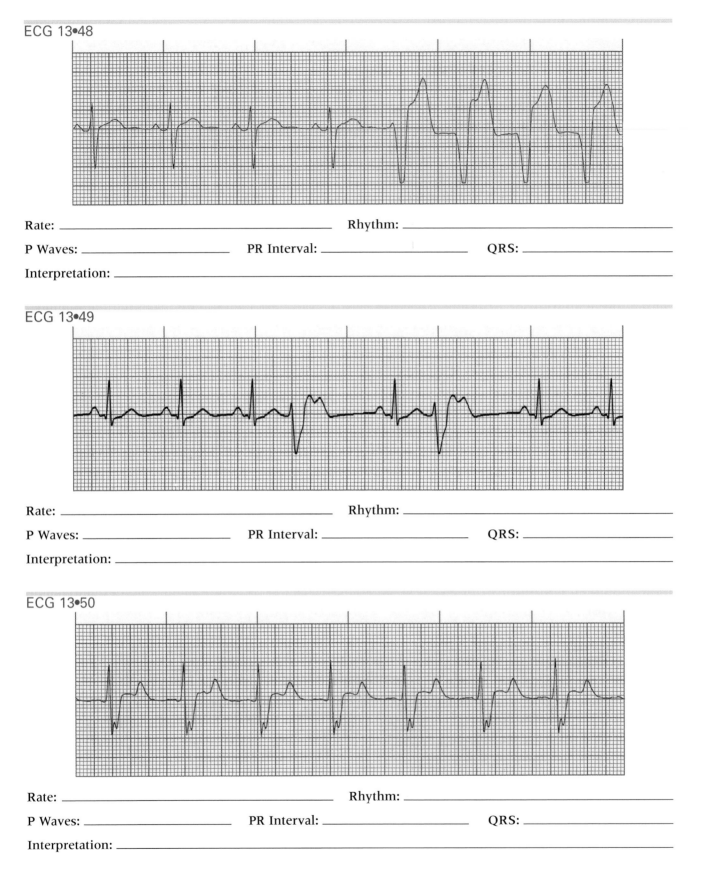

Rate: _____   Rhythm: _____

P Waves: _____   PR Interval: _____   QRS: _____

Interpretation: _____

ECG 13•49

Rate: _____   Rhythm: _____

P Waves: _____   PR Interval: _____   QRS: _____

Interpretation: _____

ECG 13•50

Rate: _____   Rhythm: _____

P Waves: _____   PR Interval: _____   QRS: _____

Interpretation: _____

ECG 13•51

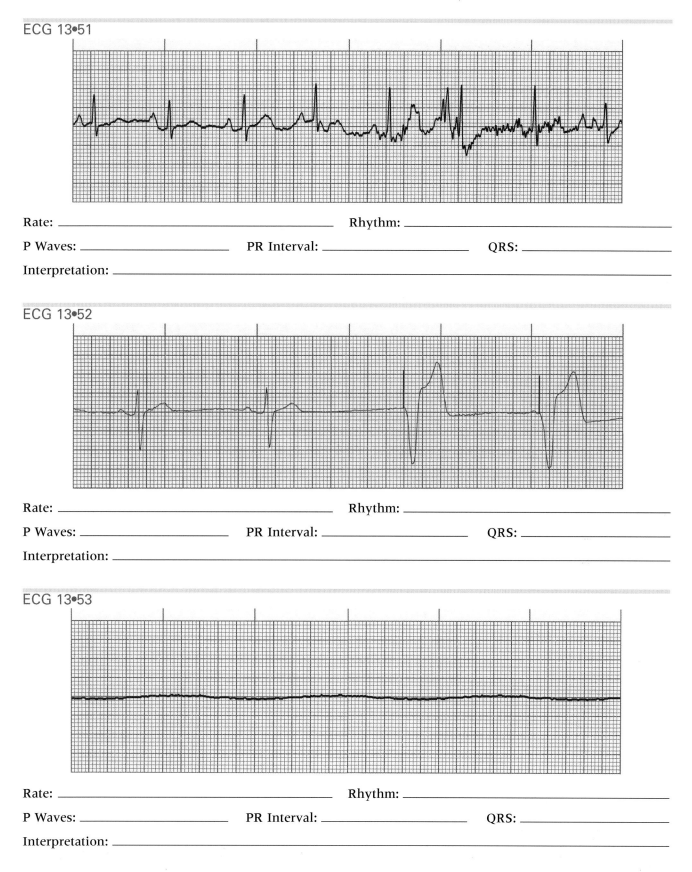

Rate: _____ Rhythm: _____

P Waves: _____ PR Interval: _____ QRS: _____

Interpretation: _____

ECG 13•52

Rate: _____ Rhythm: _____

P Waves: _____ PR Interval: _____ QRS: _____

Interpretation: _____

ECG 13•53

Rate: _____ Rhythm: _____

P Waves: _____ PR Interval: _____ QRS: _____

Interpretation: _____

ECG 13•54

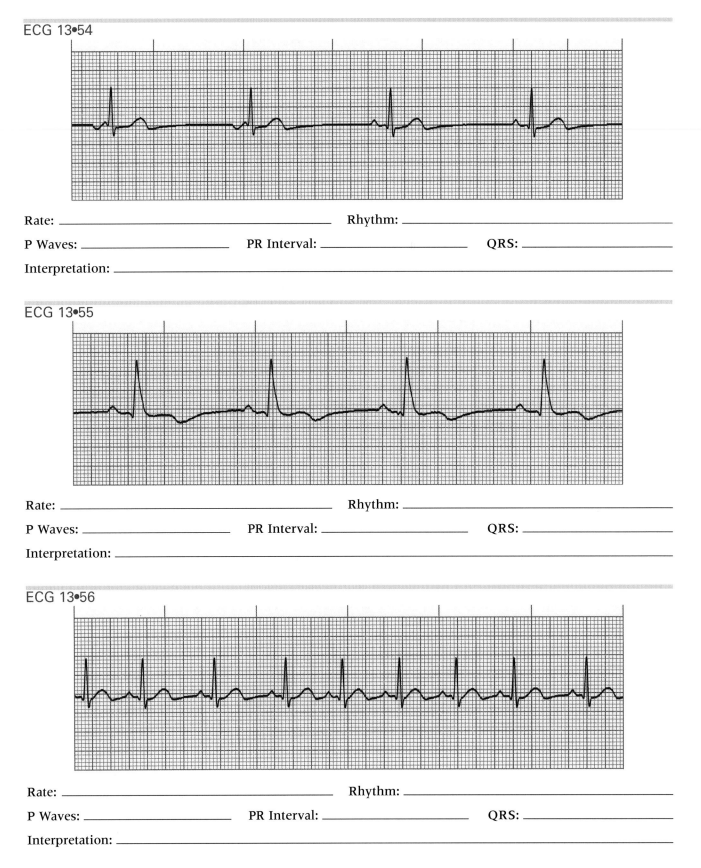

Rate: _____   Rhythm: _____

P Waves: _____   PR Interval: _____   QRS: _____

Interpretation: _____

ECG 13•55

Rate: _____   Rhythm: _____

P Waves: _____   PR Interval: _____   QRS: _____

Interpretation: _____

ECG 13•56

Rate: _____   Rhythm: _____

P Waves: _____   PR Interval: _____   QRS: _____

Interpretation: _____

ECG 13•57

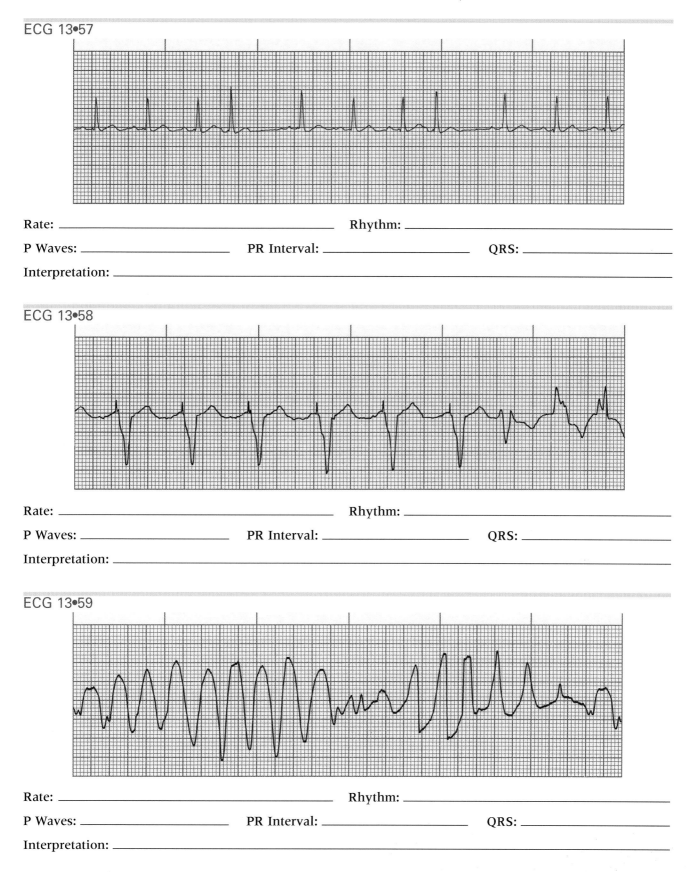

Rate: _____   Rhythm: _____

P Waves: _____   PR Interval: _____   QRS: _____

Interpretation: _____

ECG 13•58

Rate: _____   Rhythm: _____

P Waves: _____   PR Interval: _____   QRS: _____

Interpretation: _____

ECG 13•59

Rate: _____   Rhythm: _____

P Waves: _____   PR Interval: _____   QRS: _____

Interpretation: _____

174   ECG Success

ECG 13•60

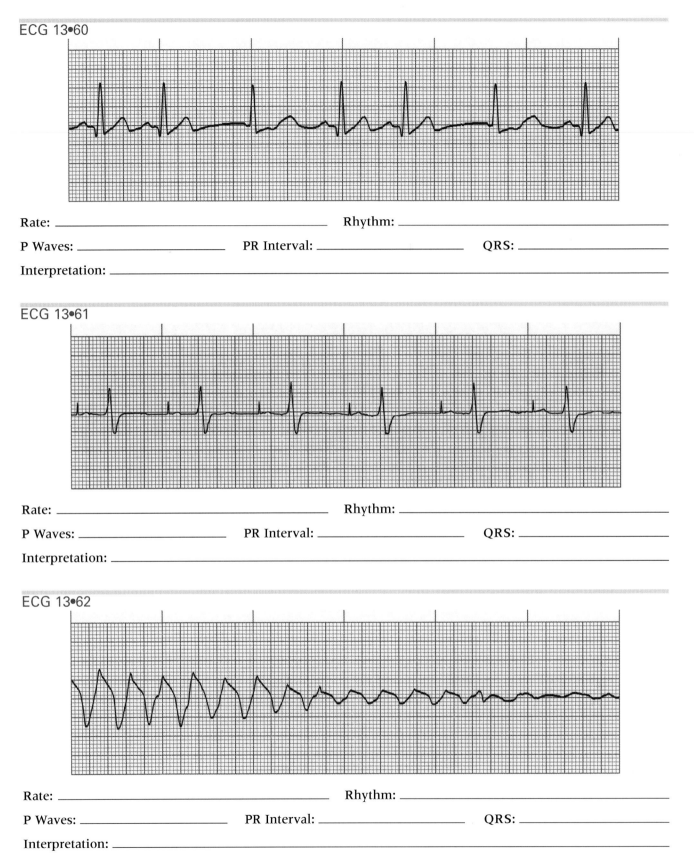

Rate: _____ Rhythm: _____

P Waves: _____ PR Interval: _____ QRS: _____

Interpretation: _____

ECG 13•61

Rate: _____ Rhythm: _____

P Waves: _____ PR Interval: _____ QRS: _____

Interpretation: _____

ECG 13•62

Rate: _____ Rhythm: _____

P Waves: _____ PR Interval: _____ QRS: _____

Interpretation: _____

ECG 13•63

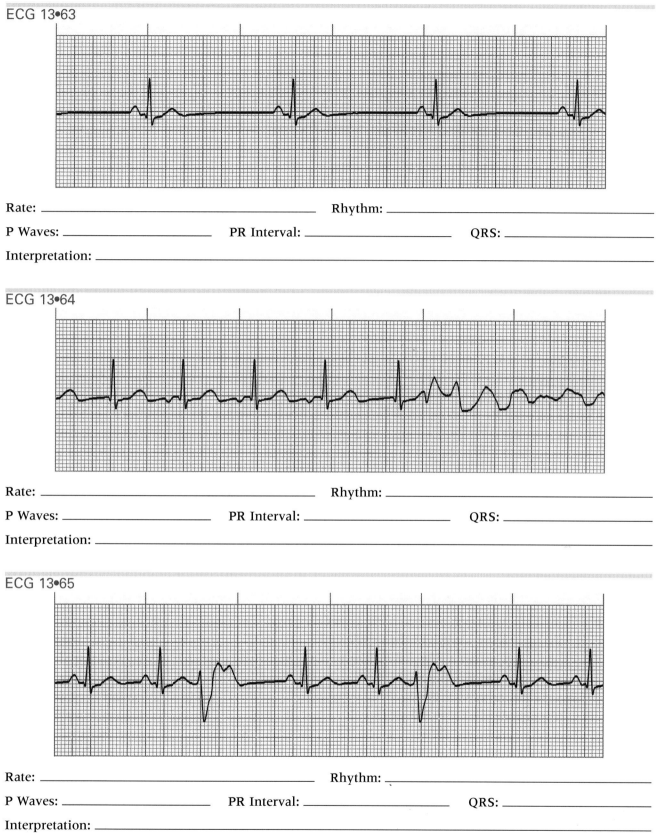

Rate: _____ Rhythm: _____

P Waves: _____ PR Interval: _____ QRS: _____

Interpretation: _____

ECG 13•64

Rate: _____ Rhythm: _____

P Waves: _____ PR Interval: _____ QRS: _____

Interpretation: _____

ECG 13•65

Rate: _____ Rhythm: _____

P Waves: _____ PR Interval: _____ QRS: _____

Interpretation: _____

ECG 13•66

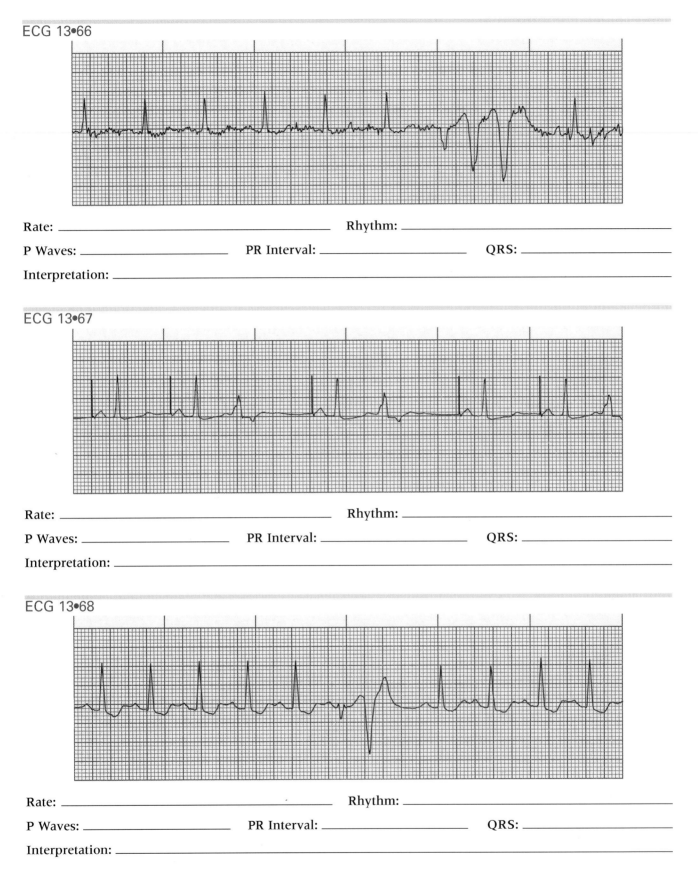

Rate: _____ Rhythm: _____

P Waves: _____ PR Interval: _____ QRS: _____

Interpretation: _____

ECG 13•67

Rate: _____ Rhythm: _____

P Waves: _____ PR Interval: _____ QRS: _____

Interpretation: _____

ECG 13•68

Rate: _____ Rhythm: _____

P Waves: _____ PR Interval: _____ QRS: _____

Interpretation: _____

ECG 13•69

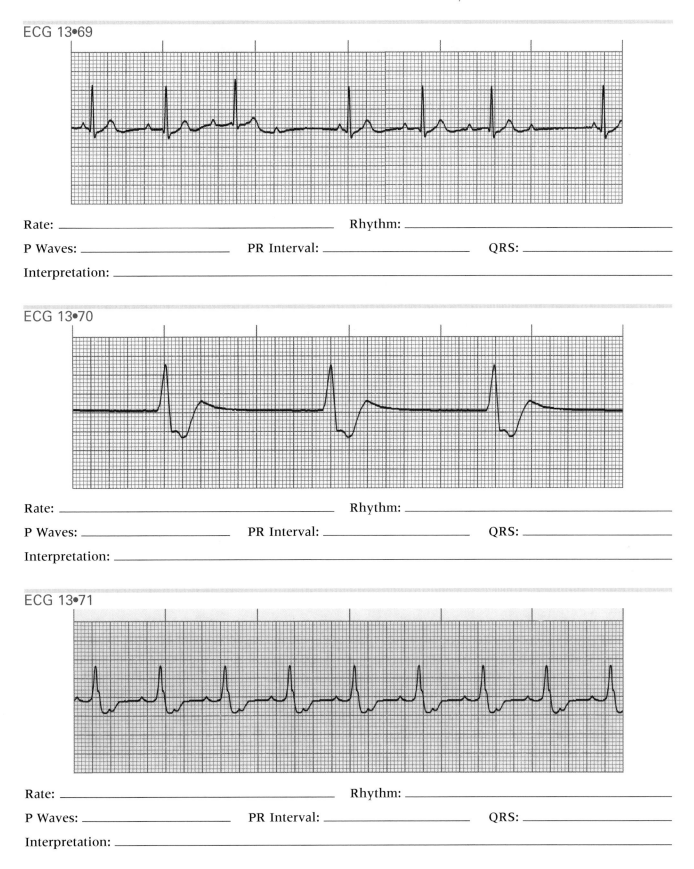

Rate: _____ Rhythm: _____

P Waves: _____ PR Interval: _____ QRS: _____

Interpretation: _____

ECG 13•70

Rate: _____ Rhythm: _____

P Waves: _____ PR Interval: _____ QRS: _____

Interpretation: _____

ECG 13•71

Rate: _____ Rhythm: _____

P Waves: _____ PR Interval: _____ QRS: _____

Interpretation: _____

ECG 13•72

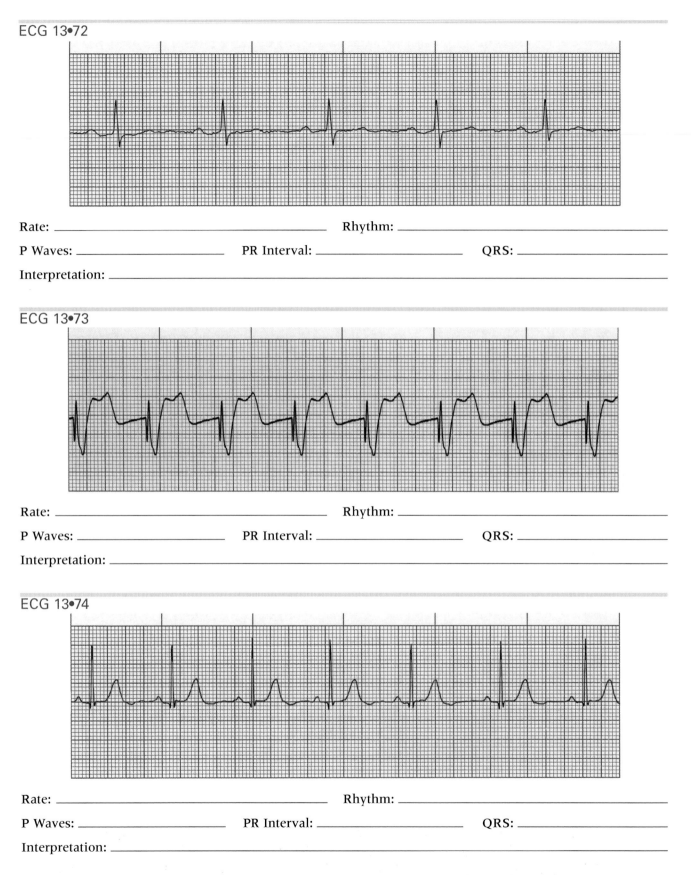

Rate: _____   Rhythm: _____

P Waves: _____   PR Interval: _____   QRS: _____

Interpretation: _____

ECG 13•73

Rate: _____   Rhythm: _____

P Waves: _____   PR Interval: _____   QRS: _____

Interpretation: _____

ECG 13•74

Rate: _____   Rhythm: _____

P Waves: _____   PR Interval: _____   QRS: _____

Interpretation: _____

ECG 13•75

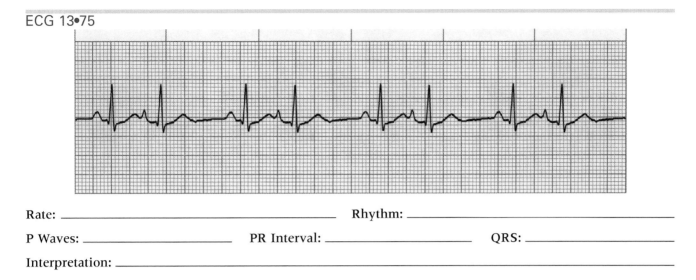

Rate: _____   Rhythm: _____

P Waves: _____ PR Interval: _____ QRS: _____

Interpretation: _____

Answers to Practice Test Three

■ **ECG 13•1**
Rate: 50 bpm
Rhythm: Irregular
P Waves: Normal
PR Interval: 0.16 sec
QRS: 0.10 sec
Interpretation: Sinus bradycardia with ST segment depression, inverted T waves, and a PAC at beat 2

■ **ECG 13•2**
Rate: 140 bpm
Rhythm: Irregular
P Waves: None
PR Interval: None
QRS: 0.08 sec
Interpretation: Atrial fibrillation with rapid ventricular response

■ **ECG 13•3**
Rate: None
Rhythm: None
P Waves: None
PR Interval: None
QRS: None
Interpretation: Loose electrode artifact

■ **ECG 13•4**
Rate: 110 bpm
Rhythm: Irregular
P Waves: Normal for beats 1, 2, and 11
PR Interval: 0.12 sec for beats 1, 2, and 11
QRS: 0.08 sec for beats 1, 2, and 11
Interpretation: Paroxysmal supraventricular tachycardia (normal sinus rhythm converting to supraventricular tachycardia and back to a sinus complex at beat 11)

■ **ECG 13•5**
Rate: 180 bpm
Rhythm: Irregular
P Waves: None
PR Interval: None
QRS: 0.08 sec
Interpretation: Atrial fibrillation with rapid ventricular response and ST segment depression

■ **ECG 13•6**
Rate: Indeterminate
Rhythm: Irregular
P Waves: None
PR Interval: None
QRS: None
Interpretation: Asystole converting to ventricular fibrillation

■ **ECG 13•7**
Rate: 60 bpm, 38 bpm in underlying rhythm
Rhythm: Irregular
P Waves: Normal
PR Interval: 0.36 sec
QRS: 0.08 sec
Interpretation: Sinus bradycardia with first-degree AV block, inverted T waves, and multiform interpolated PVCs at beats 3 and 5

■ **ECG 13•8**
Rate: 30 bpm; 48 in second half of strip
Rhythm: Irregular
P Waves: Only two visible, of same morphology
PR Interval: Variable
QRS: 0.14 sec
Interpretation: Ventricular fibrillation converting to third-degree AV block

■ ECG 13•9
Rate: 150 bpm
Rhythm: Regular
P Waves: Normal but encroaching on previous T
    waves
PR Interval: 0.12 sec
QRS: 0.08 sec
Interpretation: Sinus tachycardia

■ ECG 13•10
Rate: 50 bpm
Rhythm: Irregular
P Waves: Normal
PR Interval: 0.16 sec
QRS: 0.10 sec
Interpretation: Sinus bradycardia with PJCs at beats
    2 and 4

■ ECG 13•11
Rate: 34 bpm
Rhythm: Regular
P Waves: Flutter waves
PR Interval: None
QRS: 0.10 sec
Interpretation: Atrial flutter with 8:1 block

■ ECG 13•12
Rate: 88 bpm
Rhythm: Regular
P Waves: None
PR Interval: None
QRS: 0.16 sec following pacemaker spike
Interpretation: Pacemaker—ventricular

■ ECG 13•13
Rate: 170 bpm
Rhythm: Irregular
P Waves: None
PR Interval: None
QRS: 0.08
Interpretation: Atrial fibrillation with ST segment
    elevation and couplet PVCs

■ ECG 13•14
Rate: 80 bpm
Rhythm: Irregular
P Waves: Normal
PR Interval: 0.16 sec
QRS: 0.12 sec in postive complexes, difficult to meas-
    ure in beats 3 and 6
Interpretation: Normal sinus rhythm with bundle
    branch block and ventricular trigeminy

■ ECG 13•15
Rate: 110 bpm
Rhythm: Irregular
P Waves: Normal
PR Interval: 0.12 sec
QRS: 0.10 sec
Interpretation: Sinus tachycardia with inverted T
    waves and one PVC at beat 7

■ ECG 13•16
Rate: 48 bpm
Rhythm: Regular
P Waves: Inverted
PR Interval: 0.12 sec
QRS: 0.10 sec
Interpretation: Junctional rhythm

■ ECG 13•17
Rate: 40 bpm
Rhythm: Irregular
P Waves: Normal but not associated with QRS
PR Interval: Variable
QRS: 0.12 sec
Interpretation: Third-degree AV block

■ ECG 13•18
Rate: 70 bpm
Rhythm: Irregular
P Waves: None
PR Interval: None
QRS: 0.12 sec
Interpretation: Junctional rhythm with bundle
    branch block and bigeminal PJCs at beats 2, 4,
    and 6

■ ECG 13•19
Rate: 71 bpm
Rhythm: Regular
P Waves: Normal
PR Interval: 0.16 sec
QRS: 0.12 sec with notched appearance
Interpretation: Normal sinus rhythm with bundle
    branch block

■ ECG 13•20
Rate: 50 bpm
Rhythm: Irregular
P Waves: None
PR Interval: None
QRS: 0.12 sec
Interpretation: Atrial fibrillation with ST segment
    depression and slow ventricular response

■ ECG 13•21
Rate: 65 bpm
Rhythm: Regular
P Waves: Normal
PR Interval: 0.20 sec
QRS: 0.08 sec
Interpretation: Normal sinus rhythm with a
    U wave

■ ECG 13•22
Rate: 78 bpm
Rhythm: Regular
P Waves: None
PR Interval: None
QRS: 0.20 sec following pacemaker spike
Interpretation: Pacemaker—ventricular

■ ECG 13•23
Rate: 90 bpm (counting PVCs), 94 bpm in underlying
    rhythm
Rhythm: Irregular
P Waves: Normal
PR Interval: 0.12 sec
QRS: 0.10 sec
Interpretation: Normal sinus rhythm with
    ventricular trigeminy

■ ECG 13•24
Rate: 60 bpm, 79 bpm in underlying rhythm
Rhythm: Irregular
P Waves: Normal
PR Interval: 0.16 sec
QRS: 0.10 sec
Interpretation: Normal sinus rhythm with 2.56
    second pause (sinus arrest)

■ ECG 13•25
Rate: 40 bpm
Rhythm: Irregular
P Waves: None
PR Interval: None
QRS: 0.08 sec
Interpretation: Atrial fibrillation with slow
    ventricular response

■ ECG 13•26
Rate: 110 bpm
Rhythm: Irregular
P Waves: Fibrillatory and flutter waves
PR Interval: None
QRS: 0.08 sec
Interpretation: Atrial fibrillation converting to
    atrial flutter with 4:1 block

■ ECG 13•27
Rate: 20 bpm
Rhythm: Irregular
P Waves: None
PR Interval: None
QRS: Wide—greater than 0.10 sec
Interpretation: Idioventricular rhythm (Agonal
    rhythm)

■ ECG 13•28
Rate: 58 bpm
Rhythm: Regular
P Waves: Normal
PR Interval: 0.32 sec
QRS: 0.10 sec
Interpretation: Sinus bradycardia with first-degree
    AV block

■ ECG 13•29
Rate: 79 bpm
Rhythm: Regular
P Waves: None following pacemaker spike
PR Interval: None
QRS: 0.16 sec following pacemaker spike
Interpretation: Pacemaker—atrial and ventricular,
    with failure to capture P waves and failure to fire a
    ventricular spike at beat 4

■ ECG 13•30
Rate: 90 bpm (counting PVCs), 88 bpm in underlying
    rhythm
Rhythm: Irregular
P Waves: Normal
PR Interval: 0.12 sec
QRS: 0.08 sec
Interpretation: Normal sinus rhythm with two uni-
    form PVCs at beats 3 and 7

■ ECG 13•31
Rate: 50 bpm
Rhythm: Irregular
P Waves: Normal
PR Interval: 0.20 sec
QRS: 0.10 sec
Interpretation: Sinus bradycardia with junctional
    escape at beats 1 and 3, ST segment depression,
    and inverted T waves

■ ECG 13•32
Rate: 75 bpm
Rhythm: Regular
P Waves: Normal following pacemaker spike
PR Interval: 0.16 sec
QRS: 0.10 sec
Interpretation: Pacemaker—atrial paced, ventricular
    sensed

■ ECG 13·33
Rate: Atrial 100 bpm, ventricular 58 bpm
Rhythm: Atrial regular, ventricular regular
P Waves: Normal but not associated with
    QRS
PR Interval: Variable
QRS: 0.10 sec
Interpretation: Third-degree AV block

■ ECG 13·34
Rate: 80 bpm (counting PVCs); 38 bpm in underlying
    rhythm
Rhythm: Irregular
P Waves: Normal
PR Interval: 0.20 sec
QRS: 0.12 sec
Interpretation: Sinus bradycardia with a bundle
    branch block and bigeminal PVCs

■ ECG 13·35
Rate: 150 bpm
Rhythm: Regular
P Waves: Flutter waves
PR Interval: None
QRS: 0.08 sec
Interpretation: Atrial flutter with 2:1 block

■ ECG 13·36
Rate: 100 bpm
Rhythm: Irregular
P Waves: None
PR Interval: None
QRS: 0.08 sec
Interpretation: Atrial fibrillation

■ ECG 13·37
Rate: None
Rhythm: None
P Waves: None
PR Interval: None
QRS: None
Interpretation: Asystole

■ ECG 13·38
Rate: 80 bpm (counting PVCs), 62 bpm in underlying
    rhythm
Rhythm: Irregular
P Waves: Normal
PR Interval: 0.20 sec
QRS: 0.08 sec
Interpretation: Normal sinus rhythm with three-
    beat ventricular tachycardia (triplet PVCs at
    beats 3, 4, and 5)

■ ECG 13·39
Rate: 71 bpm
Rhythm: Regular
P Waves: Normal
PR Interval: 0.20 sec
QRS: 0.12 sec with notched appearance
Interpretation: Normal sinus rhythm with a
    bundle branch block

■ ECG 13·40
Rate: 60 bpm
Rhythm: Irregular
P Waves: None
PR Interval: None
QRS: 0.12 sec
Interpretation: Junctional rhythm with bundle
    branch block and interpolated PJC at beat 4

■ ECG 13·41
Rate: 100 bpm (counting PVCs); 75 bpm in underly-
    ing rhythm
Rhythm: Irregular
P Waves: Normal
PR Interval: 0.16 sec
QRS: 0.10 sec
Interpretation: Normal sinus rhythm with couplet
    PVCs

■ ECG 13·42
Rate: 80 bpm
Rhythm: Irregular
P Waves: Normal
PR Interval: 0.14 sec
QRS: 0.10 sec in beats 1, 4, and 8; 0.16 sec in
    beats 2, 3, 5, 6, and 7
Interpretation: Normal sinus rhythm with multiform
    PVCs at beats 2, 3, 5, 6, and 7

■ ECG 13·43
Rate: Atrial 79 bpm, ventricular 48 bpm
Rhythm: Atrial regular, ventricular regular
P Waves: Normal but not associated with QRS
PR Interval: Variable
QRS: 0.16 sec
Interpretation: Third-degree AV block

■ ECG 13·44
Rate: 115 bpm
Rhythm: Regular
P Waves: Retrograde
PR Interval: None
QRS: 0.08 sec
Interpretation: Junctional tachycardia

ECG 13·45
Rate: 140 bpm
Rhythm: Irregular
P Waves: Normal
PR Interval: 0.10 sec
QRS: 0.08 sec
Interpretation: Paroxysmal supraventricular tachycardia (sinus tachycardia converting to supraventricular tachycardia)

ECG 13·46
Rate: 50 bpm (counting PVC), 38 bpm in underlying rhythm
Rhythm: Irregular
P Waves: Normal
PR Interval: 0.16 sec
QRS: 0.10 sec
Interpretation: Sinus bradycardia with interpolated PVC at beat 4

ECG 13·47
Rate: 94 bpm
Rhythm: Regular
P Waves: Normal
PR Interval: 0.12 sec
QRS: 0.08 sec
Interpretation: Normal sinus rhythm with ST segment depression

ECG 13·48
Rate: 80 bpm; 70 bpm in underlying rhythm, 90 bpm in last section
Rhythm: Irregular
P Waves: Normal for beats 1 through 4
PR Interval: 0.16 sec for beats 1 through 4
QRS: 0.10 sec for beats 1 through 4; wide—greater than 0.10 sec—for beats 5 through 8
Interpretation: Normal sinus rhythm converting to an accelerated idioventricular rhythm

ECG 13·49
Rate: 80 bpm (counting PVCs), 75 bpm in underlying rhythm
Rhythm: Irregular
P Waves: Normal
PR Interval: 0.16 sec
QRS: 0.10 sec in beats 1, 2, 3, 5, 7, and 8; 0.20 sec in beats 4 and 6
Interpretation: Normal sinus rhythm with uniform PVCs at beats 4 and 6 with full compensatory pauses

ECG 13·50
Rate: 75 bpm
Rhythm: Regular
P Waves: Unclear, may be buried in terminal portion of QRS
PR Interval: None
QRS: 0.16 sec
Interpretation: Accelerated idioventricular rhythm

ECG 13·51
Rate: 75 bpm
Rhythm: Regular
P Waves: Normal for first four beats
PR Interval: 0.20 sec for first four beats
QRS: 0.08 sec
Interpretation: Normal sinus rhythm with muscle artifact

ECG 13·52
Rate: 40 bpm
Rhythm: Irregular
P Waves: Normal in first two beats
PR Interval: 0.20 sec for first two beats
QRS: 0.10 sec for first two beats; 0.16 sec—following pacemaker spikes at beats 3 and 4
Interpretation: Sinus bradycardia converting to a ventricular pacemaker

ECG 13·53
Rate: None
Rhythm: None
P Waves: None
PR Interval: None
QRS: None
Interpretation: Asystole

ECG 13·54
Rate: 38 bpm
Rhythm: Regular
P Waves: Inverted in first two beats, upright in last two beats
PR Interval: 0.16 sec
QRS: 0.10 sec
Interpretation: Wandering atrial pacemaker

ECG 13·55
Rate: 41 bpm
Rhythm: Regular
P Waves: Normal
PR Interval: 0.24 sec
QRS: 0.20 sec
Interpretation: Sinus bradycardia with first-degree AV block and bundle branch block

■ ECG 13•56
Rate: 90 bpm
Rhythm: Irregular
P Waves: Normal
PR Interval: 0.16 sec
QRS: 0.10 sec
Interpretation: Sinus arrhythmia

■ ECG 13•57
Rate: 110 bpm
Rhythm: Irregular
P Waves: Normal except in PACs
PR Interval: 0.14 sec
QRS: 0.08 sec
Interpretation: Sinus tachycardia with atrial
   quadrigeminy (PACs at beats 4 and 8)

■ ECG 13•58
Rate: 90 bpm; 88 bpm in paced section
Rhythm: Regular in paced section, then irregular
P Waves: None
PR Interval: None
QRS: 0.16 sec
Interpretation: Pacemaker—ventricular, with
   polymorphic ventricular tachycardia at end
   of strip

■ ECG 13•59
Rate: Indeterminate
Rhythm: Irregular
P Waves: None
PR Interval: None
QRS: Wide—greater than 0.10 sec—with bizarre
   appearance
Interpretation: Torsade de pointes

■ ECG 13•60
Rate: 70 bpm
Rhythm: Irregular
P Waves: Different forms
PR Interval: Variable
QRS: 0.10 sec
Interpretation: Wandering atrial pacemaker

■ ECG 13•61
Rate: 60 bpm
Rhythm: Regular
P Waves: Normal following pacemaker spike
PR Interval: 0.28 sec
QRS: 0.14 sec
Interpretation: Pacemaker—atrial paced with
   first-degree AV block and ventricular sensed

■ ECG 13•62
Rate: Indeterminate
Rhythm: Irregular
P Waves: None
PR Interval: None
QRS: Wide—greater than 0.10 sec
Interpretation: Ventricular tachycardia deteriorating
   to ventricular fibrillation

■ ECG 13•63
Rate: 38 bpm
Rhythm: Regular
P Waves: Normal
PR Interval: 0.16 sec
QRS: 0.10 sec
Interpretation: Sinus bradycardia

■ ECG 13•64
Rate: 50 bpm; 78 bpm in underlying rhythm
Rhythm: Irregular
P Waves: None or inverted for first five beats
PR Interval: 0.16 sec for beats 2 through 4
QRS: 0.10 sec for first five beats
Interpretation: Junctional rhythm converting to ven-
   tricular fibrillation

■ ECG 13•65
Rate: 80 bpm (counting PVCs), 75 bpm in underlying
   rhythm
Rhythm: Irregular
P Waves: Normal
PR Interval: 0.16 sec
QRS: 0.10 sec
Interpretation: Normal sinus rhythm with ventricular
   trigeminy

■ ECG 13•66
Rate: 100 bpm (counting PVCs), 92 bpm in underly-
   ing rhythm
Rhythm: Irregular
P Waves: Present, but distorted due to muscle artifact
PR Interval: 0.20 sec
QRS: 0.08 sec
Interpretation: Normal sinus rhythm with three-beat
   ventricular tachycardia (triplet PVCs) and muscle
   artifact

■ ECG 13•67
Rate: 86 bpm (counting PVCs), 68 bpm in underlying
   rhythm
Rhythm: Irregular
P Waves: Normal following pacemaker spike
PR Interval: 0.20 sec
QRS: 0.08 sec
Interpretation: Pacemaker—atrial paced, ventricular
   sensed, with PVCs at beats 3, 5, and 8

■ ECG 13•68
Rate: 110 bpm (counting PVCs), 115 bpm in under-
   lying rhythm
Rhythm: Irregular
P Waves: Normal
PR Interval: 0.16 sec
QRS: 0.10 sec
Interpretation: Sinus tachycardia with ST segment
   depression and ventricular couplet at beats 6 and 7

■ ECG 13•69
Rate: 70 bpm
Rhythm: Irregular
P Waves: Normal
PR Interval: Variable
QRS: 0.08 sec
Interpretation: Second-degree AV block Type I
   (Wenckebach)

■ ECG 13•70
Rate: 33 bpm
Rhythm: Regular
P Waves: None
PR Interval: None
QRS: 0.14 sec
Interpretation: Idioventricular rhythm

■ ECG 13•71
Rate: 88 bpm
Rhythm: Regular
P Waves: Normal
PR Interval: 0.16 sec
QRS: Wide—greater than 0.10 sec—notched appear-
   ance
Interpretation: Normal sinus rhythm with a bundle
   branch block

■ ECG 13•72
Rate: 50 bpm
Rhythm: Regular
P Waves: Normal
PR Interval: 0.28 sec
QRS: 0.08 sec
Interpretation: Sinus bradycardia with first-degree
   AV block

■ ECG 13•73
Rate: 75 bpm
Rhythm: Regular
P Waves: None
PR Interval: None
QRS: 0.16 sec
Interpretation: Pacemaker—ventricular

■ ECG 13•74
Rate: 68 bpm
Rhythm: Regular
P Waves: Normal
PR Interval: 0.16 sec
QRS: 0.06 sec
Interpretation: Normal sinus rhythm

■ ECG 13•75
Rate: 80 bpm
Rhythm: Irregular
P Waves: Normal
PR Interval: 0.16 sec
QRS: 0.10 sec
Interpretation: Normal sinus rhythm with bigeminal
   PACs

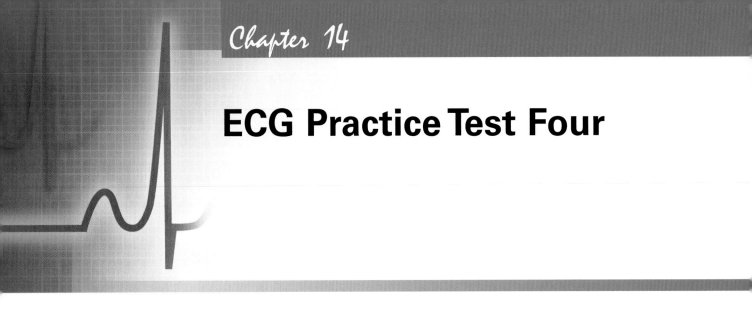

Chapter 14

ECG Practice Test Four

For instructions on analyzing these practice test strips, please see the guidelines given at the end of chapter 2.

TEST STRIP SECTION FOUR

ECG 14•1

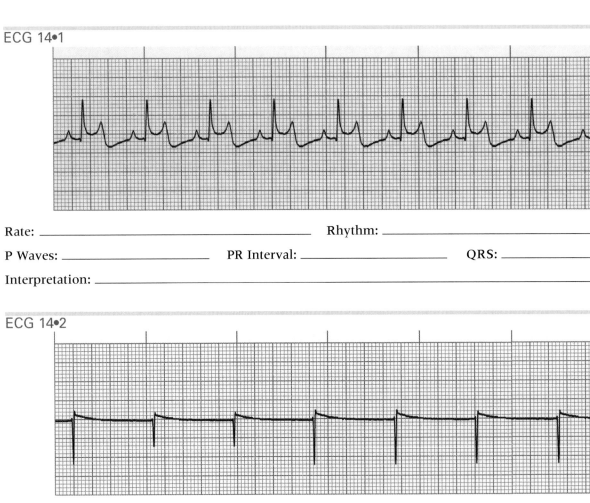

Rate: _____ Rhythm: _____

P Waves: _____ PR Interval: _____ QRS: _____

Interpretation: _____

ECG 14•2

Rate: _____ Rhythm: _____

P Waves: _____ PR Interval: _____ QRS: _____

Interpretation: _____

186

ECG 14•3

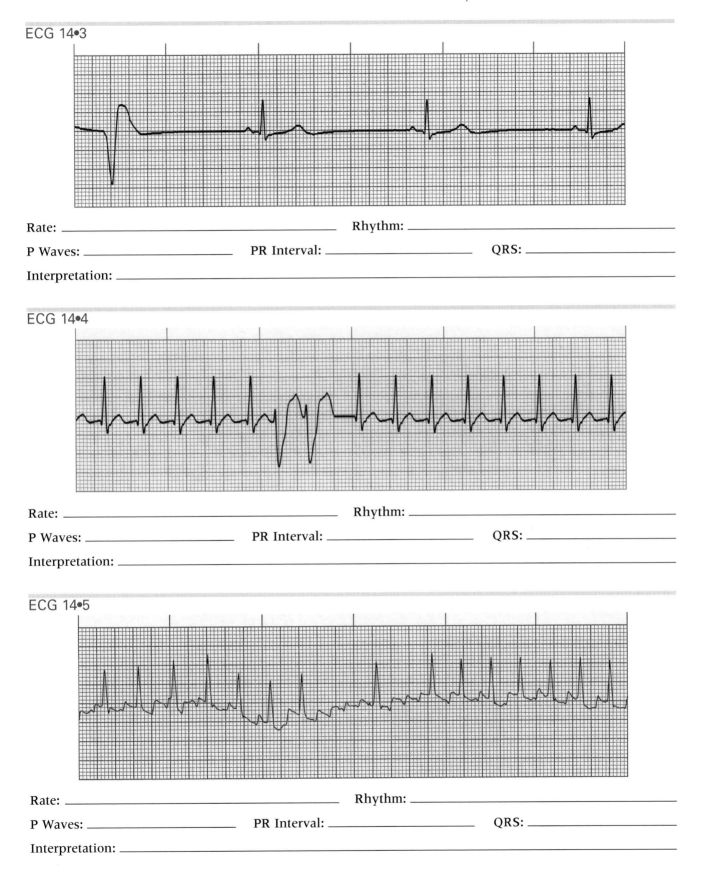

Rate: _____ Rhythm: _____

P Waves: _____ PR Interval: _____ QRS: _____

Interpretation: _____

ECG 14•4

Rate: _____ Rhythm: _____

P Waves: _____ PR Interval: _____ QRS: _____

Interpretation: _____

ECG 14•5

Rate: _____ Rhythm: _____

P Waves: _____ PR Interval: _____ QRS: _____

Interpretation: _____

ECG 14•6

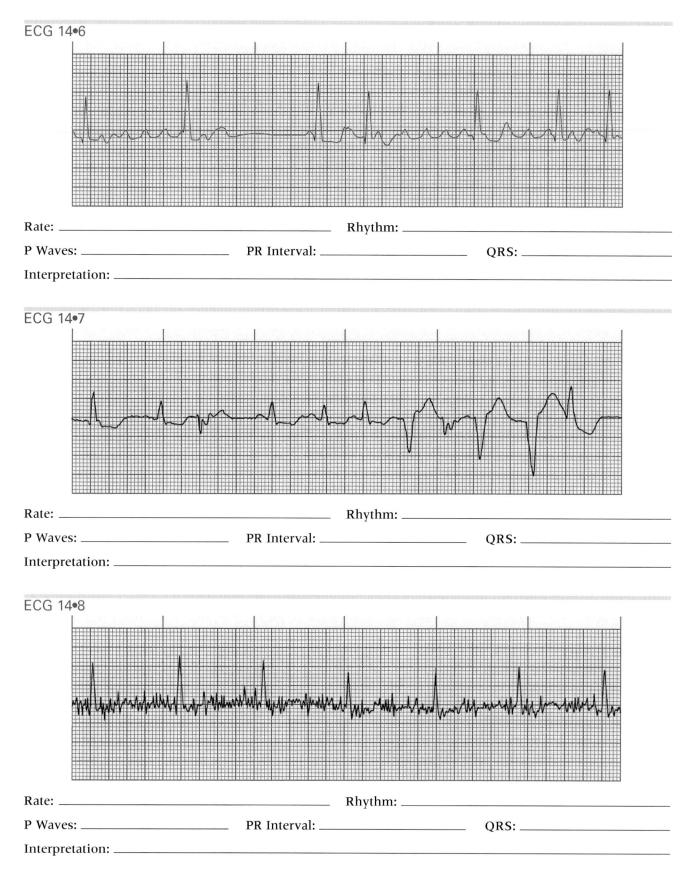

Rate: _____   Rhythm: _____

P Waves: _____   PR Interval: _____   QRS: _____

Interpretation: _____

ECG 14•7

Rate: _____   Rhythm: _____

P Waves: _____   PR Interval: _____   QRS: _____

Interpretation: _____

ECG 14•8

Rate: _____   Rhythm: _____

P Waves: _____   PR Interval: _____   QRS: _____

Interpretation: _____

ECG 14•9

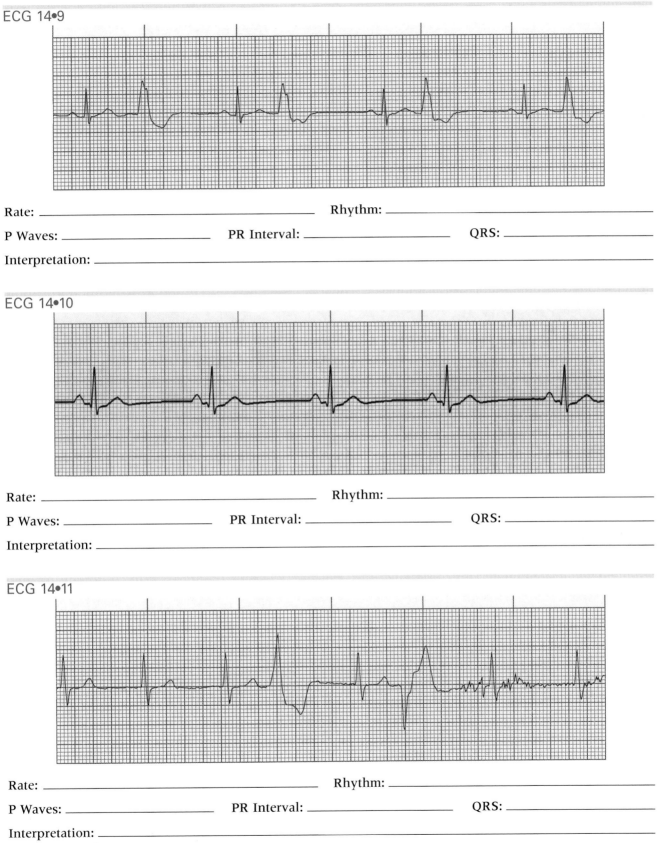

Rate: _____ Rhythm: _____

P Waves: _____ PR Interval: _____ QRS: _____

Interpretation: _____

ECG 14•10

Rate: _____ Rhythm: _____

P Waves: _____ PR Interval: _____ QRS: _____

Interpretation: _____

ECG 14•11

Rate: _____ Rhythm: _____

P Waves: _____ PR Interval: _____ QRS: _____

Interpretation: _____

ECG 14•12

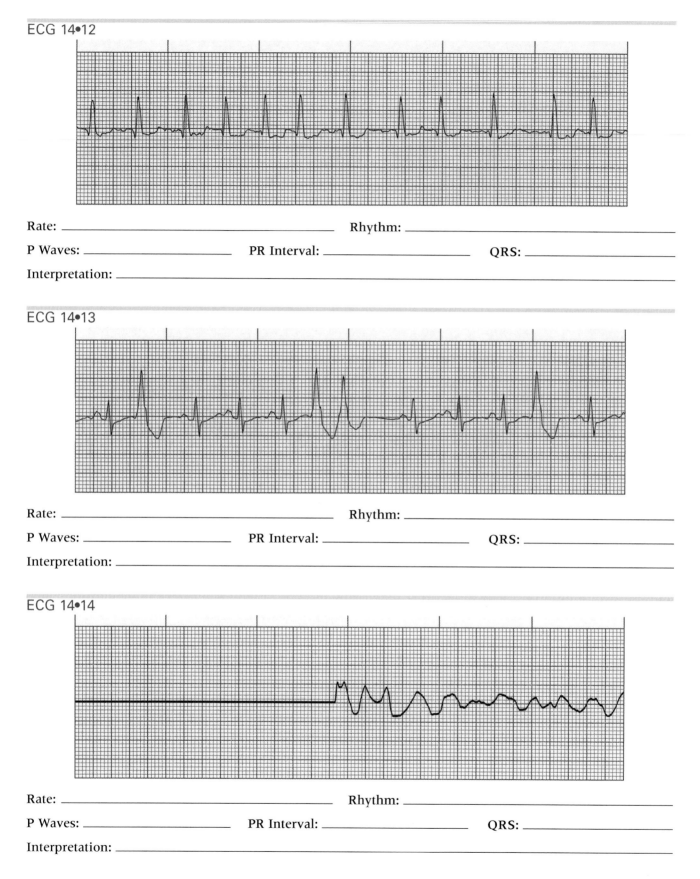

Rate: _____   Rhythm: _____

P Waves: _____   PR Interval: _____   QRS: _____

Interpretation: _____

ECG 14•13

Rate: _____   Rhythm: _____

P Waves: _____   PR Interval: _____   QRS: _____

Interpretation: _____

ECG 14•14

Rate: _____   Rhythm: _____

P Waves: _____   PR Interval: _____   QRS: _____

Interpretation: _____

ECG 14•15

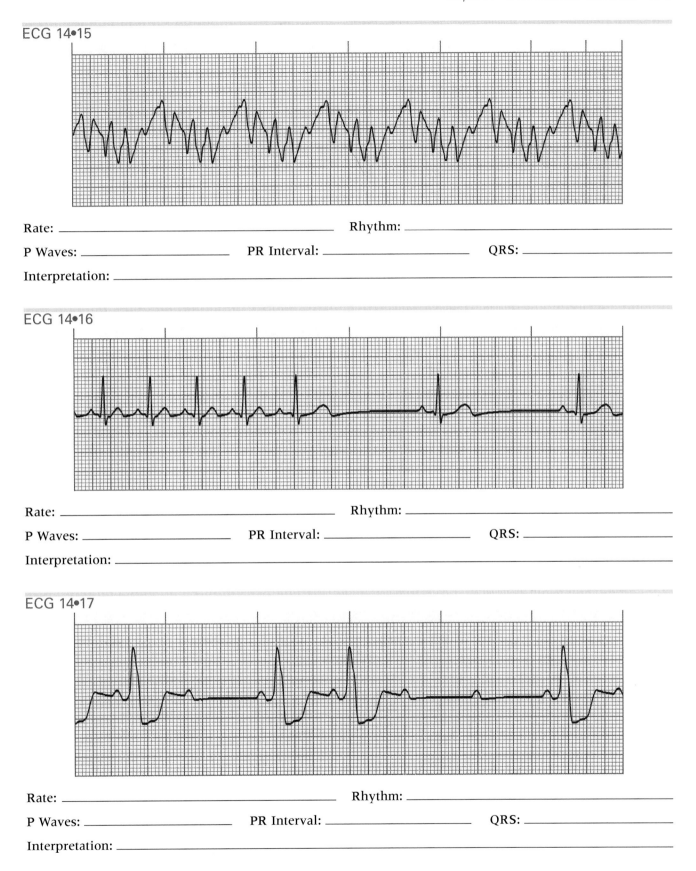

Rate: _____ Rhythm: _____

P Waves: _____ PR Interval: _____ QRS: _____

Interpretation: _____

ECG 14•16

Rate: _____ Rhythm: _____

P Waves: _____ PR Interval: _____ QRS: _____

Interpretation: _____

ECG 14•17

Rate: _____ Rhythm: _____

P Waves: _____ PR Interval: _____ QRS: _____

Interpretation: _____

ECG 14•18

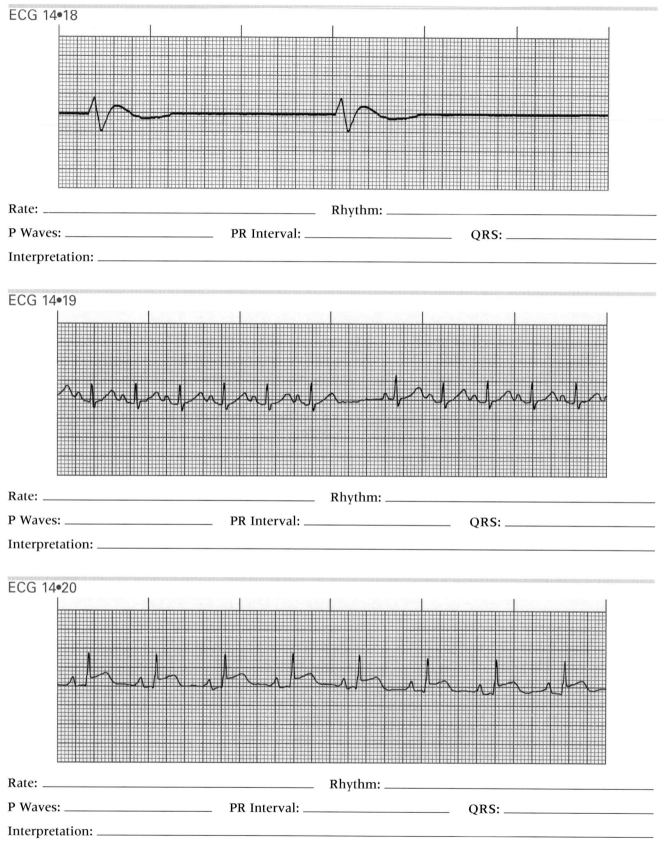

Rate: _____   Rhythm: _____

P Waves: _____   PR Interval: _____   QRS: _____

Interpretation: _____

ECG 14•19

Rate: _____   Rhythm: _____

P Waves: _____   PR Interval: _____   QRS: _____

Interpretation: _____

ECG 14•20

Rate: _____   Rhythm: _____

P Waves: _____   PR Interval: _____   QRS: _____

Interpretation: _____

ECG 14•21

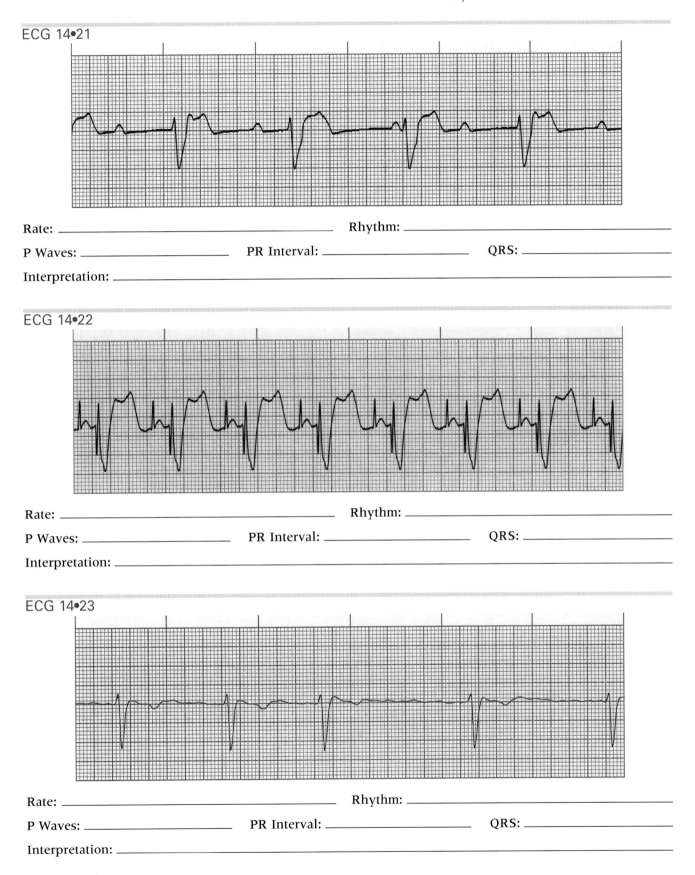

Rate: _____ Rhythm: _____

P Waves: _____ PR Interval: _____ QRS: _____

Interpretation: _____

ECG 14•22

Rate: _____ Rhythm: _____

P Waves: _____ PR Interval: _____ QRS: _____

Interpretation: _____

ECG 14•23

Rate: _____ Rhythm: _____

P Waves: _____ PR Interval: _____ QRS: _____

Interpretation: _____

ECG 14•24

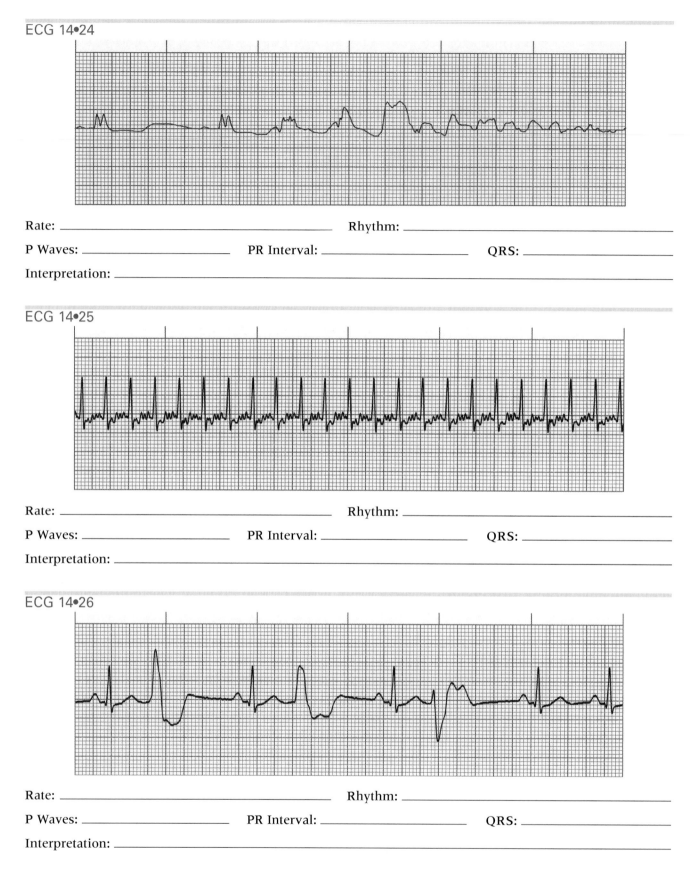

Rate: _____ Rhythm: _____

P Waves: _____ PR Interval: _____ QRS: _____

Interpretation: _____

ECG 14•25

Rate: _____ Rhythm: _____

P Waves: _____ PR Interval: _____ QRS: _____

Interpretation: _____

ECG 14•26

Rate: _____ Rhythm: _____

P Waves: _____ PR Interval: _____ QRS: _____

Interpretation: _____

ECG 14•27

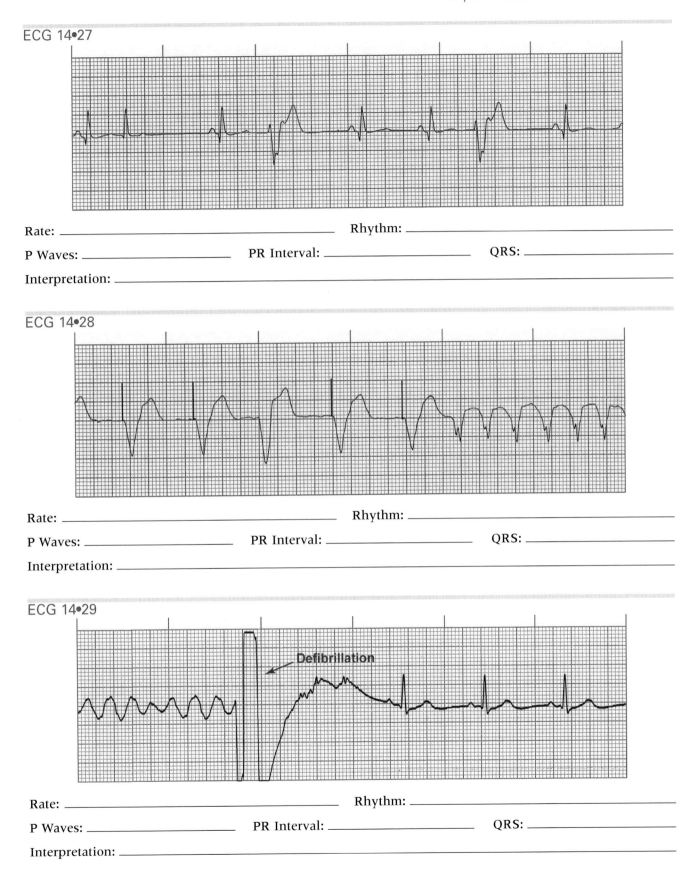

Rate: _____   Rhythm: _____

P Waves: _____ PR Interval: _____ QRS: _____

Interpretation: _____

ECG 14•28

Rate: _____   Rhythm: _____

P Waves: _____ PR Interval: _____ QRS: _____

Interpretation: _____

ECG 14•29

Defibrillation

Rate: _____   Rhythm: _____

P Waves: _____ PR Interval: _____ QRS: _____

Interpretation: _____

ECG 14•30

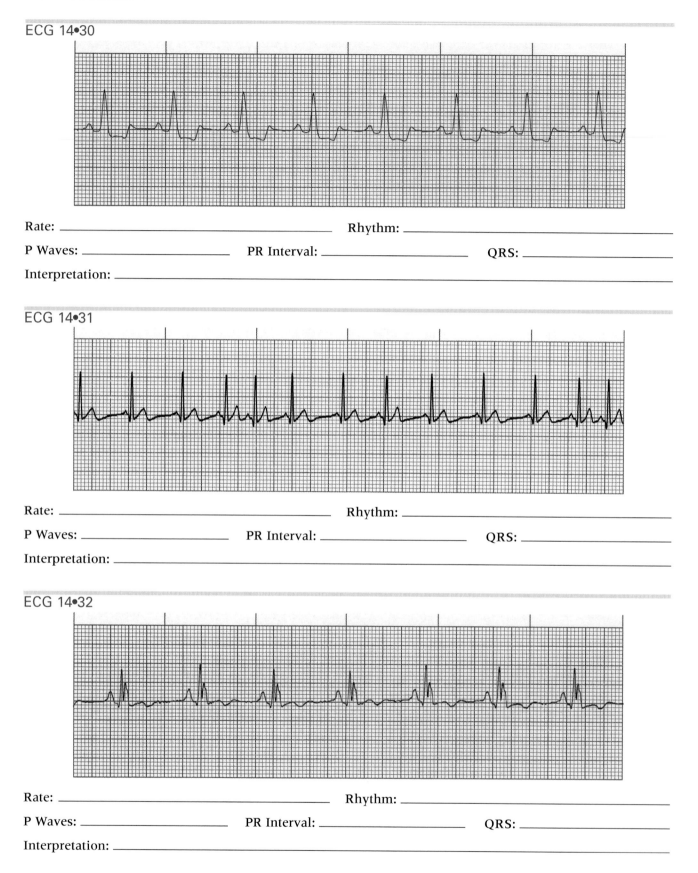

Rate: _____   Rhythm: _____

P Waves: _____   PR Interval: _____   QRS: _____

Interpretation: _____

ECG 14•31

Rate: _____   Rhythm: _____

P Waves: _____   PR Interval: _____   QRS: _____

Interpretation: _____

ECG 14•32

Rate: _____   Rhythm: _____

P Waves: _____   PR Interval: _____   QRS: _____

Interpretation: _____

ECG 14•33

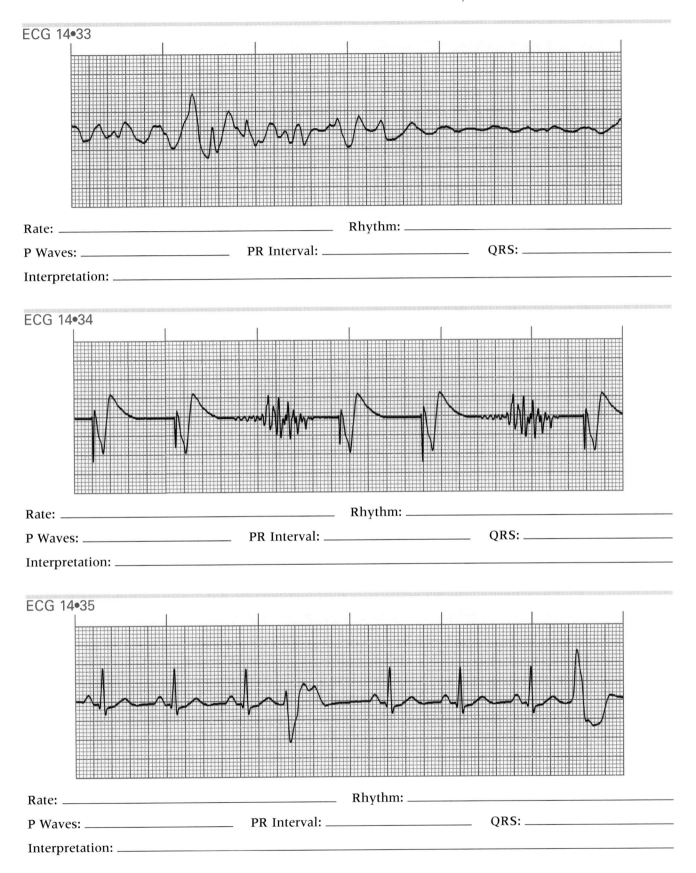

Rate: _____ Rhythm: _____

P Waves: _____ PR Interval: _____ QRS: _____

Interpretation: _____

ECG 14•34

Rate: _____ Rhythm: _____

P Waves: _____ PR Interval: _____ QRS: _____

Interpretation: _____

ECG 14•35

Rate: _____ Rhythm: _____

P Waves: _____ PR Interval: _____ QRS: _____

Interpretation: _____

ECG 14•36

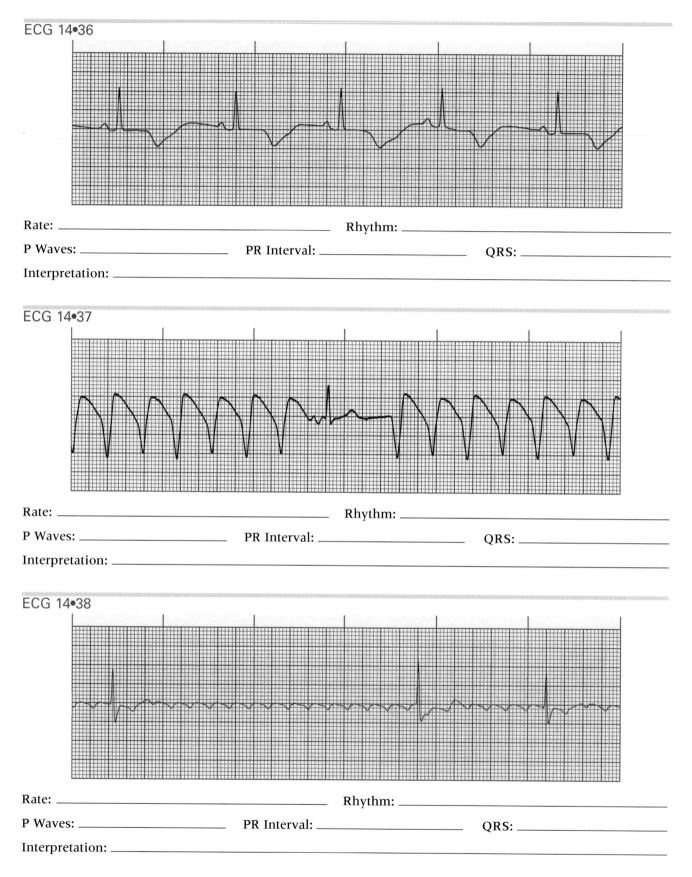

Rate: _____   Rhythm: _____

P Waves: _____   PR Interval: _____   QRS: _____

Interpretation: _____

ECG 14•37

Rate: _____   Rhythm: _____

P Waves: _____   PR Interval: _____   QRS: _____

Interpretation: _____

ECG 14•38

Rate: _____   Rhythm: _____

P Waves: _____   PR Interval: _____   QRS: _____

Interpretation: _____

ECG 14•39

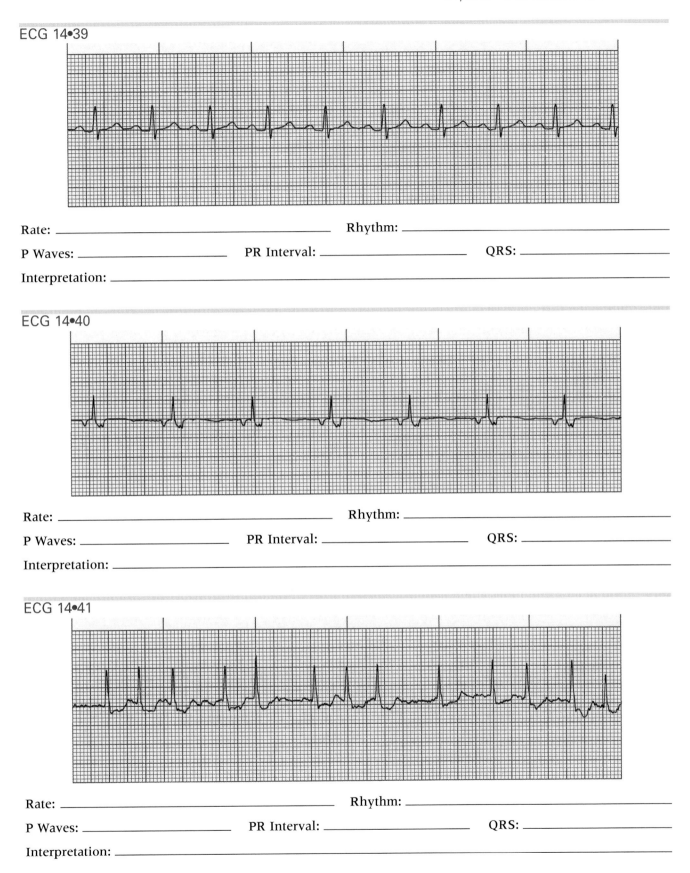

Rate: _____ Rhythm: _____

P Waves: _____ PR Interval: _____ QRS: _____

Interpretation: _____

ECG 14•40

Rate: _____ Rhythm: _____

P Waves: _____ PR Interval: _____ QRS: _____

Interpretation: _____

ECG 14•41

Rate: _____ Rhythm: _____

P Waves: _____ PR Interval: _____ QRS: _____

Interpretation: _____

ECG 14•42

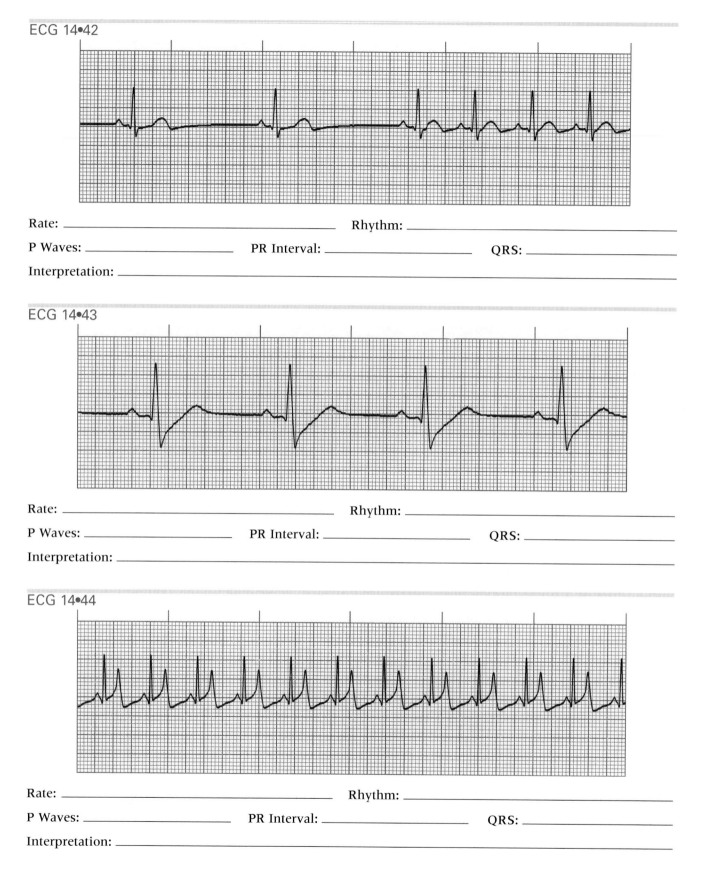

Rate: _____   Rhythm: _____

P Waves: _____   PR Interval: _____   QRS: _____

Interpretation: _____

ECG 14•43

Rate: _____   Rhythm: _____

P Waves: _____   PR Interval: _____   QRS: _____

Interpretation: _____

ECG 14•44

Rate: _____   Rhythm: _____

P Waves: _____   PR Interval: _____   QRS: _____

Interpretation: _____

ECG 14•45

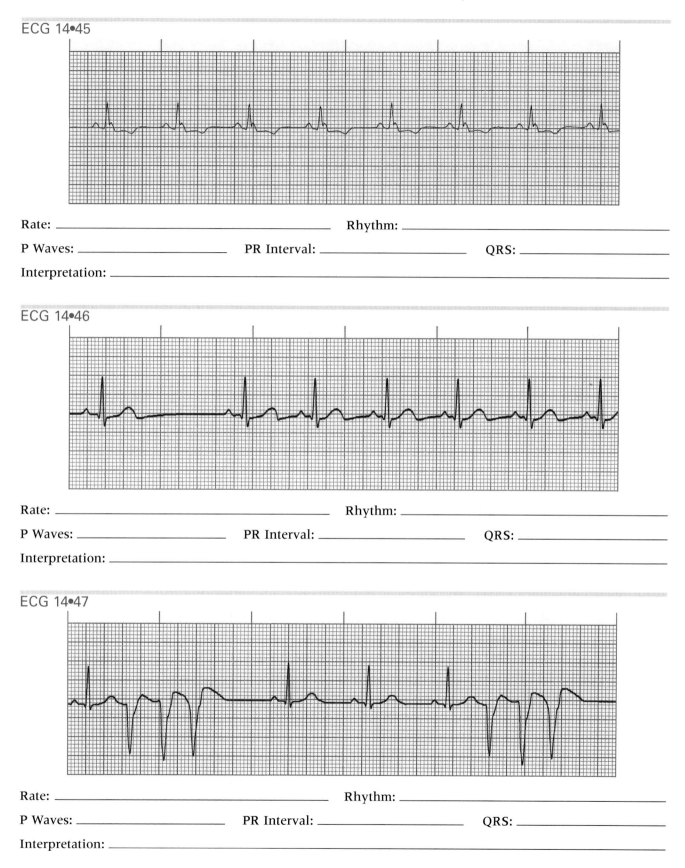

Rate: _____ Rhythm: _____

P Waves: _____ PR Interval: _____ QRS: _____

Interpretation: _____

ECG 14•46

Rate: _____ Rhythm: _____

P Waves: _____ PR Interval: _____ QRS: _____

Interpretation: _____

ECG 14•47

Rate: _____ Rhythm: _____

P Waves: _____ PR Interval: _____ QRS: _____

Interpretation: _____

ECG 14•48

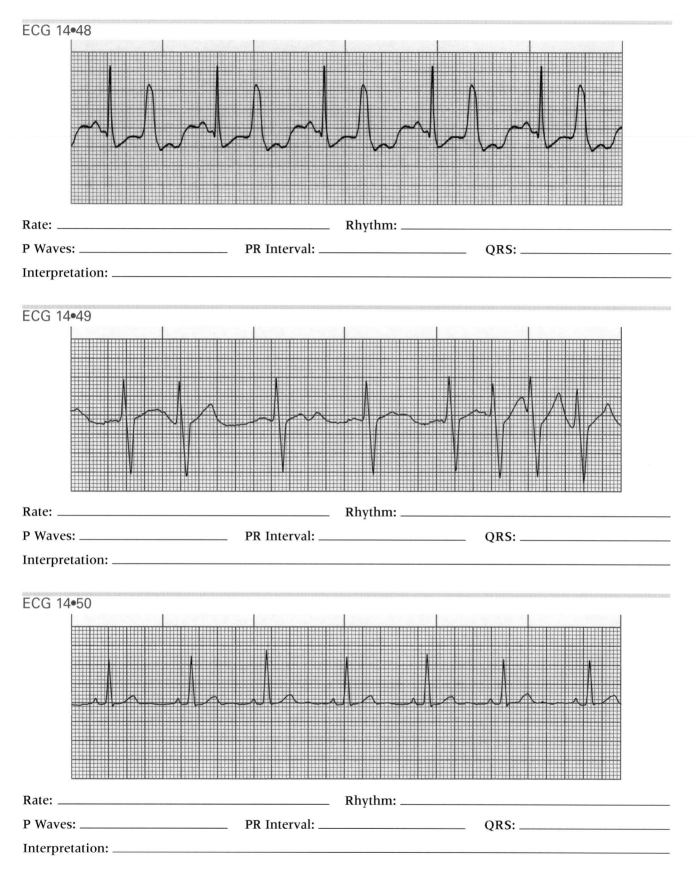

Rate: _____   Rhythm: _____

P Waves: _____   PR Interval: _____   QRS: _____

Interpretation: _____

ECG 14•49

Rate: _____   Rhythm: _____

P Waves: _____   PR Interval: _____   QRS: _____

Interpretation: _____

ECG 14•50

Rate: _____   Rhythm: _____

P Waves: _____   PR Interval: _____   QRS: _____

Interpretation: _____

ECG 14•51

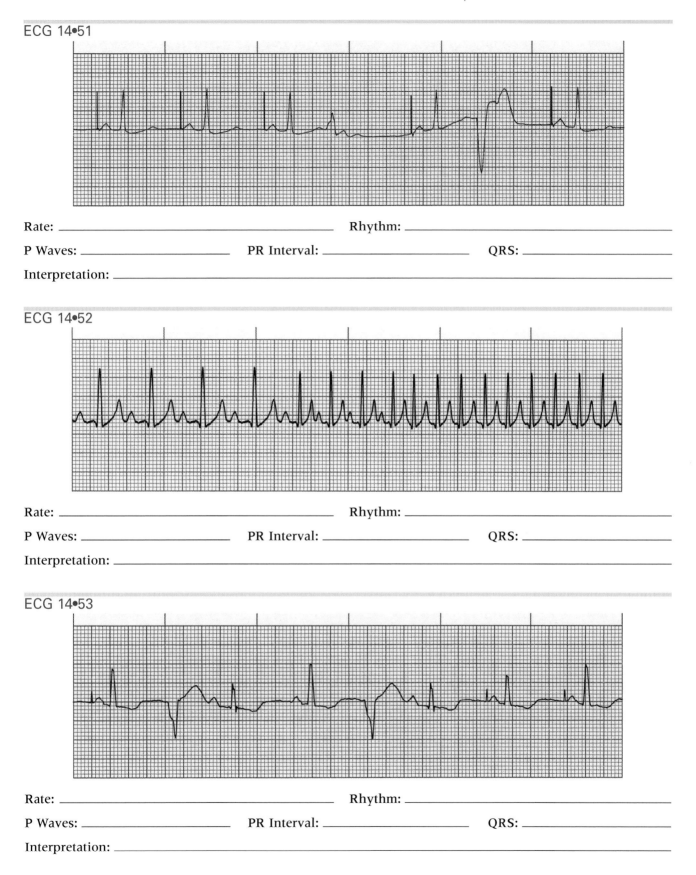

Rate: _____ Rhythm: _____

P Waves: _____ PR Interval: _____ QRS: _____

Interpretation: _____

ECG 14•52

Rate: _____ Rhythm: _____

P Waves: _____ PR Interval: _____ QRS: _____

Interpretation: _____

ECG 14•53

Rate: _____ Rhythm: _____

P Waves: _____ PR Interval: _____ QRS: _____

Interpretation: _____

ECG 14•54

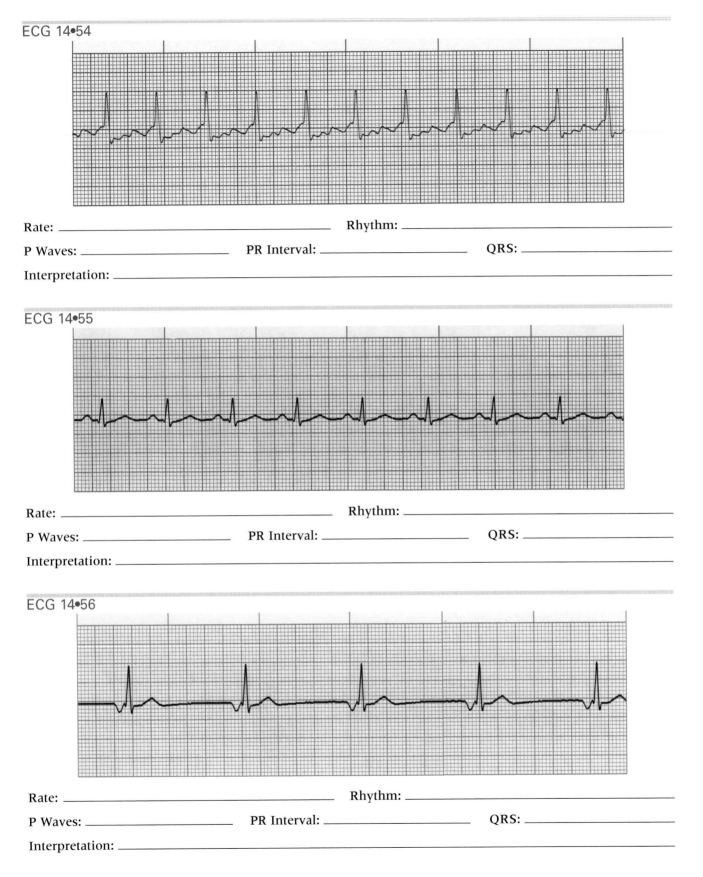

Rate: _____ Rhythm: _____

P Waves: _____ PR Interval: _____ QRS: _____

Interpretation: _____

ECG 14•55

Rate: _____ Rhythm: _____

P Waves: _____ PR Interval: _____ QRS: _____

Interpretation: _____

ECG 14•56

Rate: _____ Rhythm: _____

P Waves: _____ PR Interval: _____ QRS: _____

Interpretation: _____

ECG 14•57

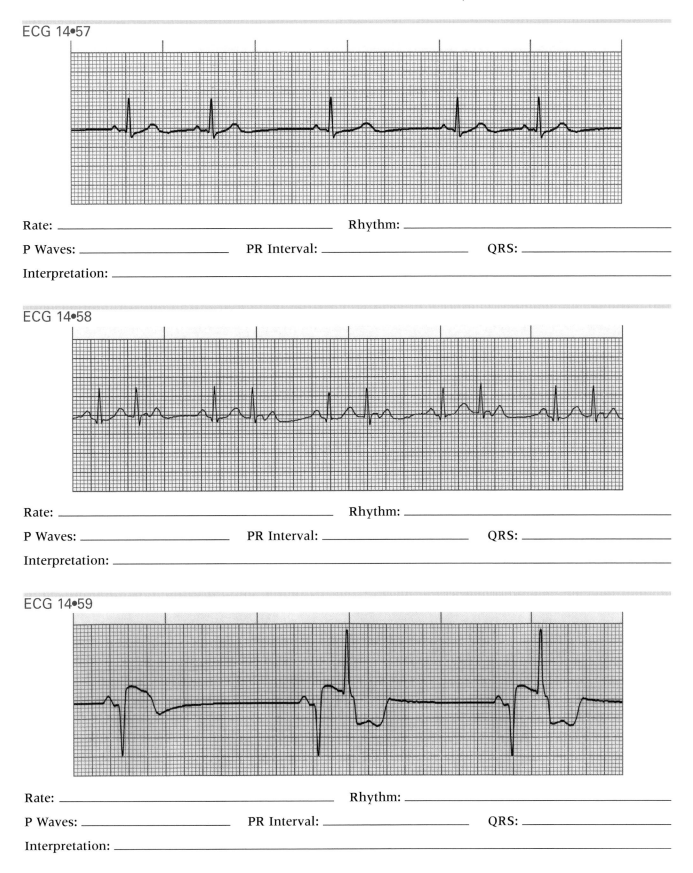

Rate: _____   Rhythm: _____

P Waves: _____   PR Interval: _____   QRS: _____

Interpretation: _____

ECG 14•58

Rate: _____   Rhythm: _____

P Waves: _____   PR Interval: _____   QRS: _____

Interpretation: _____

ECG 14•59

Rate: _____   Rhythm: _____

P Waves: _____   PR Interval: _____   QRS: _____

Interpretation: _____

ECG 14•60

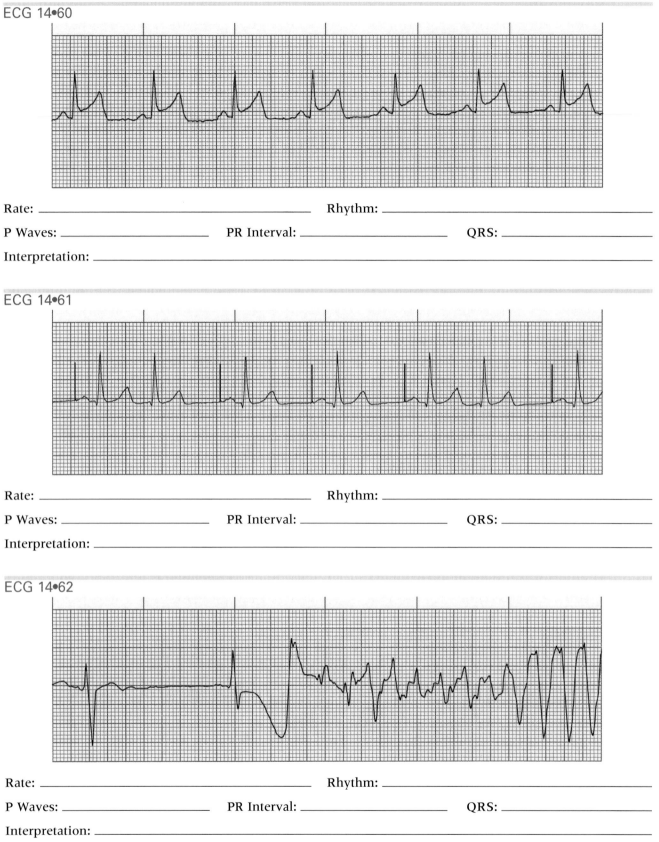

Rate: _____   Rhythm: _____

P Waves: _____   PR Interval: _____   QRS: _____

Interpretation: _____

ECG 14•61

Rate: _____   Rhythm: _____

P Waves: _____   PR Interval: _____   QRS: _____

Interpretation: _____

ECG 14•62

Rate: _____   Rhythm: _____

P Waves: _____   PR Interval: _____   QRS: _____

Interpretation: _____

ECG 14•63

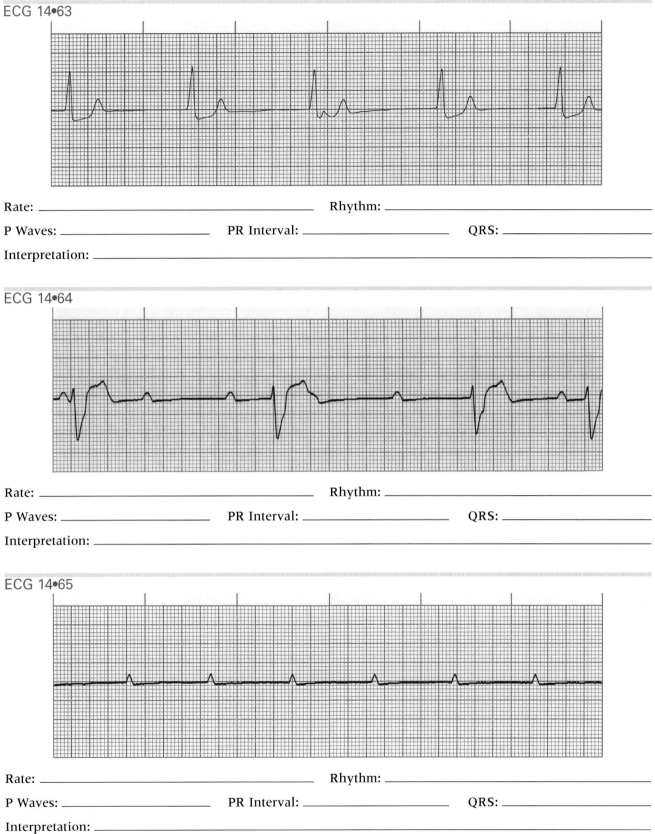

Rate: _____ Rhythm: _____

P Waves: _____ PR Interval: _____ QRS: _____

Interpretation: _____

ECG 14•64

Rate: _____ Rhythm: _____

P Waves: _____ PR Interval: _____ QRS: _____

Interpretation: _____

ECG 14•65

Rate: _____ Rhythm: _____

P Waves: _____ PR Interval: _____ QRS: _____

Interpretation: _____

ECG 14•66

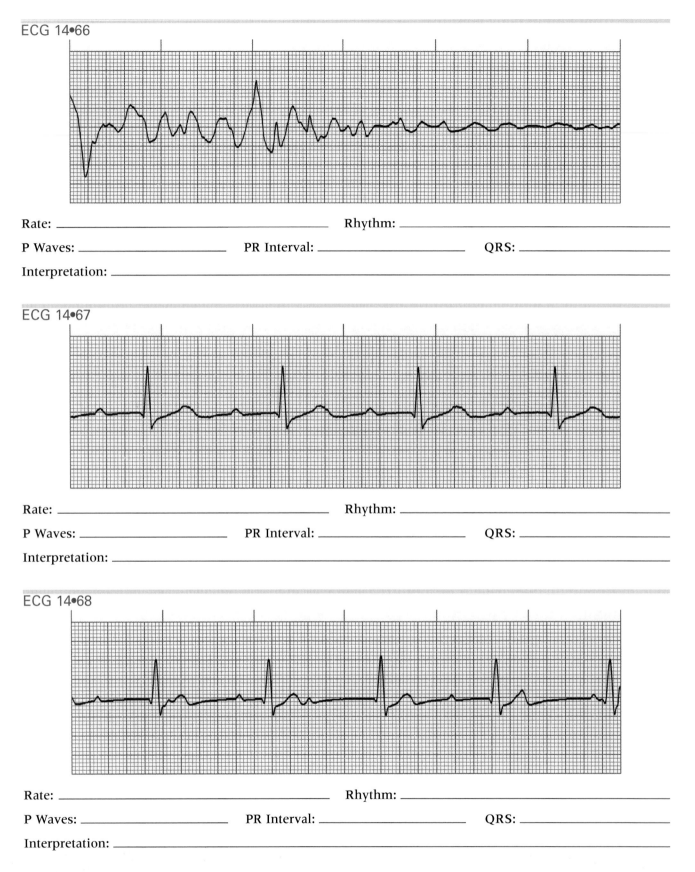

Rate: _____   Rhythm: _____

P Waves: _____   PR Interval: _____   QRS: _____

Interpretation: _____

ECG 14•67

Rate: _____   Rhythm: _____

P Waves: _____   PR Interval: _____   QRS: _____

Interpretation: _____

ECG 14•68

Rate: _____   Rhythm: _____

P Waves: _____   PR Interval: _____   QRS: _____

Interpretation: _____

ECG 14•69

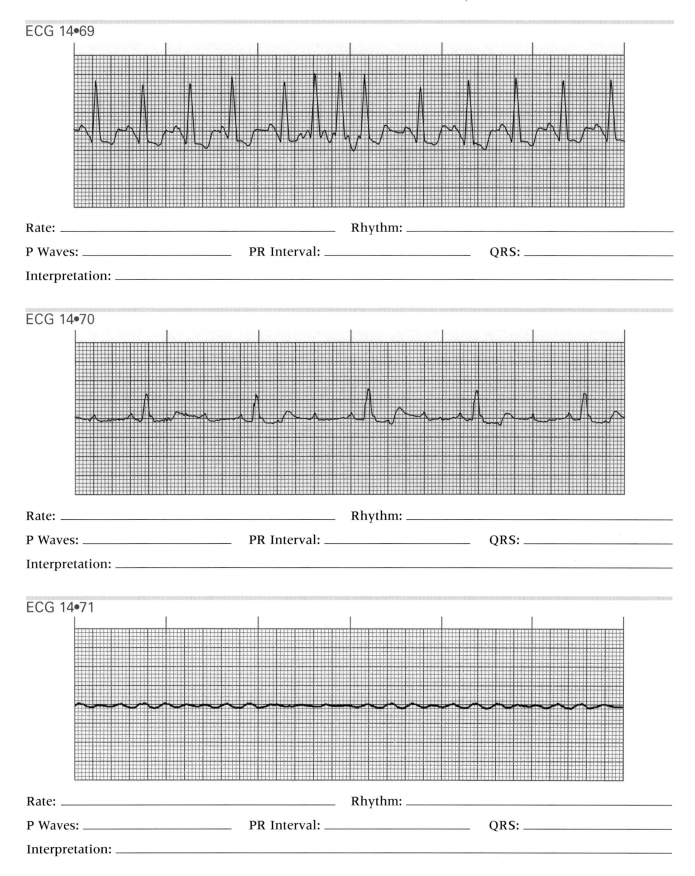

Rate: _____ Rhythm: _____

P Waves: _____ PR Interval: _____ QRS: _____

Interpretation: _____

ECG 14•70

Rate: _____ Rhythm: _____

P Waves: _____ PR Interval: _____ QRS: _____

Interpretation: _____

ECG 14•71

Rate: _____ Rhythm: _____

P Waves: _____ PR Interval: _____ QRS: _____

Interpretation: _____

ECG 14•72

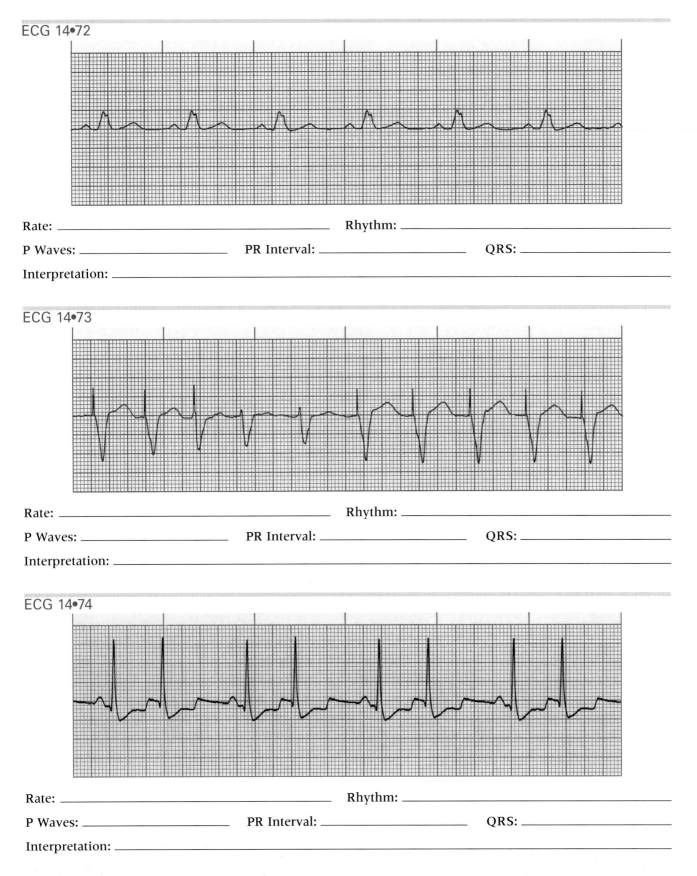

Rate: _____   Rhythm: _____

P Waves: _____   PR Interval: _____   QRS: _____

Interpretation: _____

ECG 14•73

Rate: _____   Rhythm: _____

P Waves: _____   PR Interval: _____   QRS: _____

Interpretation: _____

ECG 14•74

Rate: _____   Rhythm: _____

P Waves: _____   PR Interval: _____   QRS: _____

Interpretation: _____

ECG 14•75

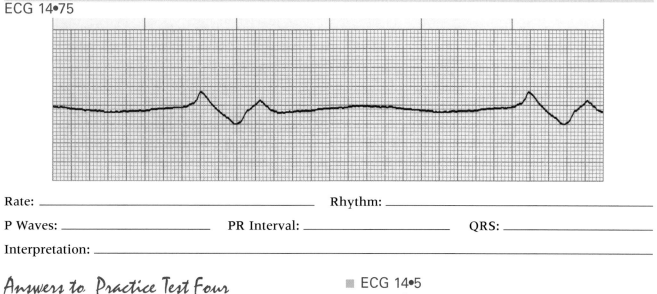

Rate: _____ Rhythm: _____

P Waves: _____ PR Interval: _____ QRS: _____

Interpretation: _____

Answers to Practice Test Four

■ ECG 14•1
Rate: 88 bpm
Rhythm: Regular
P Waves: Normal
PR Interval: 0.18 sec
QRS: 0.08 sec
Interpretation: Normal sinus rhythm with ST
   segment elevation

■ ECG 14•2
Rate: None
Rhythm: None
P Waves: None
PR Interval: None
QRS: None
Interpretation: Asystole and pacemaker with failure
   to capture

■ ECG 14•3
Rate: 40 bpm (counting PVCs), 34 bpm in underlying
   rhythm
Rhythm: Irregular, regular in underlying rhythm
P Waves: Normal
PR Interval: 0.16 sec
QRS: 0.16 sec in first beat, 0.08 sec in remaining
   beats
Interpretation: Sinus bradycardia with a PVC at beat 1

■ ECG 14•4
Rate: 150 bpm (counting PVCs), 150 bpm in under-
   lying rhythm
Rhythm: Irregular, regular in underlying rhythm
P Waves: None
PR Interval: None
QRS: 0.08 sec
Interpretation: Junctional tachycardia with couplet
   PVCs

■ ECG 14•5
Rate: 150 bpm
Rhythm: Irregular
P Waves: None
PR Interval: None
QRS: 0.08 sec
Interpretation: Atrial fibrillation with rapid
   ventricular response

■ ECG 14•6
Rate: 70 bpm
Rhythm: Irregular
P Waves: Flutter waves
PR Interval: None
QRS: 0.10 sec
Interpretation: Atrial flutter with variable
   block with atrial fibrillation from beats
   2 to 4

■ ECG 14•7
Rate: 110 bpm
Rhythm: Irregular
P Waves: Variable
PR Interval: Variable
QRS: 0.10 sec in beats 1, 2, 4, 5, 6; 0.12 sec in beats
   3, 7, and remaining beats
Interpretation: Possible sinus tachycardia with
   ST segment depression and PVC in beat 3
   and polymorphic ventricular tachycardia

■ ECG 14•8
Rate: 63 bpm
Rhythm: Regular
P Waves: Buried in artifact
PR Interval: Indeterminate
QRS: 0.08 sec
Interpretation: Indeterminate rhythm; possibly
   normal sinus rhythm with muscle artifact

■ ECG 14•9
Rate: 80 bpm
Rhythm: Irregular
P Waves: Normal
PR Interval: 0.16 sec
QRS: 0.08 sec
Interpretation: Normal sinus rhythm with ventricular bigeminy

■ ECG 14•10
Rate: 47 bpm
Rhythm: Regular
P Waves: Normal
PR Interval: 0.16 sec
QRS: 0.10 sec
Interpretation: Sinus bradycardia

■ ECG 14•11
Rate: 80 bpm (counting PVCs), 69 bpm in underlying rhythm
Rhythm: Irregular
P Waves: None
PR Interval: None
QRS: 0.12 sec
Interpretation: Junctional rhythm with a bundle branch block two multiform PVCs at beats 4 and 6 and muscle artifact at the end of the rhythm

■ ECG 14•12
Rate: 120 bpm
Rhythm: Irregular
P Waves: None
PR Interval: None
QRS: 0.10 sec
Interpretation: Atrial fibrillation with rapid ventricular response and ST segment depression

■ ECG 14•13
Rate: 120 bpm (counting PVCs), 125 in underlying rhythm
Rhythm: Irregular
P Waves: Normal
PR Interval: 0.16 sec
QRS: 0.08 sec in narrow beats, 0.12 sec in wide beats
Interpretation: Sinus tachycardia with ST segment depression and PVCs at beats 2, 6, 7, and 11

■ ECG 14•14
Rate: Indeterminate
Rhythm: Flat line, then chaotic
P Waves: None
PR Interval: None
QRS: None
Interpretation: Asystole converting to ventricular fibrillation

■ ECG 14•15
Rate: Indeterminate
Rhythm: Irregular
P Waves: None
PR Interval: None
QRS: Wide—greater than 0.10 sec with bizarre appearance
Interpretation: Possible ventricular tachycardia or CPR artifact or other artifact

■ ECG 14•16
Rate: 70 bpm; 120 bpm in initial section, then 39 bpm in remaining section
Rhythm: Irregular
P Waves: Normal
PR Interval: 0.16 sec
QRS: 0.10 sec
Interpretation: Sinus tachycardia changing to sinus bradycardia

■ ECG 14•17
Rate: Atrial 75 bpm, ventricular 40 bpm
Rhythm: Atrial regular, ventricular irregular
P Waves: Normal
PR Interval: 0.16 sec
QRS: 0.12 sec
Interpretation: Second-degree AV block Type II

■ ECG 14•18
Rate: 20 bpm
Rhythm: Irregular
P Waves: None
PR Interval: None
QRS: Wide—greater than 0.10 sec
Interpretation: Idioventricular rhythm (agonal rhythm)

■ ECG 14•19
Rate: 110 bpm
Rhythm: Irregular
P Waves: Normal
PR Interval: 0.16 sec
QRS: 0.08 sec
Interpretation: Sinus tachycardia with 0.92 second pause (sinoatrial block)

■ ECG 14•20
Rate: 79 bpm
Rhythm: Regular
P Waves: Normal
PR Interval: 0.20 sec
QRS: 0.08 sec
Interpretation: Normal sinus rhythm with ST segment elevation

■ ECG 14•21
Rate: Atrial 75 bpm, ventricular 48 bpm
Rhythm: Atrial regular, ventricular regular
P Waves: Normal, some obscured by QRS complexes
PR Interval: Variable, not associated with QRS complexes
QRS: 0.20 sec
Interpretation: Third-degree AV block

■ ECG 14•22
Rate: 75 bpm
Rhythm: Regular
P Waves: Normal following pacemaker spike
PR Interval: 0.20 sec
QRS: 0.20 sec following pacemaker spike
Interpretation: Pacemaker—atrial and ventricular

■ ECG 14•23
Rate: 50 bpm
Rhythm: Irregular
P Waves: None
PR Interval: None
QRS: 0.12 sec
Interpretation: Atrial fibrillation with bundle branch block and slow ventricular response

■ ECG 14•24
Rate: Indeterminate
Rhythm: Irregular
P Waves: Present, low amplitude in first two beats only
PR Interval: 0.20 sec in first two beats only
QRS: Wide—0.16 sec in first two beats
Interpretation: Sinus bradycardia with a bundle branch block deteriorating into ventricular fibrillation

■ ECG 14•25
Rate: 214 bpm
Rhythm: Regular
P Waves: None visible
PR Interval: None
QRS: 0.06 sec
Interpretation: Supraventricular tachycardia with muscle artifact

■ ECG 14•26
Rate: 80 bpm
Rhythm: Irregular
P Waves: Normal
PR Interval: 0.16 sec
QRS: 0.10 sec in normal beats, 0.16 sec in wide beats
Interpretation: Normal sinus rhythm with bigeminal multiform PVCs

■ ECG 14•27
Rate: 80 bpm
Rhythm: Irregular
P Waves: Normal
PR Interval: 0.12 sec
QRS: 0.10 sec
Interpretation: Normal sinus rhythm with PJC at beat 2, and uniform PVCs at beats 4 and 7

■ ECG 14•28
Rate: 110 bpm; 80 bpm in paced portion
Rhythm: Irregular
P Waves: None
PR Interval: None
QRS: 0.20 sec
Interpretation: Pacemaker—ventricular, with PVC at beat 3 and the rhythm deteriorates into monomorphic ventricular tachycardia

■ ECG 14•29
Rate: 68 bpm after defibrillation
Rhythm: Irregular
P Waves: Normal in last three beats
PR Interval: 0.16 sec in last three beats
QRS: 0.08 sec in last three beats
Interpretation: Ventricular fibrillation defibrillated and converting to normal sinus rhythm

■ ECG 14•30
Rate: 79 bpm
Rhythm: Regular
P Waves: Normal
PR Interval: 0.16 sec
QRS: 0.08 sec
Interpretation: Normal sinus rhythm with ST segment depression

■ ECG 14•31
Rate: 130 bpm
Rhythm: Irregular
P Waves: Different forms
PR Interval: Variable
QRS: 0.06 sec
Interpretation: Multifocal atrial tachycardia

■ ECG 14•32
Rate: 75 bpm
Rhythm: Regular
P Waves: Normal
PR Interval: 0.12 sec
QRS: 0.12 sec with notched appearance
Interpretation: Normal sinus rhythm with a bundle branch block

■ ECG 14•33
Rate: Indeterminate
Rhythm: Chaotic
P Waves: None
PR Interval: None
QRS: None
Interpretation: Ventricular fibrillation—coarse fibril-
  latory waves transitioning to fine fibrillatory waves

■ ECG 14•34
Rate: 50 bpm
Rhythm: Irregular
P Waves: None
PR Interval: None
QRS: Wide—greater than 0.10 sec following pace-
  maker spike
Interpretation: Pacemaker—ventricular, with over-
  sensing of muscle artifact after beats 2 and 4

■ ECG 14•35
Rate: 80 bpm (counting PVCs), 75 bpm in underlying
  rhythm
Rhythm: Irregular
P Waves: Normal
PR Interval: 0.16 sec
QRS: 0.10 sec in normal beats, 0.16 sec in wide beats
Interpretation: Normal sinus rhythm with ventricular
  quadrigeminy

■ ECG 14•36
Rate: 50 bpm
Rhythm: Irregular
P Waves: Normal
PR Interval: 0.16 sec
QRS: 0.08 sec
Interpretation: Sinus bradycardia with sinus arrhyth-
  mia with inverted T waves

■ ECG 14•37
Rate: 144 bpm
Rhythm: Irregular
P Waves: Inverted at beat 7
PR Interval: 0.16 sec
QRS: Wide—greater than 0.10 sec except for beat
  7, which is 0.10 sec
Interpretation: Monomorphic ventricular tachycardia
  with one supraventricular complex at beat 7

■ ECG 14•38
Rate: 30 bpm
Rhythm: Irregular
P Waves: Flutter waves
PR Interval: None
QRS: 0.08 sec
Interpretation: Atrial flutter with variable block and
  slow ventricular response

■ ECG 14•39
Rate: 94 bpm
Rhythm: Regular
P Waves: Normal
PR Interval: 0.20 sec
QRS: 0.08 sec
Interpretation: Normal sinus rhythm

■ ECG 14•40
Rate: 68 bpm
Rhythm: Regular
P Waves: Inverted
PR Interval: 0.12 sec
QRS: 0.04 sec
Interpretation: Accelerated junctional rhythm
  with ST segment depression and flattened
  T waves

■ ECG 14•41
Rate: 130 bpm
Rhythm: Irregular
P Waves: None
PR Interval: None
QRS: 0.08 sec
Interpretation: Atrial fibrillation with rapid ventricu-
  lar response

■ ECG 14•42
Rate: 60 bpm; 38 bpm in first section, 98 bpm
  in second section
Rhythm: Irregular
P Waves: Normal
PR Interval: 0.16 sec
QRS: 0.10 sec
Interpretation: Sinus bradycardia changing to
  normal sinus rhythm

■ ECG 14•43
Rate: 41 bpm
Rhythm: Regular
P Waves: Normal
PR Interval: 0.20 sec
QRS: 0.12 sec
Interpretation: Sinus bradycardia with bundle
  branch block

■ ECG 14•44
Rate: 115 bpm
Rhythm: Regular
P Waves: Normal
PR Interval: 0.12 sec
QRS: 0.06 sec
Interpretation: Sinus tachycardia with peaked T
  waves

■ ECG 14•45
Rate: 79 bpm
Rhythm: Regular
P Waves: Normal
PR Interval: 0.16 sec
QRS: 0.12 sec with notched appearance
Interpretation: Normal sinus rhythm with a bundle branch block

■ ECG 14•46
Rate: 70 bpm; 75 bpm in underlying rhythm
Rhythm: Irregular, regular starting with second beat
P Waves: Normal
PR Interval: 0.16 sec
QRS: 0.10 sec
Interpretation: Normal sinus rhythm with a 1.52 second pause (sinoatrial block)

■ ECG 14•47
Rate: 100 bpm; 75 bpm in underlying rhythm
Rhythm: Irregular
P Waves: Normal
PR Interval: 0.16 sec
QRS: 0.10 sec
Interpretation: Normal sinus rhythm with two runs of three-beat ventricular tachycardia (sets of triplet PVCs)

■ ECG 14•48
Rate: 100 bpm
Rhythm: Irregular
P Waves: Normal
PR Interval: 0.16 sec
QRS: 0.10 sec in normal beats, 0.16 sec in wide beats
Interpretation: Normal sinus rhythm with ST segment depression and bigeminal uniform PVCs

■ ECG 14•49
Rate: 80 bpm
Rhythm: Irregular
P Waves: None
PR Interval: None
QRS: 0.12 sec
Interpretation: Atrial fibrillation with bundle branch block and controlled ventricular response

■ ECG 14•50
Rate: 70 bpm
Rhythm: Irregular
P Waves: Normal
PR Interval: 0.16 sec
QRS: 0.08 sec
Interpretation: Sinus arrhythmia

■ ECG 14•51
Rate: 70 bpm
Rhythm: Irregular
P Waves: Normal following pacemaker spike
PR Interval: 0.20 sec
QRS: 0.08 sec
Interpretation: Pacemaker—atrial paced and ventricular sensed, with ST segment depression and PVCs at beats 4 and 6

■ ECG 14•52
Rate: 170 bpm; 110 bpm in first section, 240 bpm in last section
Rhythm: Irregular
P Waves: Normal for beats 1 through 8; buried in T wave in beats 9 through 17
PR Interval: 0.22 sec in first section; thereafter not measurable
QRS: 0.08 sec
Interpretation: Paroxysmal supraventricular tachycardia (normal sinus rhythm changing to a supraventricular tachycardia)

■ ECG 14•53
Rate: 80 bpm
Rhythm: Irregular
P Waves: Normal, some following pacemaker spike
PR Interval: 0.20 sec in paced beats, 0.24 sec in beats 3 and 6, 0.16 sec in beat 4
QRS: 0.06 sec in narrow complexes, 0.12 sec in wide complexes
Interpretation: Pacemaker—atrial paced and ventricular sensed in beats 1, 7, and 8; intrinsic sinus complexes at beats 3, 4, and 6 with T wave inversion; PVCs at beats 2 and 5

■ ECG 14•54
Rate: 107 bpm
Rhythm: Regular
P Waves: Flutter waves
PR Interval: None
QRS: 0.08 sec
Interpretation: Atrial flutter with 3:1 conduction

■ ECG 14•55
Rate: 83 bpm
Rhythm: Regular
P Waves: Normal
PR Interval: 0.20 sec
QRS: 0.10 sec
Interpretation: Normal sinus rhythm

■ ECG 14•56
Rate: 47 bpm
Rhythm: Regular
P Waves: Inverted
PR Interval: 0.10 sec
QRS: 0.10 sec
Interpretation: Junctional rhythm

■ ECG 14•57
Rate: 50 bpm
Rhythm: Irregular
P Waves: Normal
PR Interval: 0.12 sec
QRS: 0.08 sec
Interpretation: Sinus bradycardia with sinus
    arrhythmia

■ ECG 14•58
Rate: 100 bpm
Rhythm: Irregular
P Waves: Normal
PR Interval: 0.16 sec
QRS: 0.08 sec
Interpretation: Normal sinus rhythm with bigeminal
    PJCs

■ ECG 14•59
Rate: 50 bpm (counting PVCs), 28 bpm in underlying
    rhythm
Rhythm: Irregular
P Waves: Normal
PR Interval: 0.16 sec
QRS: 0.10 sec
Interpretation: Sinus bradycardia with ST elevation,
    T wave inversion, and interpolated PVCs (R on T)
    at beats 3 and 5

■ ECG 14•60
Rate: 65 bpm
Rhythm: Regular
P Waves: Normal
PR Interval: 0.16 sec
QRS: 0.08 sec
Interpretation: Normal sinus rhythm with ST seg-
    ment elevation

■ ECG 14•61
Rate: 70 bpm; 60 bpm in underlying paced rhythm
Rhythm: Irregular
P Waves: Normal following pacemaker spike
PR Interval: 0.20 sec
QRS: 0.10 sec
Interpretation: Pacemaker—atrial paced, ventricular
    sensed, with PJCs at beats 2 and 6

■ ECG 14•62
Rate: Indeterminate
Rhythm: Irregular
P Waves: None
PR Interval: None
QRS: Wide—greater than 0.10 sec
Interpretation: Sinus pause (sinus arrest) deteriorat-
    ing into ventricular tachycardia

■ ECG 14•63
Rate: 46 bpm
Rhythm: Regular
P Waves: None
PR Interval: None
QRS: 0.08 sec
Interpretation: Junctional rhythm with ST segment
    depression

■ ECG 14•64
Rate: Atrial 65 bpm, ventricular 40 bpm (28 bpm in
    first three complexes)
Rhythm: Atrial regular, ventricular irregular
P Waves: Normal
PR Interval: Variable, not associated with QRS
    complexes
QRS: 0.18 sec
Interpretation: Third-degree AV block

■ ECG 14•65
Rate: None; atrial 68 bpm
Rhythm: None
P Waves: Present and regular
PR Interval: None
QRS: None
Interpretation: Ventricular asystole

■ ECG 14•66
Rate: Indeterminate
Rhythm: Chaotic
P Waves: None
PR Interval: None
QRS: None
Interpretation: Ventricular fibrillation—coarse chang-
    ing to fine fibrillatory waves

■ ECG 14•67
Rate: 40 bpm
Rhythm: Regular
P Waves: Normal
PR Interval: 0.52 sec
QRS: 0.10 sec
Interpretation: Sinus bradycardia with first-degree
    AV block

ECG 14•68
Rate: Atrial 75 bpm, ventricular 48 bpm
Rhythm: Atrial regular, ventricular regular
P Waves: Variable (some upright, buried in QRS or in T wave)
PR Interval: Variable, not associated with QRS complexes
QRS: 0.12 sec
Interpretation: Third-degree AV block

ECG 14•69
Rate: 130 bpm; 110 bpm in underlying rhythm
Rhythm: Irregular
P Waves: Normal in first three beats and in beats 9 to 13; different in beat 4 and not visible in beats 5 to 8
PR Interval: 0.12 sec in first three beats and in beats 9 to 13; 0.08 sec in beat 4
QRS: 0.08 sec
Interpretation: Sinus tachycardia with ST segment depression and inverted T waves with a PAC in beat 4 and a short run of supraventricular tachycardia in beats 5 to 8

ECG 14•70
Rate: 50 bpm
Rhythm: Regular
P Waves: Normal
PR Interval: 0.16 sec
QRS: 0.12 sec
Interpretation: Second-degree AV block type II with 3:1 block and a bundle branch block

ECG 14•71
Rate: Indeterminate
Rhythm: Chaotic
P Waves: None
PR Interval: None
QRS: None
Interpretation: Ventricular fibrillation—fine fibrillatory waves

ECG 14•72
Rate: 63 bpm
Rhythm: Regular
P Waves: Normal
PR Interval: 0.20 sec
QRS: 0.16 sec with notched appearance
Interpretation: Normal sinus rhythm with a bundle branch block

ECG 14•73
Rate: 100 bpm
Rhythm: Irregular
P Waves: None
PR Interval: None
QRS: 0.16 sec following pacemaker spike and in intrinsic beats
Interpretation: Pacemaker—ventricular, with a pseudo-fusion beat in beat 3 and wide intrinsic complexes in beats 4 and 5

ECG 14•74
Rate: 80 bpm
Rhythm: Irregular
P Waves: Normal except for PJCs
PR Interval: 0.16 sec
QRS: 0.10 sec
Interpretation: Normal sinus rhythm with ST segment depression, inverted T waves, and bigeminal PJCs

ECG 14•75
Rate: 20 bpm
Rhythm: Irregular
P Waves: None
PR Interval: None
QRS: Wide—greater than 0.10 sec
Interpretation: Idioventricular rhythm (agonal rhythm)

Case Studies

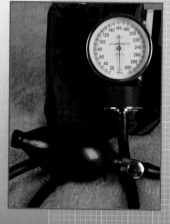

Chapter 15

ECG Case Studies One

To illustrate medical standards, the following case studies are based on the medical protocols (guidelines and medications) presented in Appendices A through D. Choose the most appropriate answer to each question according to the case scenario. All of the ECG strips were recorded in lead II.

CASE STUDY ONE

A 70-year-old woman was admitted to the hospital 2 days ago and underwent a right total hip replacement. The patient has a history of hypertension, degenerative joint disease, arthritis, pulmonary embolism, and coronary artery disease. She just finished a physical therapy session and has been resting in her hospital room. When you walk into the room to check your patient, you notice that she is unresponsive with no respiration or pulse. You immediately call a code and begin cardiopulmonary resuscitation (CPR). When the emergency team arrives, the patient is attached to the ECG monitor, which displays the rhythm shown in ECG 15–1.

ECG 15•1

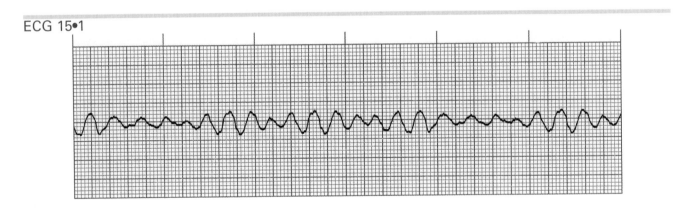

1. The interpretation of ECG 15–1 is
   A. Ventricular fibrillation.
   B. Ventricular tachycardia.
   C. Accelerated idioventricular.
   D. Asystole.

2. Your initial treatment of the patient is to
   A. Administer 300 mg of amiodarone.
   B. Defibrillate at 360 J (or equivalent biphasic energy).

   C. Consider 1 mg of atropine.
   D. Administer synchronized cardioversion at 360 J.

3. Following the appropriate treatment in question 2, ECG 15–2 now shows on the monitor as
   A. Ventricular tachycardia.
   B. Atrial tachycardia.
   C. Ventricular fibrillation.
   D. Atrial fibrillation.

ECG 15•2

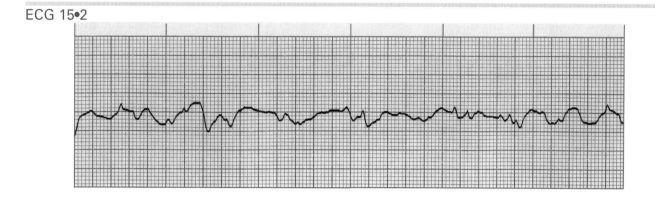

4. Your next appropriate treatment of choice for this patient is to

   A. Provide five cycles (2 min) of CPR.
   B. Defibrillate at 360 J (or equivalent biphasic energy).
   C. Consider 1–2 g of magnesium sulfate.
   D. Defibrillate at 200 J (or equivalent biphasic energy).

5. Following the appropriate treatment in question 4, ECG 15–3 shows on the monitor as

   A. Torsade de pointes.
   B. Asystole.
   C. Ventricular fibrillation.
   D. Ventricular tachycardia.

ECG 15•3

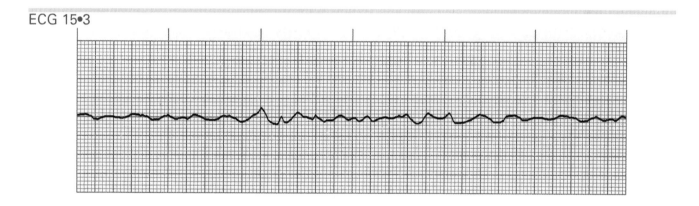

6. Your next appropriate treatment for this patient is to

   A. Defibrillate at 360 J (or equivalent biphasic energy).
   B. Administer epinephrine 1 mg (10 mL of 1:1000).
   C. Administer vasopressin 40 U.
   D. Either A or C.

7. Following the appropriate treatment in question 6, ECG 15–4 shows on the monitor as

   A. Atrial fibrillation.
   B. Ventricular fibrillation.
   C. Torsade de pointes.
   D. Ventricular tachycardia.

ECG 15•4

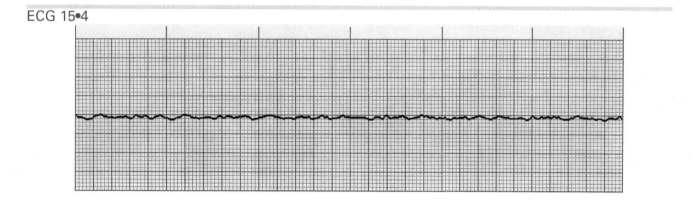

8. The patient is still pulseless with no respiration and has not responded to any treatments given so far. Now your most appropriate treatment choice is to administer

    A. Epinephrine 1 mg (10 mL of 1:10,000).
    B. Vasopressin 40 U.
    C. Epinephrine 1 mg (10 mL of 1:1000).
    D. Either A or B.

9. Following the appropriate treatment in question 8, there is no pulse. After 2 minutes of CPR you defibrillate at 360 J, the rhythm (ECG 15–5) shows on the monitor as

    A. Ventricular fibrillation converting to a sinus rhythm.
    B. Ventricular tachycardia converting to asystole.
    C. Torsade de pointes.
    D. Atrial tachycardia converting to a sinus rhythm.

ECG 15•5

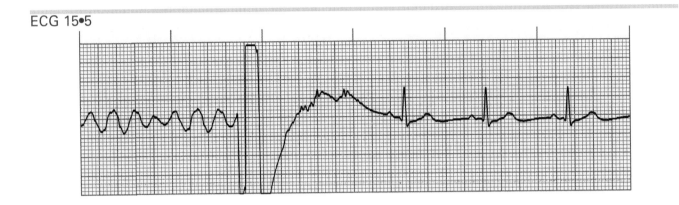

10. The patient is still not responsive but now has spontaneous respirations of 12 breaths per minute, a palpable carotid pulse, and a blood pressure (BP) of 100/70 mm Hg. Please identify the last rhythm in this case study that shows on the monitor (ECG 15–6):

    A. Sinus rhythm at 75 bpm.
    B. Atrial fibrillation at 70 bpm.
    C. Junctional tachycardia at 80 bpm.
    D. Sinus arrhythmia at 90 bpm.

ECG 15•6

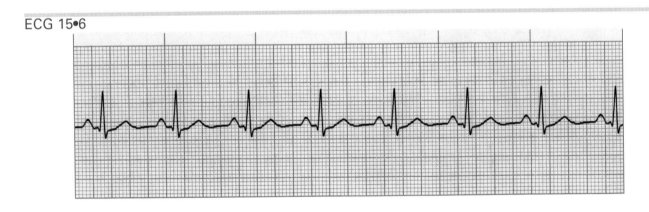

CASE STUDY TWO

You are at a public beach and suddenly notice an 8-year-old boy floating face down close to shore. At first you wonder if he is breathing through a snorkel, but you see no sign of either a snorkel or a mask. You become concerned for his safety because he is not lifting his head to breathe. You swim out about 10 feet and bring the boy back to the beach. You lay him on his back. There is no apparent trauma. You later find out that the boy, who is not a good swimmer, had ventured out dangerously far from shore.

1. What is your first plan of action?

    A. Turn the child on his side to expel any water he may have swallowed.
    B. Hit the child firmly between the shoulder blades to expel any water he may have swallowed.
    C. Check for responsiveness.
    D. Begin CPR.

2. After you perform the proper step in question 1, the boy is still not moving. The boy's parents are not around, but you see several bystanders. You

A. Send a bystander to summon help, phone 911, and get an automated external defibrillator (AED) if one is available.
B. Wait until the parents arrive before you do anything else.
C. Wait for the lifeguard, who is 10 minutes away.
D. Begin rescue breathing.

3. **You have already placed the boy supine on a flat surface and found him to be unresponsive. There are no signs of trauma or spinal injury. Your next step is to**

A. Open the airway by using the jaw thrust method.
B. Begin rescue breathing.
C. Check for a pulse.
D. Open the airway by using the head tilt–chin lift method.

4. **Following the correct procedure in question 3, your next step is to**

A. Begin chest compressions.
B. Begin rescue breathing.
C. Look, listen, and feel for adequate breathing.
D. Check for a pulse.

5. **Following the correct procedure in question 4, you find that the boy is not breathing. You**

A. Give one breath.
B. Give two breaths.
C. Check for a pulse.
D. Begin chest compressions.

6. **If the procedure in question 5 is successful, your next step is to**

A. Check for a carotid pulse.
B. Check for a pedal pulse.
C. Check for a radial pulse.
D. Check for a brachial pulse.

7. **After checking for a pulse you find none. You then begin chest compressions at a rate of**

A. 80 per minute.
B. 90 per minute.
C. 100 per minute.
D. 120 per minute.

8. **You compress the chest at**

A. 1.0–2.0 in.
B. 1.5–2.0 in.
C. One third the depth of the chest.
D. One third to one half the depth of the chest.

9. **The proper compression-to-ventilation ratio for a child with one rescuer performing CPR is**

A. 3:1.
B. 15:2.
C. 15:1.
D. 30:2.

10. **After the fifth cycle of CPR (2 min) you stop to recheck the pulse and look for any other signs of circulation. You find a pulse of 80 bpm but no respiratory rate. You then**

A. Continue rescue breathing at 10–12 breaths per minute.
B. Continue rescue breathing at 12–20 breaths per minute.
C. Continue rescue breathing at 24–30 breaths per minute.
D. None of the above.

11. **After another 4 minutes the ambulance arrives and the young boy is taken to the closest hospital. If the boy had started breathing at 16 breaths per minute with a pulse of 80 bpm before the ambulance arrived, what would have been your next step?**

A. Monitor breathing and circulation and place the child in the recovery position.
B. Leave for home.
C. Walk around and look for the boy's parents.
D. Continue CPR.

CASE STUDY THREE

An 82-year-old man arrives in the emergency department complaining of chest pain and palpitations. He has an altered level of conscious-ness, shortness of breath, and diaphoresis. There are no signs of trauma. He has a history of heart disease, hypertension, and diabetes. When the emergency team arrives, the patient is attached to the ECG monitor, which displays the rhythm shown in ECG 15–7.

ECG 15•7

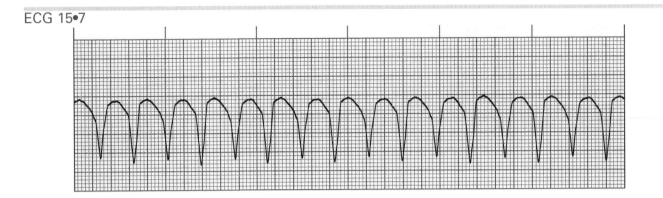

1. The interpretation of ECG 15–7 is

   A. Paroxysmal supraventricular tachycardia.
   B. Supraventricular tachycardia.
   C. Ventricular tachycardia.
   D. Atrial tachycardia.

2. Your initial assessment of the patient is to

   A. Defibrillate at 360 J (or equivalent biphasic energy).
   B. Administer 300 mg of amiodarone.
   C. Administer five cycles (2 min) of CPR.
   D. Consider and treat possible causes.

3. Following the appropriate assessment in question 2, ECG 15–8 shows on the monitor as

   A. Atrial fibrillation.
   B. Ventricular tachycardia.
   C. Sinus tachycardia.
   D. Supraventricular tachycardia.

ECG 15•8

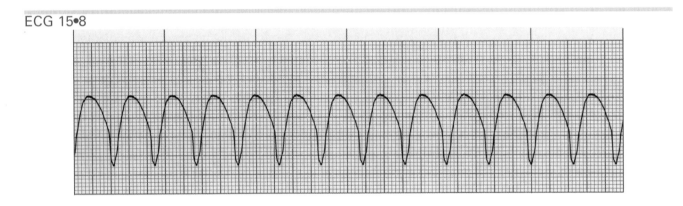

4. Your appropriate treatment choice for this patient is to

   A. Defibrillate at 360 J (or equivalent biphasic energy).
   B. Administer synchronized cardioversion at 100 J (or equivalent biphasic energy).
   C. Administer 1 mg of epinephrine.
   D. Administer 1 mg of atropine.

5. Following the appropriate treatment in question 4, the rhythm (ECG 15–9) shows on the monitor as

   A. Ventricular fibrillation.
   B. Supraventricular tachycardia.
   C. Ventricular tachycardia.
   D. Paroxysmal supraventricular tachycardia.

ECG 15•9

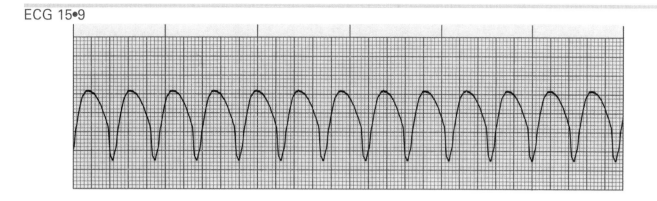

6. The patient's condition is still unstable. Your next appropriate treatment is to

   A. Administer synchronized cardioversion at 200 J (or equivalent biphasic energy).

   B. Administer 1–2 g of magnesium sulfate.

   C. Defibrillate at 360 J (or equivalent biphasic energy).

   D. Administer 1 mg of atropine.

7. Following the appropriate treatment in question 6, ECG 15–10 shows on the monitor as

   A. Ventricular fibrillation.

   B. Atrial fibrillation.

   C. Ventricular tachycardia.

   D. Sinus tachycardia.

ECG 15•10

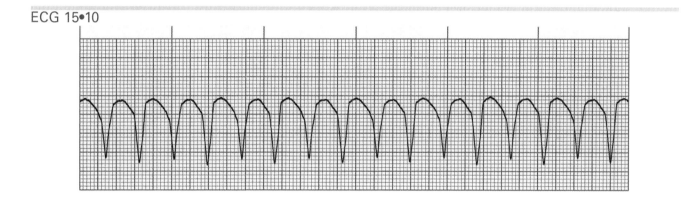

8. Your next most appropriate treatment choice would be to

   A. Administer synchronized cardioversion at 300 J (or equivalent biphasic energy).

   B. Administer synchronized cardioversion at 100 J (or equivalent biphasic energy).

   C. Administer synchronized cardioversion at 50 J (or equivalent biphasic energy).

   D. Defibrillate at 360 J (or equivalent biphasic energy).

9. Following the appropriate treatment in question 8, the rhythm (ECG 15–11) shows on the monitor as

   A. Ventricular tachycardia converting to a sinus rhythm.

   B. Ventricular tachycardia converting to agonal rhythm.

   C. Ventricular fibrillation converting to junctional rhythm.

   D. Paroxysmal supraventricular tachycardia.

ECG 15•11

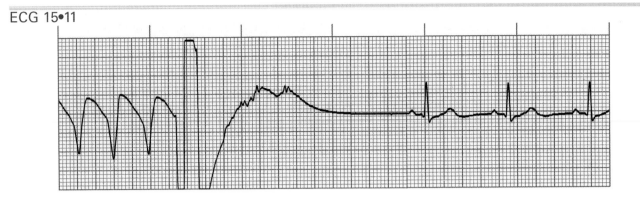

10. After about 30 minutes, the patient feels
calm and has respirations of 18 per minute,
a BP of 130/80 mm Hg, and a temperature
of 98.6° F. His rhythm (ECG 15–12) shows
on the monitor as

A. Sinus arrhythmia.
B. Sinus bradycardia.
C. Normal sinus rhythm.
D. Atrial flutter.

ECG 15•12

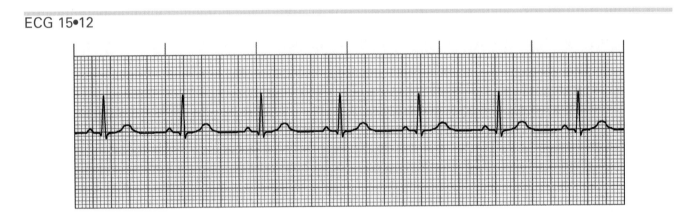

CASE STUDY FOUR

You and your Emergency Medical Services team are called to respond to an unconscious person. A 48-year-old woman has been found unresponsive, sitting in a living room chair. Her husband quickly phoned 911. When you arrive, you find him correctly administering one-person CPR to his wife. He has recently taken a CPR course at a local hospital. He tells you that his wife had an aortic valve replacement 8 months ago and has a history of hypertension. The woman remains pulseless. Once you attach the ECG monitor, ECG 15–13 shows

ECG 15•13

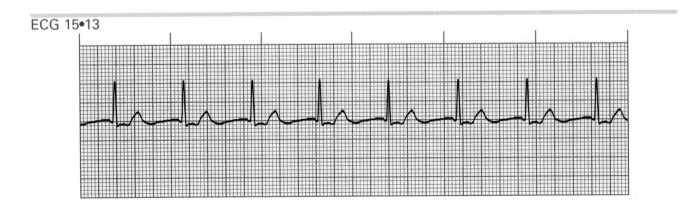

1. The interpretation of the rhythm in ECG 15–13 is

   A. Junctional tachycardia with pulseless electrical activity.
   B. Atrial tachycardia with pulseless electrical activity.
   C. Sinus tachycardia with pulseless electrical activity.
   D. Accelerated junctional rhythm with pulseless electrical activity.

2. Your initial treatment of the patient is to continue CPR and

   A. Defibrillate at 360 J (or equivalent biphasic energy).
   B. Consider and treat possible causes.
   C. Administer 300 mg of amiodarone.
   D. Administer 6 mg of adenosine.

3. Following the appropriate treatment in question 2, the patient still has no respiration or pulse and the monitor (ECG 15–14) shows

   A. Junctional tachycardia with pulseless electrical activity.
   B. Atrial tachycardia with pulseless electrical activity.
   C. Sinus tachycardia with pulseless electrical activity.
   D. Accelerated junctional rhythm with pulseless electrical activity.

ECG 15•14

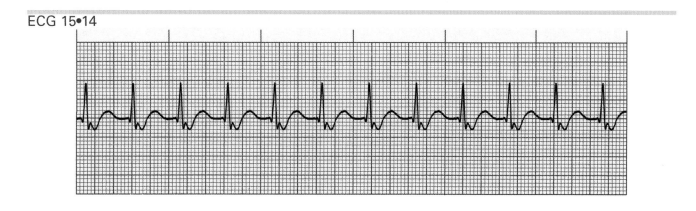

4. Your next appropriate treatment of choice is to administer

   A. Epinephrine 1 mg.
   B. Vasopressin 40 U.
   C. Vasopressin 50 U.
   D. Either A or B.

5. Following the appropriate treatment in question 4, the patient is still not breathing but does have a pulse. The monitor (ECG 15–15) shows

   A. Accelerated junctional rhythm.
   B. Atrial tachycardia.
   C. Sinus bradycardia.
   D. Junctional tachycardia.

ECG 15•15

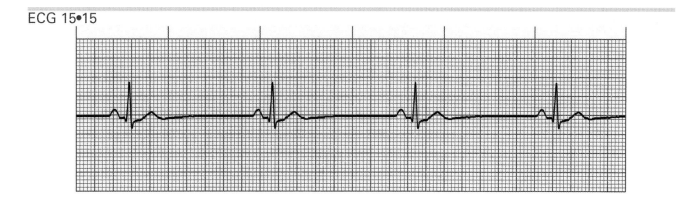

6. Your next appropriate treatment for this patient is to

   A. Administer 0.5 mg of atropine.
   B. Stop ventilating the patient.
   C. Begin chest compressions.
   D. Administer 6 mg of adenosine.

7. Following the correct treatment in question 6, the patient is now breathing on her own at

14 breaths per minute and has a BP of 110/70 mm Hg. The monitor displays the rhythm shown in ECG 15–16. The interpretation of this rhythm is

   A. Sinus tachycardia.
   B. Normal sinus rhythm.
   C. Junctional rhythm.
   D. Sinus bradycardia.

ECG 15•16

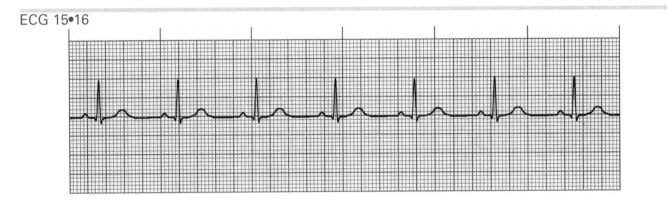

CASE STUDY FIVE

You are staffing the medical area for a 5 K marathon in your city. The ambient temperature is 81° F and the relative humidity is 46%. One of the runners, a 32-year-old man, crosses the finish line, walks over to the medical area, and asks for your help. He is sweating profusely and says he just needs to sit down and rest. He complains of some slight cramping in his legs. He says he drank water along the course. He indicates that he has no past medical problems and is not taking any medication. He has participated in marathons before. He appears to be of average height and weight and says he runs about 10 miles a day. You take his vital signs and find a temperature of 98.8° F, respirations of 20 per minute, and a BP of 118/60 mm Hg. The monitor shows the rhythm in ECG 15–17.

ECG 15•17

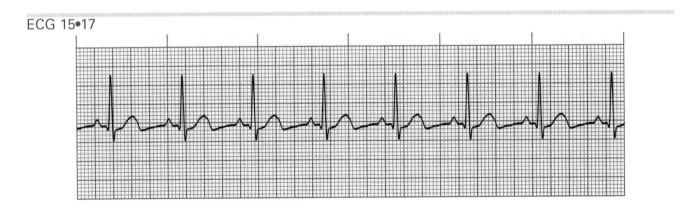

1. The interpretation of ECG 15–17 is

   A. Junctional rhythm.
   B. Normal sinus rhythm.
   C. Sinus bradycardia.
   D. Sinus tachycardia.

2. Your initial assessment of the man's vital signs and ECG indicate that they are

   A. Abnormal.
   B. Within normal limits.
   C. Outside normal limits.
   D. None of the above.

3. Your initial treatment of the man would be to

   A. Offer him water or a sports drink.
   B. Let him leave the medical area.

C. Call for an ambulance.

D. Administer 325 mg of aspirin.

4. After drinking fluids and lying down on a cot for about 30 minutes, the man has cooled off and is asking to go home. At this point he has a temperature of 98.5° F, respirations of 12 per minute, and a BP of 120/70 mm Hg. The rhythm (ECG 15–18) shows on the monitor as

A. Sinus tachycardia.

B. Normal sinus rhythm.

C. Sinus bradycardia.

D. Sinus arrhythmia.

ECG 15•18

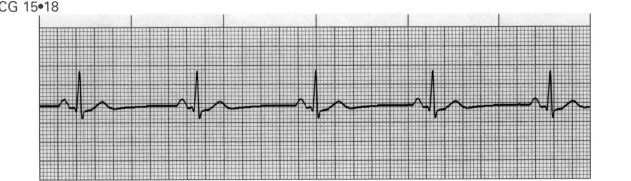

5. If the man refuses to go to the hospital your next appropriate management is to

A. Let him run the race again.

B. Administer 325 mg of aspirin.

C. Obtain a signed medical release.

D. Call the police and restrain the patient.

Answers to
CASE STUDY ONE

1. The correct answer is A.

Chaotic electrical activity occurs with no ventricular depolarization or contraction.

2. The correct answer is B.

Once the defibrillator is available, use it without delay. Defibrillate at a monophasic energy level of 360 J (or, if using a biphasic manual defibrillator, use the manufacturer's device-specific energy levels, usually 120–200 J).

3. The correct answer is C.

The rhythm is still chaotic with no organized activity.

4. The correct answer is A.

Once defibrillation is complete, CPR should resume immediately.

5. The correct answer is C.

The rhythm is still chaotic with no organized activity.

6. The correct answer is A.

Because the patient still has a shockable rhythm, defibrillate at a monophasic energy level of 360 J (or,

if using a biphasic manual defibrillator, use the manufacturer's device-specific energy levels, usually 120–200 J).

7. The correct answer is B.

The rhythm is still chaotic with no organized activity.

8. The correct answer is D.

Administer epinephrine 1 mg (10 mL of 1:10,000) by the intravenous or intraosseous (IV/IO) method; follow with 20 mL IV flush. Repeat every 3–5 minutes; give 2.0–2.5 mg diluted in 10 mL normal saline if administering by endotracheal (ET) tube; or administer a single dose of vasopressin 40 U IV/IO to replace the first or second dose of epinephrine.

9. The correct answer is A.

Your treatment choice of defibrillation converted the chaotic electrical activity into an organized rhythm.

10. The correct answer is A.

Although the patient's ECG is normal and her heart rate has stabilized, she is still not responsive and will need to undergo tests and be medically managed for her health issues.

Answers to
CASE STUDY TWO

1. The correct answer is C.

Once the child is out of the water, gently tap his shoulder, and ask, "Are you OK?" Checking for responsiveness is the first step in CPR.

2. The correct answer is A.

The bystanders can activate the EMS system while you begin immediate steps for CPR. Because the child is a victim of asphyxial arrest (e.g., drowning) if you had been alone you would have given five cycles (2 min) of CPR before you called for help.

3. The correct answer is D.

Because there is no evidence of trauma or spinal injury, the easiest way to open the airway is by using the head tilt–chin lift method.

4. The correct answer is C.

Once you have opened the airway, it is important to look for the chest to rise, listen for any breath sounds, and feel for any airflow from the child's nose or mouth. You should take no more than 10 seconds to do this.

5. The correct answer is B.

At this point in the CPR algorithm you would give two breaths, allowing 1 second for each breath.

6. The correct answer is A.

In a child (1 yr to adolescent [12–14 yr]) you would check for a carotid pulse because the carotid artery is usually the strongest pulse point. You would check for a brachial pulse in an infant (younger than 1 yr).

7. The correct answer is C.

The compression rate is the speed of the compressions, not the actual number of compressions per minute. The compression rate in a child, if uninterrupted, would be 100 per minute.

8. The correct answer is D.

For a child you would compress at one third to one half the depth of the chest.

9. The correct answer is D.

The correct ratio for a child is 30:2 for one rescuer CPR. If two rescuers were involved the ratio would be 15:2.

10. The correct answer is B.

Your efforts have been successful at reestablishing a pulse. However, the child still needs respiratory support of 12–20 breaths per minute.

11. The correct answer is A.

If the child had regained adequate breathing and circulation, he should have been placed in the recovery position (on his side) and had his breathing and circulation monitored until help arrived.

Answers to CASE STUDY THREE

1. The correct answer is C.

The patient is showing signs and symptoms of this rapid heart rate.

2. The correct answer is D.

Always check for an underlying illness or condition such as trauma, tension pneumothorax, thrombosis (pulmonary or coronary), tamponade (cardiac), toxins, hypo- or hyperkalemia, hypovolemia, hypoxia, hypoglycemia, hypothermia, or hydrogen ion (acidosis). Correcting or managing one of these issues may help with the treatment.

3. The correct answer is B.

Because this form of VT has a regular rhythm and the complexes are formed similarly, it is called monomorphic ventricular tachycardia.

4. The correct answer is B.

Because the patient is unstable and obviously symptomatic, electrical cardioversion starting at 100 J is the treatment of choice.

5. The correct answer is C.

The patient's condition is still unstable and the ECG shows VT.

6. The correct answer is A.

Since the initial synchronized cardioversion of 100 J had no effect the next synchronized electrical charge would be 200 J.

7. The correct answer is C.

The patient is still unstable and the ECG continues to show ventricular tachycardia.

8. The correct answer is A.

The correct sequence of synchronized electrical cardioversion is 100 J, 200 J, 300 J, and 360 J.

9. The correct answer is A.

The ECG shows that the last cardioversion of 300 J converted the patient's rhythm from VT to a sinus rhythm.

10. The correct answer is C.

The electrical cardioversion finally stabilized the patient's rhythm. He will now undergo tests and be medically managed for his health issues.

Answers to
CASE STUDY FOUR

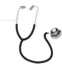

1. The correct answer is D.

The monitor shows an identifiable electrical rhythm, in this case accelerated junctional rhythm; however, no pulse is detectable. Therefore this arrhythmia is described as PEA.

2. The correct answer is B.

Always check for an underlying illness or disease such as trauma, tension pneumothorax, thrombosis (pulmonary or coronary), tamponade (cardiac), toxins, hypo- or hyperkalemia, hypovolemia, hypoxia, hypoglycemia, hypothermia, or hydrogen ion (acidosis). Correcting or managing one of these issues may help with the treatment.

3. The correct answer is A.

The ECG still shows a junctional rhythm with no pulse, but the heart rate is faster. The arrhythmia is still PEA.

4. The correct answer is D.

You can elect to use either epinephrine or vasopressin as your first vasopressor. Remember that if you begin with vasopressin it can be used only as a single dose. After that you must use epinephrine every 3–5 minutes.

5. The correct answer is C.

Sinus bradycardia is a sinus rhythm with a rate of less than 60 bpm.

6. The correct answer is A.

Consider atropine 0.5 mg IV if the heart rate is less than 60 bpm with a pulse.

7. The correct answer is B.

This is a normal sinus rhythm with a rate of 75 bpm. Although the patient's ECG is normal and her heart rate has returned, she will need to undergo tests and be medically managed for her health issues.

Answers to
CASE STUDY FIVE

1. The correct answer is B.

Regular exercise improves the heart's ability to pump blood efficiently. Drinking water during the race has kept the runner from having serious signs and symptoms from dehydration. Therefore, his heart rate has remained normal.

2. The correct answer is B.

All vital signs and the ECG are within normal limits. The runner probably became somewhat dehydrated. In summer sports, it is not the heat, but the combination of heat and humidity, that can cause potential heat-related problems.

3. The correct answer is A.

Water and light sports drinks will help the man avoid potentially dangerous dehydration. They should also be offered along the racecourse and be consumed regularly.

4. The correct answer is C.

The man has a strong pulse with good vital signs, and sinus bradycardia shows on the monitor. The man states that his heart rate normally ranges between 50 and 58 bpm.

5. The correct answer is C.

In most cases, bradycardia in healthy, well-trained athletes does not need to be treated. Once the patient has rested and is feeling back to normal, he does not need further care. It is, however, imperative to have him sign a medical release before he leaves the medical area.

Chapter 16

ECG Case Studies Two

To illustrate medical standards, the following case studies are based on the medical protocols (guidelines and medications) presented in Appendices A through D. Choose the most appropriate answer to each question according to the case scenario. All of the ECG strips were recorded in lead II.

CASE STUDY ONE

As a healthcare provider you are attending a workshop, required of all employees at your hospital, concerning workplace safety issues. During a short food break you notice that one of your coworkers, a 55-year-old man, is coughing. As you walk toward your coworker you notice that he is unable to speak and is making high-pitched crowing sounds. He has a panicked look on his face and is grabbing his throat with both hands.

1. **What is your first plan of action?**

   A. Find the instructor in charge of the workshop.
   B. Hit the man firmly between the shoulder blades.
   C. Ask, "Are you choking? Can you speak?"
   D. Perform a finger sweep.

2. **After performing the correct skill in question 1 you next**

   A. Perform a finger sweep.
   B. Stand behind the man, wrapping your hands around his waist, and firmly perform abdominal thrusts.
   C. Strike him between the shoulder blades five times.
   D. Ask him to try to cough up the obstructed object.

3. **Following the correct procedure in question 2, the airway still is obstructed and**
   your coworker suddenly slumps slowly to the floor. You first

   A. Establish unresponsiveness.
   B. Find the instructor in charge of the workshop.
   C. Perform a finger sweep.
   D. Check for a carotid pulse.

4. **After you have performed the correct procedure in question 3, you find that the man has lost consciousness. Your next step is to**

   A. Open the airway, then look, listen, and feel for breathing.
   B. Check for a pulse and then open the airway.
   C. Begin chest compressions.
   D. Begin rescue breathing.

5. **After you open the man's airway you notice a chunk of cookie at the back of his pharynx. You then**

   A. Begin rescue breathing.
   B. Begin chest compressions.
   C. Check for a pulse.
   D. Perform a finger sweep.

6. **After you successfully complete the correct step in question 5, the man coughs, begins breathing normally, and is responsive. You**

   A. Let him leave the facility and go home.
   B. Have him drink a glass of water.
   C. Call for help and ask him to stay calm.
   D. Ask him if he wants another cookie.

CASE STUDY TWO

A 65-year-old man arrives in the Emergency Department with heart palpitations. His BP is 148/84 mm Hg, his respirations are 18 per minute, his temperature is 98.6° F, and his heart rate is fast (ECG 16–1). He says he feels as though his heart were racing. He had a similar episode during the past year and says that, by using the Valsalva manueuver (bearing down), he was able to slow his heart rate on his own. However, that manueuver has not worked this time.

He is not taking any medications and has no prior medical history other than degenerative joint disease requiring a right total knee replacement 2 years ago. Once the emergency team arrives, the patient is attached to the ECG monitor (see ECG 16–1).

ECG 16•1

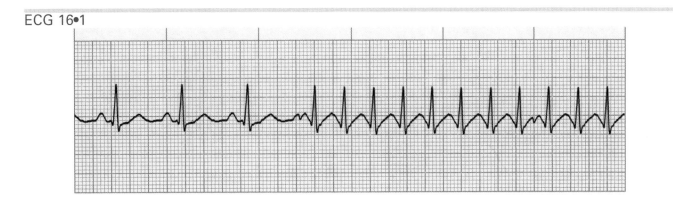

1. The interpretation of ECG 16–1 is

   A. Paroxysmal supraventricular tachycardia.
   B. Supraventricular tachycardia.
   C. Ventricular tachycardia.
   D. Atrial tachycardia.

2. Your initial treatment for this patient is to

   A. Defibrillate at 360 J (or equivalent biphasic energy).
   B. Administer 300 mg of amiodarone.
   C. Administer 5 cycles (2 min) of CPR.
   D. Supply oxygen, start an IV, and obtain a 12-lead ECG.

3. Following your treatment in question 2, you

   A. Consider and treat possible causes of the arrhythmia.
   B. Defibrillate at 360 J (or equivalent biphasic energy).
   C. Administer 300 mg of amiodarone.
   D. Administer 5 cycles (2 min) of CPR.

4. Following the appropriate assessment in question 3, the rhythm (ECG 16–2) shows on the monitor as

   A. Atrial fibrillation.
   B. Ventricular tachycardia.
   C. Sinus tachycardia.
   D. Supraventricular tachycardia.

ECG 16•2

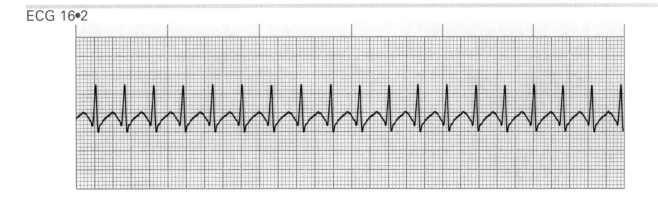

5. The patient's vital signs are still stable except for the fast heart rate. Your next appropriate treatment choice for this patient is to

   A. Defibrillate at 360 J (or equivalent biphasic energy).
   B. Administer 6.0 mg of adenosine.
   C. Administer 1.0 mg of epinephrine.
   D. Administer 1.0 mg of atropine.

6. Following the appropriate treatment in question 5, the rhythm (ECG 16–3) shows on the monitor as

   A. Ventricular fibrillation.
   B. Supraventricular tachycardia.
   C. Ventricular tachycardia.
   D. Paroxysmal supraventricular tachycardia.

ECG 16•3

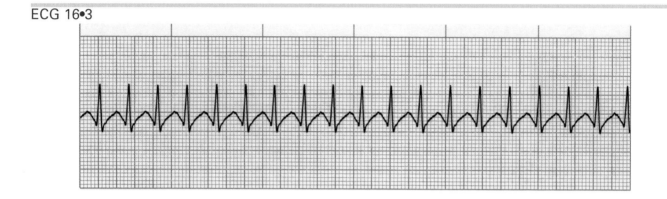

7. The patient is still responsive and stable, but after 1–2 minutes the rhythm in ECG 16–3 still shows on the monitor. Your next appropriate treatment for this patient is to

   A. Defibrillate at 360 J (or equivalent biphasic energy).
   B. Administer 1–2 g of magnesium sulfate.
   C. Administer 12 mg of adenosine.
   D. Administer 1 mg of atropine.

8. Following the appropriate treatment in question 7, the rhythm (ECG 16–4) shows on the monitor as

   A. Ventricular fibrillation.
   B. Atrial fibrillation.
   C. Supraventricular tachycardia.
   D. Sinus tachycardia.

ECG 16•4

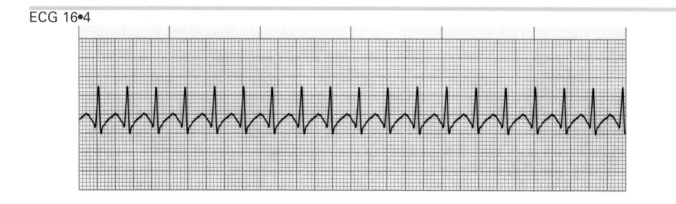

9. After another 2 minutes the rhythm in ECG 16–4 still shows up on the monitor. Now your most appropriate treatment choice is to

   A. Administer 12 mg of adenosine.
   B. Administer 6 mg of adenosine.
   C. Defibrillate at 200 J (or equivalent biphasic energy).
   D. Defibrillate at 360 J (or equivalent biphasic energy).

10. Following the appropriate treatment in question 9, the rhythm (ECG 16–5) shows on the monitor as

   A. Atrial fibrillation.
   B. Atrial tachycardia.
   C. Sinus tachycardia.
   D. Conversion to normal sinus rhythm.

ECG 16•5

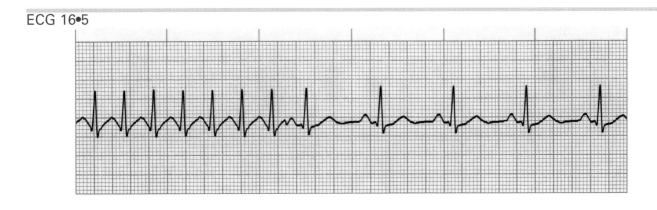

11. After about 30 minutes the patient feels calm and has a temperature of 98.6°F, respiration of 12 breaths per minute, and a BP of 130/80 mm Hg. His rhythm (ECG 16–6) shows on the monitor as

A. Sinus arrhythmia.
B. Sinus bradycardia.
C. Normal sinus rhythm.
D. Atrial flutter.

ECG 16•6

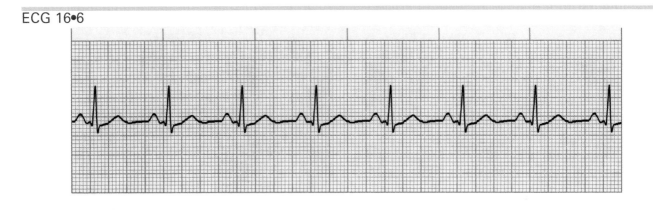

CASE STUDY THREE

As a paramedic in a rural community you arrive at the scene of an emergency, where an 80-year-old woman has been found lying in an alleyway. You establish that she has no respiration or pulse. No one at the scene knows how long she has been unresponsive. No trauma is visible and CPR was not initiated before your arrival. The weather is mild, with an ambient temperature of about 70° F. Once your Emergency Medical Services team begins CPR, you attach the ECG monitor and obtain the rhythm (ECG 16–7).

ECG 16•7

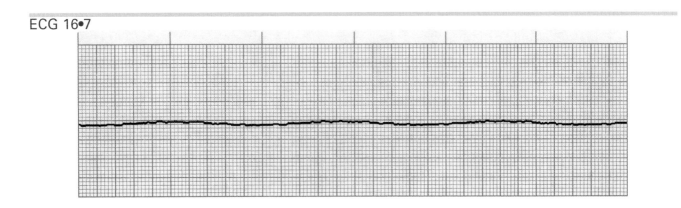

1. The interpretation of ECG 16–7 is

   A. Ventricular fibrillation.
   B. Asystole.
   C. Agonal rhythm.
   D. Third-degree block.

2. After initiating CPR you begin treatment by

   A. Administering 6 mg of adenosine.
   B. Considering and treating possible causes for the arrhythmia.
   C. Considering diltiazem or beta blockers.

   D. Defibrillating at 360 J (or equivalent biphasic energy).

3. Following the appropriate treatment in question 2, the rhythm (ECG 16–8) shows on the monitor as

   A. Atrial flutter.
   B. Ventricular tachycardia.
   C. Ventricular fibrillation.
   D. Asystole.

ECG 16•8

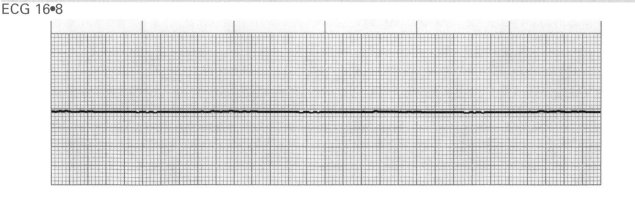

4. Your next appropriate treatment for this patient is to administer

   A. Amiodarone 300 mg.
   B. Epinephrine 1 mg or vasopressin 40 U.
   C. Magnesium sulfate 1–2 g.
   D. Amiodarone 150 mg.

5. Following the appropriate treatment in question 4, the rhythm (ECG 16–9) shows on the monitor as

   A. Asystole.
   B. Ventricular fibrillation.
   C. Ventricular tachycardia.
   D. Third-degree block.

ECG 16•9

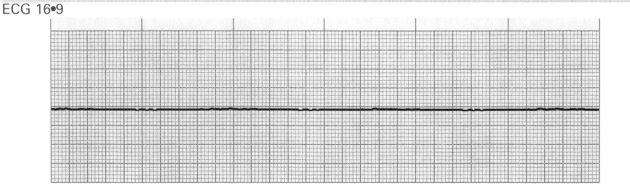

6. As your Emergency Medical Services team continues CPR your next appropriate treatment is to

   A. Administer 12 mg of adenosine.
   B. Defibrillate at 360 J (or equivalent biphasic energy).
   C. Administer 150 mg of amiodarone.
   D. Administer 1.0 mg of atropine.

7. Following the appropriate treatment in question 6, the rhythm (ECG 16–10) shows on the monitor as

   A. Ventricular fibrillation.
   B. Asystole.
   C. Atrial fibrillation.
   D. Agonal rhythm.

ECG 16•10

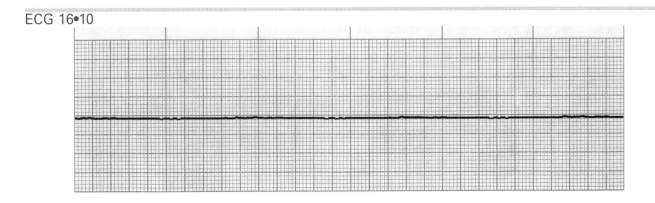

8. After 30 minutes of CPR and the right medications, the patient is still pulseless with no respiration. The next appropriate treatment choice is to

A. Continue CPR for 2 more hours.

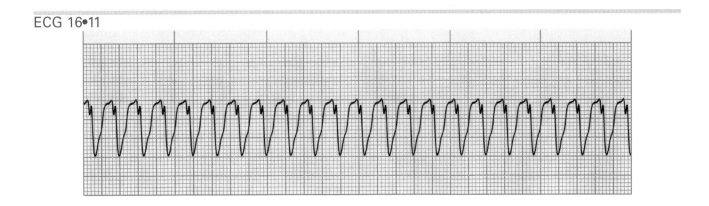

CASE STUDY FOUR

A 40-year-old female trauma patient is in a monitored room in the Intensive Care Unit of your hospital. You suddenly hear the ECG alarm go off and rush to the patient's room. You find her unre-

B. Defibrillate at 200 J (or equivalent biphasic energy).

C. Follow local policy to stop resuscitation efforts.

D. Defibrillate at 360 J (or equivalent biphasic energy).

sponsive, with no respirations and no pulse. You call a code and begin CPR. Once the code team arrives the patient, who is already attached to the ECG monitor, has the rhythm shown in ECG 16–11.

ECG 16•11

1. The interpretation of ECG 16–11 is

A. Ventricular fibrillation.
B. Agonal rhythm.
C. Ventricular tachycardia.
D. Asystole.

2. Your initial treatment of the patient is to

A. Defibrillate at 200 J (or equivalent biphasic energy).
B. Defibrillate at 360 J (or equivalent biphasic energy).

C. Defibrillate at 50 J (or equivalent biphasic energy).
D. Defibrillate at 100 J (or equivalent biphasic energy).

3. Following the appropriate treatment in question 2, ECG 16–12 now shows

A. Asystole.
B. Ventricular fibrillation.
C. Agonal rhythm.
D. Ventricular tachycardia.

ECG 16•12

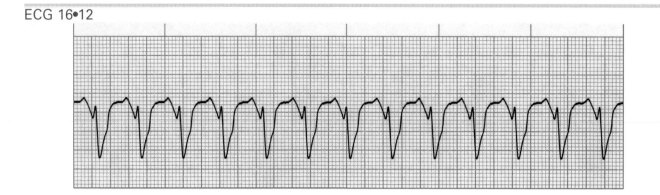

4. The patient is still unresponsive, is not breathing, and has no pulse. Your next appropriate treatment is to

A. Provide 5 cycles (2 min) of CPR.
B. Administer 1–3 g of magnesium sulfate.
C. Administer 150 mg of amiodarone.
D. Stop any further resuscitation efforts.

5. Following the appropriate treatment in question 4, ECG 16–13 shows

A. Ventricular fibrillation.
B. Ventricular tachycardia.
C. Asystole.
D. Atrial fibrillation.

ECG 16•13

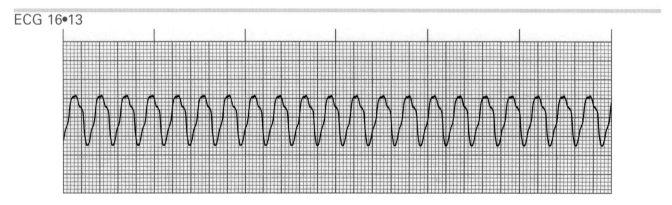

6. The patient is still unresponsive, with no respirations and no pulse. Your next appropriate treatment is to

A. Perform synchronized cardioversion at 100 J (or equivalent biphasic energy).
B. Perform synchronized cardioversion at 200 J (or equivalent biphasic energy).
C. Defibrillate at 360 J (or equivalent biphasic energy).
D. Stop any further resuscitation.

7. Following the appropriate treatment in question 6, ECG 16–14 shows

A. Ventricular tachycardia.
B. Torsade de pointes.
C. Ventricular fibrillation converting to a sinus rhythm.
D. Ventricular tachycardia converting to a sinus rhythm.

ECG 16•14

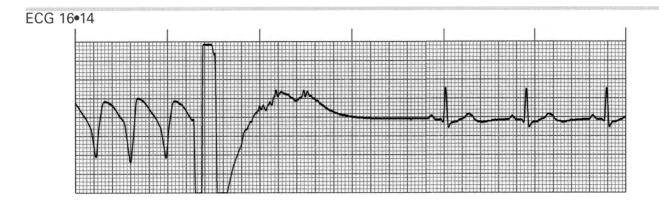

8. In about 15 minutes the patient begins breathing on her own at 12 breaths per minute. Her BP is 100/80 mm Hg and the rhythm in ECG 16–15 shows on the monitor. What is this rhythm?

A. Sinus rhythm at 60 bpm.
B. Sinus rhythm with PVCs at 70 bpm.
C. Sinus rhythm at 75 bpm.
D. Sinus rhythm with PVCs at 50 bpm.

ECG 16•15

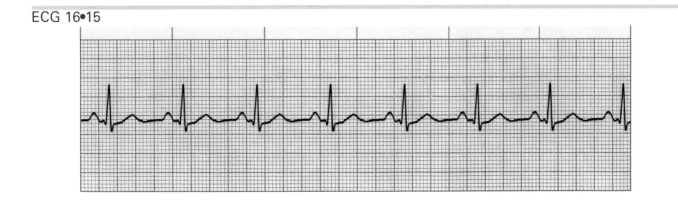

CASE STUDY FIVE

A 70-year-old woman arrives in the Emergency Department with a sudden onset of weakness, fatigue, and chest pain. She has a medical history of diabetes, hypertension, and osteoporosis. Her vital signs are: temperature 98.6°F, respiration 16 breaths per minute, BP 150/90 mm Hg, and heart rate 75 bpm. Once the patient is attached to the ECG monitor, the rhythm in ECG 16–16 is seen.

ECG 16•16

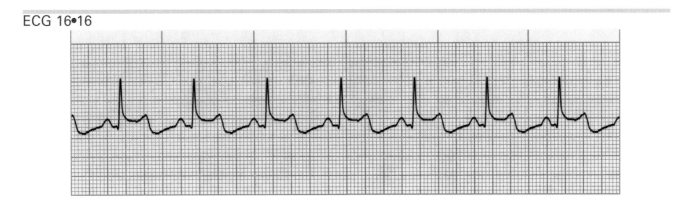

1. The interpretation of ECG 16–16 is

   A. Normal sinus rhythm.
   B. Sinus rhythm with depressed ST segment.
   C. Sinus rhythm with ST segment elevation.
   D. Junctional rhythm with ST segment elevation.

2. Your initial management of the patient is to

   A. Administer atropine 0.5 mg.
   B. Supply oxygen, start an IV, and obtain a 12-lead ECG.
   C. Begin CPR.
   D. Perform cardioversion at 100 J.

3. Your initial treatment of the patient would be to

   A. Perform cardioversion at 50 J.
   B. Begin CPR.
   C. Administer epinephrine 1 mg.
   D. Administer aspirin 160–325 mg.

4. Following the appropriate treatment in question 3, the rhythm (ECG 16–17) shows as

   A. Sinus rhythm with ST segment elevation.
   B. Normal sinus rhythm.
   C. Sinus rhythm with depressed ST segment.
   D. Junctional rhythm with ST segment elevation.

ECG 16•17

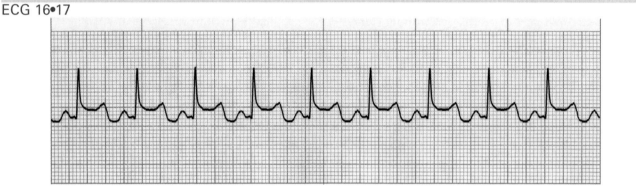

5. Your next treatment of choice for this patient is to administer

   A. Nitroglycerin by sublingual route 0.3–0.4 mg.
   B. Nitroglycerin aerosol spray for 0.5–1.0 sec.
   C. Aspirin 500 mg.
   D. Either A or B.

6. Following the appropriate treatment in question 4, the rhythm (ECG 16–18) shows as

   A. Normal sinus rhythm.
   B. Sinus rhythm with depressed ST segment.
   C. Sinus rhythm with ST segment elevation.
   D. Junctional rhythm with ST segment elevation.

ECG 16•18

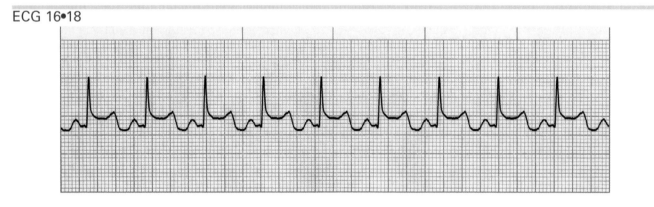

7. Your next appropriate treatment is to

   A. Administer epinephrine 1 mg.
   B. Begin the checklist for fibrinolytic therapy.
   C. Let the patient rest for an hour.
   D. Perform cardioversion at 100 J.

8. The patient is still complaining of chest pain and her BP is 110/60. Following the appropriate treatment in question 7, ECG 16–19 shows

   A. Sinus rhythm with ST segment elevation.
   B. Normal sinus rhythm.
   C. Sinus rhythm with depressed ST segment.
   D. Junctional rhythm with ST segment elevation.

ECG 16•19

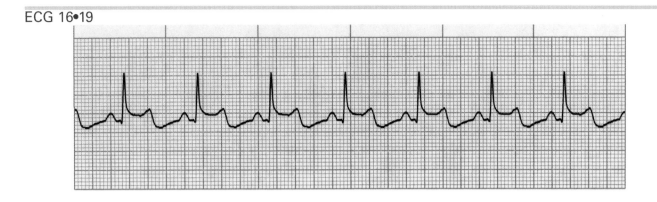

9. Your next most appropriate treatment choice would be to

    A. Administer aspirin 160–325 mg.

    B. Repeat nitroglycerin to a maximum of three doses.

    C. Administer atropine 1 mg.

    D. Administer epinephrine 1 mg.

CASE STUDY SIX

You are monitoring the medical treatment of a 58-year-old man in the Coronary Care Unit at your hospital. Three days ago the patient underwent a triple coronary artery bypass graft. He has a history of coronary artery disease, congestive heart failure, hypertension, and diabetes. You are at the nursing station and hear the patient's ECG monitor alarm go off. You rush to his bedside. He is conscious, but his mental status is altered and his BP is 80/50 mm Hg. You check the rhythm on his ECG monitor (ECG 16–20).

10. If the chest pain is still not relieved and the patient's systolic BP is above 90 mm Hg, your next treatment choice is to administer

    A. Aspirin 160–325 mg.

    B. Atropine 1 mg.

    C. Epinephrine 1 mg.

    D. Morphine 2–4 mg.

ECG 16•20

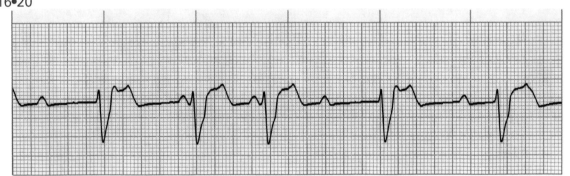

1. The interpretation of the rhythm in ECG 16–20 is

    A. Normal sinus rhythm.

    B. Sinus bradycardia.

    C. Third-degree AV block.

    D. Sinus pause (sinus arrest).

2. Your initial management of the patient is to

    A. Administer epinephrine 1 mg.

    B. Supply oxygen, start an IV, and obtain a 12-lead ECG.

    C. Begin CPR.

    D. Defibrillate at 360 J (or equivalent biphasic energy).

3. Your first drug treatment of choice would be to administer

    A. Epinephrine 5 mg.

    B. Atropine 0.5 mg.

    C. Adenosine 12 mg.

    D. Magnesium 1–2 g.

4. The patient is still conscious but symptomatic. Following the appropriate treatment in question 3, ECG 16–21 shows

    A. Sinus bradycardia.

    B. Third-degree AV block.

    C. Second-degree AV block, Type II.

    D. First-degree AV block.

ECG 16•21

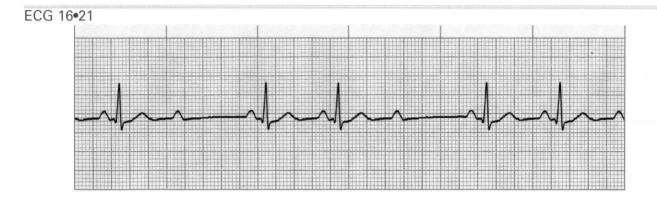

5. The patient's BP is now 90/60 mm Hg and he is still confused. Your last correct treatment in question 3 was given 4 minutes ago. Your next treatment of choice is to administer

A. Epinephrine 5 mg.
B. Atropine 0.5 mg.
C. Adenosine 12 mg.
D. Magnesium sulfate 1–2 g.

6. The patient now is alert, oriented, and able to follow commands. His BP is 140/90 mm Hg. Following the appropriate treatment in question 5, ECG 16–22 shows

A. Sinus bradycardia.
B. Sinus tachycardia.
C. Sinus rhythm at a rate of 75 bpm.
D. Sinus rhythm at a rate of 90 bpm.

ECG 16•22

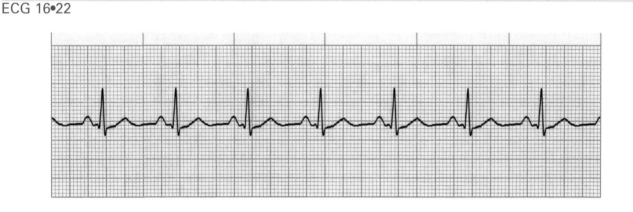

Answers to
CASE STUDY ONE

1. The correct answer is C.

When you see a person in respiratory distress displaying the universal sign for choking—one or two hands around the neck—ask, "Are you choking? Can you speak?"

2. The correct answer is B.

Stand behind the person and wrap your hands around his waist. Then make a fist with one hand. Place the thumb side of your fist in the middle of the abdomen just above the navel. Grasp your fist with your other hand. Press your fist abruptly into the abdomen using an upward, inward thrust. You have just performed the Heimlich maneuver.

3. The correct answer is A.

When a person slumps to the floor he may be losing consciousness. Before you begin any other step, establish whether the person is still responsive by gently tapping him and asking, "Are you OK?"

4. The correct answer is A.

Once you have established that the person is unresponsive, you need to open the airway and look, listen, and feel for breathing. Do not take longer than 10 seconds to perform this step.

5. The correct answer is D.

Each time the airway is opened, look for an object in the person's mouth. Only remove material you can see, in this case a piece of cookie, with a finger sweep.

Never perform a finger sweep if you do not see a foreign body in the airway.

6. The correct answer is C.

Once the foreign object is removed and the person is responsive and breathing normally, you should make sure medical help arrives and the patient is evaluated to rule out aspiration or other complications.

Answers to CASE STUDY TWO

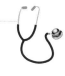

1. The correct answer is A.

The onset of PSVT in this case begins as a sinus rhythm then quickly escalates to a rapid SVT.

2. The correct answer is D.

It is important to give the patient oxygen and begin an IV to establish a route for medication administration. Obtaining a 12-lead ECG will identify any other irregularities in the patient's ECG.

3. The correct answer is A.

Always check for underlying illness or disease such as trauma, tension pneumothorax, thrombosis (pulmonary or coronary), tamponade (cardiac), toxins, hypo- or hyperkalemia, hypovolemia, hypoxia, hypoglycemia, hypothermia, or hydrogen ion (acidosis). Correcting or managing one of these issues may help with the treatment.

4. The correct answer is D.

This arrhythmia has such a fast rate that the P waves are not seen and are usually buried in the T waves.

5. The correct answer is B.

Because the patient is stable and the Valsalva maneuver was not successful, the next treatment choice would be 6 mg of adenosine IV given rapidly over 1–3 seconds followed by a 20-mL bolus of normal saline.

6. The correct answer is B.

The ECG still shows SVT.

7. The correct answer is C.

If within 1–2 minutes the SVT does not convert to a slower rate, administer 12 mg of adenosine IV given rapidly over 1–3 seconds followed by a 20-mL bolus of normal saline.

8. The correct answer is C.

The patient is still responsive but the ECG continues to show SVT.

9. The correct answer is A.

In another 1–2 minutes, if the rhythm has not converted, you may give a third dose of adenosine, 12 mg IV given rapidly over 1–3 seconds, followed by a 20-mL bolus of normal saline. You should not exceed a maximum total dose of 30 mg.

10. The correct answer is D.

The adenosine finally slowed and converted the rhythm to normal sinus rhythm.

11. The correct answer is C.

Although the patient's ECG is normal and his heart rate has stabilized, he will need to undergo tests and be medically managed for his health issues.

Answers to CASE STUDY THREE

1. The correct answer is B.

The electrical activity in the heart is completely absent.

2. The correct answer is B.

In asystole it is extremely important to check for underlying illness or disease such as trauma, tension pneumothorax, thrombosis (pulmonary or coronary), tamponade (cardiac), toxins, hypo- or hyperkalemia, hypovolemia, hypoxia, hypoglycemia, hypothermia, or hydrogen ion (acidosis). Correcting or managing one of these issues may help with the treatment.

3. The correct answer is D.

There is no change in the ECG.

4. The correct answer is B.

You can elect to use either epinephrine or vasopressin as your first vasopressor. Remember that if you begin with vasopressin it can be used only as a single dose. After that you must use epinephrine every 3–5 minutes.

5. The correct answer is A.

There is still no change in the ECG.

6. The correct answer is D.

Even with CPR and emergency medications, the time is running out for this patient. Because the rhythm still shows asystole, you should give 1 mg of atropine, repeating every 3–5 minutes as needed to a total dose of no more than 3 mg.

7. The correct answer is B.

If CPR had been started by a bystander and 911 called immediately, the outcome for this patient might have been extremely different. Unfortunately the ECG still shows asystole.

8. The correct answer is C.

All localities have different policies to terminate resuscitation efforts. Make sure you know your local protocols. To follow up on the case, you talk to your medical director the next day. She tells you that the autopsy report showed a ruptured aortic aneurysm. The patient had died suddenly even before you began resuscitative efforts.

Answers to

CASE STUDY FOUR

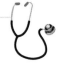

1. The correct answer is C.

It is important in VT to confirm the presence or absence of pulses because ventricular tachycardia may be perfusing or nonperfusing.

2. The correct answer is B.

Do not delay defibrillation. Defibrillate at a monophasic energy level of 360 J. If using a biphasic manual defibrillator, use the manufacturer's device-specific energy levels, usually 120–200 J.

3. The correct answer is D.

The ventricular rate has decreased.

4. The correct answer is A.

Between each defibrillation, it is important to provide 5 cycles (2 min) of CPR.

5. The correct answer is B.

The ventricular rate has increased.

6. The correct answer is C.

If the rhythm is still shockable, defibrillate at a monophasic energy level of 360 J. If using a biphasic manual defibrillator, use the manufacturer's device-specific energy levels, usually 120–200 J.

7. The correct answer is D.

The last defibrillation converted the patient's rhythm to a sinus rhythm.

8. The correct answer is C.

This is a normal sinus rhythm with a rate of 75 bpm. Although the patient's ECG is normal and her heart rate has stabilized, she will need to undergo tests and be medically managed for her health issues.

Answers to

CASE STUDY FIVE

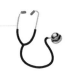

1. The correct answer is C.

ST segment elevation is significant for myocardial injury and must be managed immediately.

2. The correct answer is B.

Oxygen is essential for the heart to survive, an IV allows immediate administration of medications, and a 12-lead ECG is essential in diagnosing an acute MI.

3. The correct answer is D.

Aspirin is the first choice for a patient with the initial signs of acute coronary syndrome. It must be given within minutes of the onset of signs and symptoms.

4. The correct answer is A.

Although the rate may be a little faster, there is still no change in the ECG.

5. The correct answer is D.

Nitroglycerin can be given by either an aerosol or a sublingual route.

6. The correct answer is C.

There is still no change in the ECG.

7. The correct answer is B.

The key to successful fibrinolysis is to start early.

8. The correct answer is A.

There is still no change in the ECG.

9. The correct answer is B.

Nitroglycerin administration requires a systolic blood pressure greater than 90 mm Hg.

10. The correct answer is D.

Administer morphine 2–4 mg (over 1–5 min) every 5–30 minutes until the chest pain is relieved or the patient's blood pressure falls below 90 mm Hg.

Answers to

CASE STUDY SIX

1. The correct answer is C.

Notice that the P waves are not associated with the QRS complexes.

2. The correct answer is B.

Oxygen is critical, an IV will allow immediate administration of medications, and a 12-lead ECG is essential in diagnosing an acute MI.

3. The correct answer is B.

While awaiting a pacemaker, consider atropine 0.5 mg IV every 3–5 minutes (maximum dose not to exceed 3 mg).

4. The correct answer is C.

Notice that the rhythm has changed from a third-degree AV block to a second-degree AV block Type II.

5. The correct answer is B.

Atropine appears to have stabilized the patient's condition, eliminating the need for a transcutaneous pacemaker.

6. The correct answer is C.

Although the patient's ECG is normal and his heart rate has stabilized, he will need to undergo tests and be medically managed for his health issues.

Healthcare Provider Guidelines for Cardiopulmonary Resuscitation (CPR)

CPR HEALTHCARE PROVIDER SKILL PERFORMANCE

CPR Method	Compression/ Ventilation Ratio	Rate of Compressions (min)	Depth of Compressions	Pulse Check (artery)	Hand Position for Compressions
Adult, 1 rescuer	30:2	At least 100	2.0 in	Carotid	Heels of 2 hands over center of chest; lower half of sternum
Adult, 2 rescuers	30:2	At least 100	2.0 in	Carotid	Heels of 2 hands over center of chest; lower half of sternum
Child, 1 rescuer	30:2	At least 100	1/3 Depth of chest (about 2 in)	Carotid	Heel of 1 or 2 hands over center of chest; lower half of sternum
Child, 2 rescuers	15:2	At least 100	1/3 Depth of chest (about 2 in)	Carotid	Heel of 1 or 2 hands over center of chest; lower half of sternum
Infant, 1 rescuer	30:2	At least 100	1/3 Depth of chest (about 1½ in)	Brachial	2 Fingers over center of chest; lower half of sternum
Infant, 2 rescuers	15:2	At least 100	1/3 Depth of chest (about 1½ in)	Brachial	Two thumb-encircling hands technique over lower half of sternum
Newborn	3:1	At least 120	1/3 Depth of chest (about 1½ in)	Brachial	Two thumb-encircling hands technique over lower third of sternum

CPR: Adult (Age of puberty or older)

1. Ensure that the scene is safe. **Check for unresponsiveness.** Gently tap the person's shoulder. Ask, "Are you OK?"
2. **Check for breathing.** Is the breathing normal, no breathing, or abnormal (only agonal gasps)?
3. **In a sudden collapse, if there is no response with no breathing or abnormal breathing (only agonal gasps) and you are alone, summon help, call a code, or phone 911 and get an automated external defibrillator (AED), if available.** Send a second rescuer, if available, for help.
4. **Position the person supine** on a hard, flat surface.
5. **Assess the carotid pulse and look for other signs of circulation (no more than 10 sec).** If signs of circulation are present but the person is still not breathing, give rescue breaths at the rate of 10–12 breaths/min (one breath every 5–6 sec).

6. If a pulse and signs of circulation are not present, **begin chest compressions.** Place the heel of one hand on the center of the chest over the lower half of the breastbone; place the heel of your other hand over the first. **Firmly compress the chest at least 2.0 in. Push hard and fast. Give 30 compressions. Compress at a rate of at least 100/min. Ensure complete chest recoil after each compression.**

7. If the person is not breathing, **begin rescue breaths.** Open the airway by the head tilt-chin lift method or, if spinal injury is suspected, use the jaw thrust method, if possible.

8. Using a face mask or barrier device, **give 2 breaths (1 sec each) with sufficient volume to cause the chest to rise. Do not overventilate.** Note: If the chest does not rise, reposition the head, chin, and jaw, and give 2 more breaths. **If the chest still does not rise, follow instructions for unconscious adult with an obstructed airway.**

9. **Continue to give 30 compressions followed by 2 breaths.** After the fifth cycle of 30:2 (2 min), use the AED. Follow the instructions on how to use an AED in Appendix D: Emergency Medical Skills. If an AED is unavailable, continue to give 30 compressions followed by 2 breaths. After each fifth cycle of 30:2 (2 min), recheck the pulse and look for other signs of circulation (no more than 10 sec).

10. If circulation resumes but breathing does not or is inadequate, continue rescue breathing at 10–12 breaths/min.

11. If adequate breathing and circulation resume, place the person in the recovery position and monitor until help arrives.

 Clinical Tip:

Victims of asphyxial arrest (e.g., drowning, drug overdose, respiratory failure) should receive five cycles (2 min) of CPR before the lone rescuer calls for help (activates the EMS system).

Clinical Tip:

When two rescuers are available, give cycles of 30 compressions and 2 breaths for adult CPR. If available, a bag-valve-mask device can be used with two person CPR.

CPR: Child (1 yr to age of puberty)

1. Ensure that the scene is safe. **Check for unresponsiveness.** Gently tap child's shoulder. Ask, "Are you okay?"

2. **Check for breathing.** Is the breathing normal, no breathing, or abnormal (only agonal gasps)?

3. If **there is no response with no breathing or abnormal breathing (only agonal gasps)** send a second rescuer, if available, for help and to get an AED, if available.

4. If you are alone, begin the steps for CPR.

5. **Position the child supine** on a hard, flat surface.

6. **Assess the carotid pulse and look for other signs of circulation (no more than 10 sec).** If signs of circulation are present but the child is still not breathing, give rescue breaths at the rate of 12–20 breaths/min (one breath every 3–5 sec).

7. If a pulse and signs of circulation are not present, **begin chest compressions.** One hand: Place the heel of one hand on the center of the chest over the lower half of the breastbone. Two hands: Place the heel of one hand on the center of the chest over the lower half of the breast-bone; place the heel of your other hand over the first. **Firmly compress the chest at least one third the depth of the chest (at least 2.0 in). Push hard and fast. Give 30 compressions. Compress at a rate of at least 100/min. Ensure complete chest recoil after each compression.**

8. If the child is not breathing, **begin rescue breaths.** Open the airway by the head tilt-chin lift method or, if spinal injury is suspected, use the jaw thrust method, if possible.

9. Using a face mask or barrier device, **give 2 breaths (1 sec each) with sufficient volume to cause the chest to rise. Do not overventilate.** Note: If the chest does not rise, reposition the head, chin, and jaw, and give 2 more breaths. **If the chest still does not rise, follow instructions for unconscious child with an obstructed airway.**

10. **Continue cycles of 30 compressions followed by 2 breaths.** After the fifth cycle of 30:2 (2 min), if you are still alone and no signs of circulation are present, **summon help, call a code, or phone 911 and get an AED, if available.**

11. If circulation is still not present, continue CPR starting with chest compressions until an AED is available. Follow the instructions on how to use an AED in Appendix D: Emergency Medical Skills. If an AED is unavailable, continue to give 30 compressions followed by 2 breaths.

12. If circulation resumes but breathing does not or is inadequate, continue rescue breathing at 12–20 breaths/min.

13. If adequate breathing and circulation resume, place the child in the recovery position and monitor until help arrives.

13. If adequate breathing and circulation resume, place the child in the recovery position and monitor until help arrives.

♡ | *Clinical Tip:*

If you are alone and know a child or infant has had a **sudden collapse** due to heart failure, request immediate help including an AED. Do not delay defibrillation.

♡ | *Clinical Tip:*

When two rescuers are available, give cycles of 15 compressions and 2 breaths for child CPR.

CPR: Infant (Younger than 1 yr)

1. Ensure that the scene is safe. **Check for unresponsiveness.** Gently rub the infant's back or tap the feet.
2. **Check for breathing.** Is the breathing normal, no breathing, or abnormal (only agonal gasps)?
3. If **there is no response with no breathing or abnormal breathing (only agonal gasps)** send a second rescuer, if available, for help and an AED, if available.
4. If you are alone, begin the steps for CPR.
5. **Position the infant supine** on a hard, flat surface.
6. **Assess the brachial pulse and look for other signs of circulation (no more than 10 sec).** If signs of circulation are present but the infant is still not breathing, give rescue breaths at the rate of 12–20 breaths/min (one breath every 3–5 sec).
7. If a pulse and signs of circulation are not present, **begin chest compressions.** Place two fingers of one hand over the center of the chest just below the nipple line. **Firmly compress the chest at least one third the depth of the chest (at least 1.5 in). Push hard and fast. Give 30 compressions. Compress at a rate of at least 100/min. Ensure complete chest recoil after each compression.**
8. If the infant is not breathing, **begin rescue breaths.** Open the airway by the head tilt-chin lift method or, if spinal injury is suspected, use the jaw thrust method, if possible.
9. Using a face mask or barrier device, **give 2 breaths (1 sec each) with sufficient volume to cause the chest to rise. Do not overventilate.** Note: If the chest does not rise, reposition the head, chin, and jaw, and give

2 more breaths. **If the chest still does not rise, follow instructions for unconscious infant with an obstructed airway.**
10. **Continue to give 30 compressions followed by 2 breaths.** After the fifth cycle of 30:2 (2 min), if you are still alone and no signs of circulation are present, **summon help, call a code, or phone 911 and get an AED, if available.**
11. If circulation is still not present, continue CPR until the AED is available. Follow the instructions on how to use an AED in Appendix D: Emergency Medical Skills. If an AED is unavailable, continue to give 30 compressions followed by 2 breaths.
12. If circulation resumes but breathing does not or is inadequate, continue rescue breathing at 12–20 breaths/min.
13. If adequate breathing and circulation resume, place the infant in the recovery position and monitor until help arrives.

♡ | *Clinical Tip:*

When two rescuers are available, give cycles of 15 compressions and 2 breaths for infant CPR. Use the two thumb-encircling hands technique for chest compressions. If available, a bag-valve-mask device can be used with two person CPR.

OBSTRUCTED AIRWAY: Conscious Adult or Child (1 yr or older)

Signs and Symptoms

- Grabbing at the throat with one or both hands
- Inability to speak; high-pitched crowing sounds
- Wheezing, gagging, ineffective coughing
1. **Determine that the airway is obstructed.** Ask, "Are you choking? Can you speak?"
2. Let the person know you are going to help.
3. **Stand behind the choking person and wrap your arms around the person's waist.** For someone who is obese or pregnant, wrap your arms around the chest.
4. **Make a fist. Place the thumb side of your fist in the middle of the person's abdomen, just above the navel.** Locate the middle of the sternum for obese or pregnant persons.
5. Grasp your fist with your other hand.
6. **Press your fist abruptly into the person's abdomen using an upward, inward thrust.** Use a straight chest thrust back for someone who is obese or pregnant.
7. Continue abdominal or chest thrusts until the object is dislodged or the person loses consciousness.

7. Continue abdominal or chest thrusts until the object is dislodged or the person loses consciousness.

8. If the person loses consciousness, treat as an unconscious adult or a child with an obstructed airway.

8. **Continue the sequence of five back slaps and five chest thrusts until the object is dislodged or the infant loses consciousness.** If the infant loses consciousness, treat as an unconscious infant with an obstructed airway.

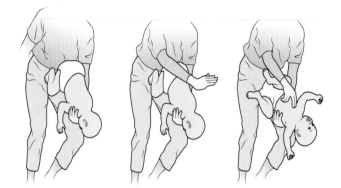

OBSTRUCTED AIRWAY: Unconscious Adult (Age of puberty or older)

Signs and Symptoms

- Failure to breathe, cyanosis
- Inability to move air into lungs with rescue breaths
  1. Ensure that the scene is safe. **Check for unresponsiveness.** Gently tap the person's shoulder. Ask, "Are you OK?"
  2. **Check for breathing.** Is the breathing normal, no breathing, or abnormal (only agonal gasps)?
  3. **In a sudden collapse, if there is no response with no breathing or abnormal breathing (only agonal gasps) and you are alone, summon help, call a code, or phone 911 and get an automated external defibrillator (AED), if available.** Send a second rescuer, if available, for help.
  4. **Position the person supine** on a hard, flat surface.
  5. **Assess the carotid pulse and look for other signs of circulation (no more than 10 sec).** If signs of circulation are present but the person is still not breathing, give rescue breaths at the rate of 10–12 breaths/min (one breath every 5–6 sec).
  6. If a pulse and signs of circulation are not present, **begin chest compressions.** Place the heel of one hand on the center of the chest over the lower half of the breastbone; place the heel of your other hand over the first. **Firmly compress the chest at least 2.0 in. Push hard and fast. Give 30 compressions. Compress at a rate of at least 100/min. Ensure complete chest recoil after each compression.**
  7. If the person is not breathing, **begin rescue breaths.** Open the airway by the head tilt-chin lift method or, if spinal injury is suspected, use the jaw thrust method, if possible.

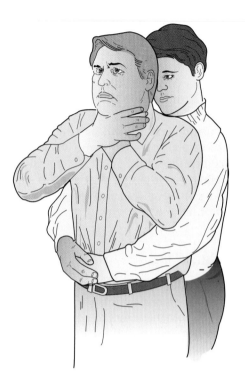

OBSTRUCTED AIRWAY: Conscious Infant (younger than 1 yr)

Signs and Symptoms

- Inability to breathe or cry
- High-pitched crowing sounds
- Sudden wheezing or noisy breathing
  1. **Determine that the airway is obstructed. Notice if air exchange is poor or does not occur.**
  2. Lay the infant down on your forearm, supporting the jaw between your thumb and index finger and the chest supported by your hand and forearm.
  3. Using your thigh or lap for support, keep the infant's head lower than the body.
  4. **Give five quick, forceful slaps between the shoulder blades** with the heel of your hand.
  5. Turn the infant over to be face up on your other arm. Using your thigh or lap for support, keep the infant's head lower than the body.
  6. Place two fingers of one hand over the center of the chest just below the nipple line.
  7. **Give five quick thrusts downward, depressing the chest by 1/3 (1.5 in) its depth** each time.

8. Using a face mask or barrier device, **give 2 breaths (1 sec each) with sufficient volume to cause the chest to rise. Do not overventilate.**

9. If the chest does not rise, reposition the head, chin, and jaw, and give 2 more breaths. **If the chest still does not rise,** each time the airway is opened, look for an object in the person's mouth. **Only use a finger sweep to remove material you see obstructing the airway. Never perform a finger sweep if you do not see a foreign body in the airway.**

10. **Continue to give 30 compressions followed by opening the airway, looking for an object, performing a finger sweep if object is visible, and attempt to give 2 breaths.** After the fifth cycle of 30:2 (2 min), **recheck the pulse** and look for other signs of circulation (no more than 10 sec). If circulation is not present, use the AED. Follow the instructions on how to use an AED in Appendix D: Emergency Medical Skills. If an AED is unavailable, continue to give 30 compressions followed by 2 breaths. After each fifth cycle of 30:2 (2 min), recheck the pulse and look for other signs of circulation (no more than 10 sec).

11. If circulation resumes but breathing does not or is inadequate, continue rescue breathing at 10–12 breaths/min.

12. If adequate breathing and circulation resume, place the person in the recovery position and monitor until help arrives.

♡ | *Clinical Tip:*

An airway obstruction is successfully removed if you see and remove the object or feel air movement and see the chest rise when you give breaths.

OBSTRUCTED AIRWAY: Unconscious Child (1 yr to age of puberty)

Signs and Symptoms

• Failure to breathe, cyanosis
• Inability to move air into lungs with rescue breaths

1. Ensure that the scene is safe. **Check for unresponsiveness.** Gently tap child's shoulder. Ask, "Are you okay?"

2. **Check for breathing.** Is the breathing normal, no breathing, or abnormal (only agonal gasps)?

3. If **there is no response with no breathing or abnormal breathing (only agonal gasps)** send a second rescuer, if available, for help and an AED, if available.

4. If you are alone, begin the steps for CPR.

5. **Position the child supine** on a hard, flat surface.

6. **Assess the carotid pulse and look for other signs of circulation (no more than 10 sec).** If signs of circulation are present but the child is still not breathing, give rescue breaths at the rate of 12–20 breaths/min (one breath every 3–5 sec).

7. If a pulse and signs of circulation are not present, **begin chest compressions.** One hand: Place the heel of one hand on the center of the chest over the lower half of the breastbone. Two hands: Place the heel of one hand on the center of the chest over the lower half of the breastbone; place the heel of your other hand over the first. **Firmly compress the chest at least one third the depth of the chest (at least 2.0 in). Push hard and fast. Give 30 compressions. Compress at a rate of at least 100/min. Ensure complete chest recoil after each compression.**

8. If the child is not breathing, **begin rescue breaths.** Open the airway by the head tilt-chin lift method or, if spinal injury is suspected, use the jaw thrust method, if possible.

9. Using a face mask or barrier device, **give 2 breaths (1 sec each) with sufficient volume to cause the chest to rise. Do not overventilate.**

10. **If the chest does not rise, reposition the head, chin, and jaw, and give two more breaths.** Each time the airway is opened, look for an object in the child's mouth. **Only use a finger sweep to remove material you see obstructing the airway. Never perform a finger sweep if you do not see a foreign body in the airway.**

11. **Continue to give 30 compressions followed by opening the airway, looking for an object, performing a finger sweep if object is visible, and attempt to give 2 breaths.** After the fifth cycle of 30:2 (2 min), **recheck the pulse** and look for other signs of circulation (no more than 10 sec). If you are still alone and no signs of circulation are present, **summon help, call a code, or phone 911 and get an AED, if available.**

12. If circulation is still not present, continue CPR until the AED is available. Follow the instructions on how to use an AED in Appendix D: Emergency Medical Skills. If an AED is unavailable, continue to give 30 compressions followed by 2 breaths. After each fifth cycle of 30:2 (2 min), recheck the pulse and look for other signs of circulation (no more than 10 sec).

13. If circulation resumes but breathing does not or is inadequate, continue rescue breathing at 12–20 breaths/min.

14. If adequate breathing and circulation resume, place the child in the recovery position and monitor until help arrives.

❤ *Clinical Tip:*

Never perform a blind finger sweep.

OBSTRUCTED AIRWAY: Unconscious Infant (younger than 1 yr)

- Inability to breathe, high-pitched noises
- Inability to move air into lungs with rescue breaths
- Cyanosis
  1. Ensure that the scene is safe. **Check for unresponsiveness.** Gently rub the infant's back or tap the feet.
  2. **Check for breathing.** Is the breathing normal, no breathing, or abnormal (only agonal gasps)?
  3. If **there is no response with no breathing or abnormal breathing (only agonal gasps)** send a second rescuer, if available, for help.
  4. If you are alone, begin the steps for CPR.
  5. **Position the infant supine** on a hard, flat surface.
  6. **Assess the brachial pulse and look for other signs of circulation (no more than 10 sec).** If signs of circulation are present but the infant is still not breathing, give rescue breaths at the rate of 12–20 breaths/min (one breath every 3–5 sec).
  7. If a pulse and signs of circulation are not present, **begin chest compressions.** Place two fingers of one hand over the center of the chest just below the nipple line. **Firmly compress the chest at least one third the depth of the chest (at least 1.5 in). Push hard and fast. Give 30 compressions. Compress at a rate of at least 100/min. Ensure complete chest recoil after each compression.**
  8. If the infant is not breathing, **begin rescue breaths.** Open the airway by the head tilt-chin lift method or, if spinal injury is suspected, use the jaw thrust method, if possible.
  9. Using a face mask or barrier device, **give 2 breaths (1 sec each) with sufficient volume to cause the chest to rise. Do not overventilate.**
  10. **If the chest does not rise, reposition the head, chin, and jaw, and give two more breaths.** Each time the airway is opened, look for an object in the infant's mouth. **Only use a finger sweep to remove material you see obstructing the airway. Never perform a finger sweep if you do not see a foreign body in the airway.**
  11. **Continue to give 30 compressions followed by opening the airway, looking for an object, performing a finger sweep if object is visible, and attempt to give 2 breaths.** After the fifth cycle of 30:2 (2 min), **recheck the pulse** and look for other signs of circulation (no more than 10 sec). If you are still alone and no signs of circulation

are present, **summon help, call a code, or phone 911 and get an AED, if available.**
  12. If circulation is still not present, continue CPR until the AED is available. Follow the instructions on how to use an AED in Appendix D: Emergency Medical Skills. If an AED is unavailable, continue to give 30 compressions followed by 2 breaths. After each fifth cycle of 30:2 (2 min), recheck the pulse and look for other signs of circulation (no more than 10 sec).
  13. If circulation resumes but breathing does not or is inadequate, continue rescue breathing at 12–20 breaths/min.
  14. If adequate breathing and circulation resume, place the infant in the recovery position and monitor until help arrives.

❤ *Clinical Tip:*

When you open an infant's airway by the head tilt–chin lift method, do not overextend the head or the airway will become obstructed.

CPR AND OBSTRUCTED AIRWAY POSITIONS

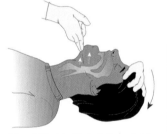
Head tilt-chin lift (adult or child).

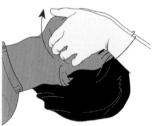
Jaw thrust maneuver.

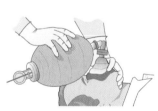
Bag-valve-mask.

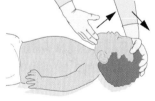
Head tilt-chin lift (infant).

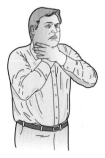
Universal choking sign.

Advanced Cardiac Life Support Protocols

VENTRICULAR FIBRILLATION (VF) OR PULSELESS VENTRICULAR TACHYCARDIA (VT)

Clinical Presentation

- Unresponsive state
- No respiration, pulse, or blood pressure (BP)
  1. Establish unresponsiveness with no respiration or pulse. Call for help.
  2. Begin CPR, provide oxygen and attach AED or monitor-defibrillator when available without interrupting CPR.
  3. When device is attached, stop CPR and assess rhythm. If shock is advised when using an AED, defibrillate following AED prompts. If using a manual monitor-defibrillator and rhythm is ventricular fibrillation or pulseless ventricular tachycardia, defibrillate at 120–200 J if using a biphasic defibrillator following manufacturer's device-specific energy levels if known, or 200 J if unknown, or defibrillate at 360 J if using a monophasic defibrillator.
  4. Immediately resume CPR, beginning with compressions. Provide five cycles (2 min) of uninterrupted CPR. During CPR, establish IV or IO access. Prepare vasopressor dose (epinephrine or vasopressin).
  5. Assess rhythm. If the rhythm is shockable, follow AED prompts or defibrillate at same or higher energy for biphasic manual defibrillator or at 360 J for a monophasic manual defibrillator.
  6. Immediately resume CPR beginning with compressions and using five cycles of 30 compressions and 2 breaths.
  7. Consider insertion of an advanced airway (ET tube, LMA, King LT, or Combitube) if basic airway management is inadequate. Once an advanced airway is in place, compressions should be uninterrupted at a rate of at least 100/min and ventilations should be 8 to 10 breaths/min (1 breath every 6-8 sec). Use waveform capnography to confirm and monitor ET tube placement.
  8. Administer epinephrine 1 mg (10 mL of 1:10,000) by the intravenous or intraosseous (IV/IO) method; follow with 20 mL IV flush. Repeat every 3–5 minutes. A single dose of vasopressin 40 U IV/IO can be administered to replace the first or second dose of epinephrine. If no IV/IO access is available; give 2.0–2.5 mg (1:1,000) epinephrine diluted in 5–10 mL normal saline or sterile water and administer by endotracheal (ET) tube every 3–5 minutes until IV/IO access is available.
  9. Continue CPR; check the rhythm every 2 minutes.
  10. If the rhythm is still shockable, defibrillate as in step 5.
  11. Immediately resume CPR, check the rhythm every 2 minutes.

Consider antiarrhythmics for shock-refractory VF or pulseless VT:

  12. Administer amiodarone 300 mg IV/IO or lidocaine 1.0–1.5 mg/kg IV/IO. Lidocaine should only be used as an alternative if the patient is allergic to amiodarone or amiodarone is unavailable.
  13. Repeat antiarrhythmic therapy for shock-refractory VF or VT: amiodarone 150 mg IV/IO in 3–5 minutes (use only one time); or lidocaine 0.5–0.75 mg/kg IV/IO. Repeat lidocaine every 5–10 minutes, maximum dose 3 mg/kg. Lidocaine should only be used as an alternative if the patient is allergic to amiodarone or amiodarone is unavailable.
  14. Consider magnesium sulfate 1–2 g (2–4 mL of a 50% solution) diluted in 10 mL of D5W IV/IO, given over 1–2 minutes for cardiac arrest due to hypomagnesemia or Torsade de Pointes.

♡ | *Clinical Tip:*

Do not delay defibrillation for a witnessed arrest. For an unwitnessed arrest with a down time greater than 4–5 minutes, perform two minutes of CPR prior to defibrillation.

♡ | *Clinical Tip:*

Airway must be secured and placement verified with observation of chest rise and auscultation of breath sounds plus a confirmatory device (exhaled CO_2 detector). Monitor tube for displacement during transport or whenever patient is moved.

PULSELESS ELECTRICAL ACTIVITY (PEA)

Clinical Presentation

- Unresponsive state
- No respiration, pulse, or BP
- Identifiable organized electrical rhythm on monitor but no pulse
  1. Establish unresponsiveness with no respiration or pulse. Call for help.
  2. Begin CPR, provide oxygen and attach manual monitor-defibrillator when available without interrupting CPR.
  3. When device is attached, stop CPR to assess rhythm. If organized rhythm noted on monitor, immediately resume CPR beginning with compressions. Establish IV/IO access.
  4. During CPR, consider and treat possible causes:

Tension pneumothorax	Hypokalemia/hyperkalemia
Thrombosis (pulmonary or coronary)	Hypovolemia
	Hypoxia
Tamponade, cardiac	Hypothermia
Toxins	Hydrogen ion (acidosis)

  5. Continue CPR using five cycles of 30 compressions and 2 breaths; check the rhythm every 2 minutes.
  6. Consider insertion of an advanced airway (ET tube, LMA, King LT, or Combitube) if basic airway management is inadequate. Once an advanced airway is in place, compressions should be uninterrupted at a rate of at least 100/min and ventilations should be 8 to 10 breaths/min (1 breath every 6-8 sec). Use waveform capnography to confirm and monitor ET tube placement.
  7. If PEA persists, administer epinephrine 1 mg (10 mL of 1:10,000) by the intravenous or intraosseous (IV/IO) method; follow with 20 mL IV flush. Repeat every 3–5 minutes. A single dose of vasopressin 40 U IV/IO can be administered to replace the first or second dose of

epinephrine. If no IV/IO access is available; give 2.0–2.5 mg (1:1,000) epinephrine diluted in 5–10 mL normal saline or sterile water and administer by endotracheal (ET) tube every 3–5 minutes until IV/IO access is available.
  8. Continue CPR; check the rhythm every 2 minutes.
  9. If the rhythm is shockable with no pulse, follow VF/VT protocol.
  10. If the rhythm is not shockable with no pulse, resume CPR and repeat steps 4–8.
  11. If a stable ECG rhythm returns with adequate breathing and circulation, monitor and reevaluate the patient.

♡ | *Clinical Tip:*

PEA is frequently caused by potentially reversible conditions and can be treated successfully if those conditions are identified and corrected easily.

ASYSTOLE

Clinical Presentation

- Unresponsive state, no respiration, pulse, or BP
- ECG shows flat line; no electrical activity
  1. Establish unresponsiveness with no respiration or pulse. Call for help.
  2. Begin CPR, provide oxygen and attach manual monitor-defibrillator when available without interrupting CPR.
  3. When device is attached, stop CPR to assess rhythm. If no electrical activity (flat line or asystole) is noted on monitor, immediately resume CPR beginning with compressions. Establish IV/IO access.
  4. During CPR consider and treat possible causes:

Tension pneumothorax	Hypokalemia/hyperkalemia
Thrombosis (pulmonary or coronary)	Hypovolemia
	Hypoxia
Tamponade, cardiac	Hypothermia
Toxins	Hydrogen ion (acidosis)

  5. Continue CPR beginning with compressions and using five cycles of 30 compressions and 2 breaths; check the rhythm every 2 minutes.
  6. Consider insertion of an advanced airway (ET tube, LMA, King LT, or Combitube) if basic airway management is inadequate. Once an advanced airway is in place, compressions should be uninterrupted at a rate of at least 100/min and ventilations should be 8 to 10 breaths/min (1 breath every 6-8 sec). Use waveform capnography to confirm and monitor ET tube placement.

7. If asystole persists, administer epinephrine 1 mg (10 mL of 1:10,000) by the intravenous or intraosseous (IV/IO) method; follow with 20 mL IV flush. Repeat every 3–5 minutes. A single dose of vasopressin 40 U IV/IO can be administered to replace the first or second dose of epinephrine. If no IV/IO access is available, give 2.0–2.5 mg (1:1,000) epinephrine diluted in 5–10 mL normal saline or sterile water and administer by endotracheal (ET) tube every 3–5 minutes until IV/IO access is available.

8. Continue CPR; check the rhythm every 2 minutes.

9. If the rhythm is shockable with no pulse, follow VF/VT protocol.

10. If the rhythm is not shockable with no pulse, resume CPR and repeat steps 4–8.

11. If asystole persists, consider whether proper resuscitation protocols were followed and reversible causes identified. If procedures were performed correctly, follow local criteria for terminating resuscitation efforts.

 Clinical Tip:

Transcutaneous pacing is not recommended for asystolic cardiac arrest.

 Clinical Tip:

Study local policy to learn established criteria for stopping resuscitation efforts.

ACUTE CORONARY SYNDROME (ACS)

Clinical Presentation

- History of coronary artery disease, angina, or acute MI
- Chest pain or discomfort
- Pain spreading to neck, shoulders, arms, jaw, or upper back
- Sudden unexplained shortness of breath, weakness, fatigue with or without chest pain/discomfort
- Associated nausea, diaphoresis, lightheadedness, fainting.
  1. Establish responsiveness.
  2. Perform primary ABCD survey.
  3. Measure vital signs, including oxygen saturation.
  4. Administer oxygen if oxygen saturation is <94%. Titrate to effect.
  5. Administer aspirin 160–325 mg orally (PO) if no history of aspirin allergy. Aspirin 81 mg (times 4 tablets) is commonly given. Chewing the tablet(s) is preferable; use non–enteric-coated tablets for antiplatelet effect. Give within minutes of onset.

6. Start an IV and attach a cardiac monitor. Obtain a 12 lead ECG.

7. If the 12-lead ECG shows ST segment elevation, notify the attending physician. Begin the checklist for fibrinolytic therapy. If possible, prehospital providers should transport the patient to the closest facility with rapid coronary intervention capabilities.

8. Administer nitroglycerin by the sublingual route 0.3–0.4 mg (1 tablet), repeated every 3–5 minutes for a total of three doses over a 15-minute interval, or administer aerosol spray for 0.5–1.0 second at 3–5 minute intervals (provides 0.4 mg per dose) not to exceed three sprays in 15 minutes. Nitroglycerin administration requires a systolic BP greater than 90 mm Hg.

9. Repeat nitroglycerin (see step 8) until chest pain is relieved, systolic BP falls below 90 mm Hg, or signs of ischemia or infarction are resolved.

10. If chest pain is not relieved by nitroglycerin, administer morphine 2–4 mg IV (over 1–5 min). If symptoms are not resolved, administer 2–8 mg every 5–15 min if hemodynamically stable. Do not administer morphine if systolic BP is less than 90 mm Hg.

 Clinical Tip:

Do not delay rapid transport to a Cardiac Catheterization Lab for reperfusion. Consider fibrinolytic therapy within 30 minutes if a cardiac catheterization lab is not immediately available.

Clinical Tip:

Patients should not be given nitroglycerin if they have taken sildenafil (**Viagra**), or vardenafil (**Levitra**) in the last 24 hours or tadalafil (**Cialis**), within 48 hours. The use of nitroglycerin with these medication may cause irreversible hypotension.

Clinical Tip:

Nitroglycerin should be used with caution in patients with an inferior MI with possible right ventricular involvement. It is contraindicated with right ventricular MI, tachycardia, and bradycardia.

Clinical Tip:

Diabetic patients, the elderly, and women frequently present with atypical symptoms (e.g., weakness, fatigue, complaints of indigestion).

BRADYCARDIA

Clinical Presentation

- Heart rate less than 50 bpm in symptomatic patient.
- Sinus bradycardia, junctional escape rhythm, or AV block
- Symptoms of chest discomfort/pain, lightheadedness, dizziness, dyspnea, tachypnea, presyncope, syncope.
- Signs of hypoxemia, hypotension, diaphoresis, altered mental status, congestive heart failure (CHF), shock
    1. Establish responsiveness.
    2. Perform primary ABCD survey.
    3. Measure vital signs, including oxygen saturation.
    4. Administer oxygen if oxygen saturation is <94%. Titrate to effect. Start an IV and attach cardiac monitor to identify rhythm.
    5. Obtain a 12-lead ECG.
    6. If the patient is stable and asymptomatic with a heart rate less than 50 bpm, monitor and observe for any changes.
    7. If the patient is symptomatic with signs of poor perfusion, initiate treatment.
    8. Administer atropine 0.5 mg IV every 3–5 minutes, maximum total dose 3 mg. In sinus bradycardia, junctional escape rhythm, or second-degree AV block Wenckebach/Mobitz type I, atropine is usually effective. In second-degree Mobitz type II or third-degree AV block, atropine is likely to be ineffective; prepare for transcutaneous pacing.
    9. If the patient fails to respond to atropine in step 8, sedate and begin transcutaneous pacing (TCP) as a temporizing measure if IV access is not available. TCP is painful and will require sedation/analgesia in the conscious patient.
    10. If the patient is hypotensive with severe bradycardia, or if TCP is unavailable or ineffective, initiate drug therapy with a continuous dopamine infusion starting at 2–10 mcg/kg/min (chronotropic or heart rate dose) and titrate to patient response. Mix 400 mg/250 mL in normal saline, lactated Ringer's solution, or D5W (1,600 mcg/mL). An alternative may be an epinephrine infusion, 2–10 mcg/min IV (add 1 mg of 1:1,000 in 500 mL normal saline and infuse at 1–5 mL/min). Seek expert consultation and prepare for transvenous pacing.

Clinical Tip:

If the patient is symptomatic, do not delay transcutaneous pacing while waiting for atropine to take effect or for IV access.

Clinical Tip:

Use atropine with caution in a suspected acute MI; atropine may lead to rate-induced ischemia.

TACHYCARDIA—UNSTABLE

Clinical Presentation

- Altered level of consciousness (LOC)
- Symptoms of shortness of breath, diaphoresis, weakness, fatigue, syncope or presyncope, chest discomfort or pain, palpitations
- Signs of hypotension, shock, congestive heart failure, ischemic ECG changes, poor peripheral perfusion
- Heart rate typically ≥ 150 bpm
    1. Establish responsiveness.
    2. Perform primary ABCD survey.
    3. Measure vital signs, including oxygen saturation.
    4. Administer oxygen if oxygen saturation is <94%. Titrate to effect. Start an IV, and begin cardiac monitoring.
    5. Establish that serious signs and symptoms are related to the tachycardia.
    6. If the patient is **unstable and symptomatic** with a heart rate ≥150 bpm, prepare for immediate synchronized cardioversion (patients with a healthy heart are unlikely to be unstable if the ventricular rate is less than 150 bpm; however patients with cardiac disease may be unstable with heart rates less than 150 bpm). It is important to look at the patient's stability in addition to monitoring heart rate as criteria for cardioversion.
    7. Premedicate with a sedative plus an analgesic whenever possible.
    8. Place the defibrillator in synchronized (sync) mode.
    9. Administer synchronized cardioversion at: **Narrow regular rhythm (supraventricular tachyarrhythmia [SVT])**—generally requires less energy, 50 to 100 J either biphasic or monophasic is often sufficient; **narrow irregular rhythm (atrial fibrillation)**—120 to 200 J biphasic or 200 J monophasic. If the initial cardioversion shock fails, the energy should be increased in a stepwise fashion. **Wide regular rhythm (monomorphic ventricular tachycardia)**—usually responds well to biphasic or monophasic initial energies of 100 J. If there is no response to the first shock, it may be reasonable to increase the dose in a stepwise fashion.
    10. If **a regular narrow complex tachycardia** is seen in an unstable patient, consider administering adenosine prior to cardioversion.

Adenosine—6mg IV in the antecubital or other large vein given rapidly over 1–3 seconds followed by a 20-ml bolus of normal saline. If the rhythm has not converted in 1–2 minutes, repeat adenosine at 12 mg IV. If the rhythm still does not convert, a third dose of 12 mg IV may be given after another 1–2 minutes, maximum 30 mg.

11. If pulseless arrest develops, identify arrhythmia and follow algorithm for VF/VT, PEA, or asystole.

Clinical Tip:

Reactivate the "sync" mode before each attempted cardioversion.

Clinical Tip:

The "sync" mode delivers energy synchronizing with the timing of the QRS complex to avoid stimulation during the refractory, or vulnerable, period of the cardiac cycle when a shock could potentially produce VF.

Clinical Tip:

Synchronized cardioversion **must not be used** for treatment of VF because the device is unlikely to sense a QRS wave, and thus a shock may not be delivered. Synchronized cardioversion should also not be used for pulseless VT or polymorphic VT (irregular VT). These rhythms require delivery of high-energy unsynchronized shocks (i.e., defibrillation doses).

NARROW-COMPLEX TACHYCARDIA— STABLE REGULAR RHYTHM

Clinical Presentation

- No *serious* signs or symptoms related to the tachycardia
- Regular ECG rhythm
- QRS narrow (<0.12 sec)
- Heart rate typically ≥150 bpm
  1. Establish responsiveness.
  2. Perform primary ABCD survey.
  3. Measure vital signs, including oxygen saturation.
  4. Administer oxygen if oxygen saturation is <94%. Titrate to effect. Start an IV, and attach cardiac monitor to identify rhythm. Obtain a 12-lead ECG.

5. Attempt vagal maneuvers such as ice to the face (diving reflex), holding the breath while bearing down (Valsalva maneuver), or blowing through an obstructed straw.
6. If rhythm has not converted to sinus rhythm, administer adenosine 6 mg IV in the antecubital or other large vein given rapidly over 1–3 seconds followed by a 20-mLbolus of normal saline.
7. If the rhythm has not converted in 1–2 minutes, repeat adenosine at 12 mg IV. If the rhythm still does not convert, a third dose of 12 mg IV may be given after another 1–2 minutes, maximum 30 mg.
8. If the rhythm still does not convert, it may be atrial flutter, atrial tachycardia, multifocal atrial tachycardia, or junctional tachycardia. Consider rate control using diltiazem or beta blockers. Obtain expert consultation.
9. If the rhythm converts, observe the patient and treat any recurrence with adenosine, diltiazem, or beta blockers. Obtain expert consultation.

Clinical Tip:

If the patient's condition becomes unstable during the tachycardia, perform immediate synchronized cardioversion.

Clinical Tip:

Use beta blockers with caution in patients with obstructive pulmonary disease or congestive heart failure. Avoid use in patients with bronchospastic disease.

WIDE-COMPLEX TACHYCARDIA— STABLE REGULAR RHYTHM

Clinical Presentation

- No *serious* signs and symptoms related to the tachycardia
- Regular ECG rhythm
- QRS wide (>0.12 sec)
- Heart rate typically ≥150 bpm
  1. Establish responsiveness.
  2. Perform primary ABCD survey.
  3. Measure vital signs, including oxygen saturation.
  4. Administer oxygen if oxygen saturation is <94%. Titrate to effect. Start an IV, and attach cardiac monitor to identify rhythm. Obtain a 12-lead ECG.

5. If the arrhythmia is VT, administer amiodarone 150 mg IV/IO over 10 minutes. May repeat every 10 minutes and start infusion at 1 mg/min for 6 hours, followed by 0.5 mg/min for 18 hours. Do not exceed 2.2 g in 24 hours.

6. If the wide-complex tachycardia is regular, monomorphic, and suspected to be SVT with aberrancy, administer adenosine 6 mg IV in the antecubital or other large vein given rapidly over 1–3 seconds followed by a 20-mL bolus of normal saline.

7. If the rhythm transiently slows or converts to a sinus rhythm, it likely was SVT. However, if there was no effect after adenosine, the rhythm is likely monomorphic VT or atrial fibrillation with preexcitation and should be treated with amiodarone.

8. If pulseless arrest develops, identify arrhythmia and follow algorithm for VF/VT.

Appendix C

Emergency Medications

This list is a reference list only. It is not meant to be exhaustive in clinical content.

- Always consult an authoritative, current reference about dose, dilution, route and rate of administration, and interactions before administering medications, especially IV medications. Have a second licensed person independently check dose calculations, preparation, original orders, and infusion pump programming.

❖ ACE INHIBITORS
Class: Angiotensin-Converting Enzyme Inhibitors
Common Agents: Captopril, Enalapril, Lisinopril, Ramipril.
Indications: Myocardial infarction, especially with ST elevation and with left ventricular dysfunction, hypertension, heart failure without hypotension.
Dose: See individual order and drug for route and dosage. Usually not started in the Emergency Department for an acute MI, but within 24 hours after reperfusion therapy has been completed and BP has stabilized.
Contraindications: Lactation, pregnancy, angioedema, hypersensitivity to ACE inhibitors, serum potassium more than 5 mEq/L, angioedema, hypotension.
Side Effects: Cough, dizziness, headache, fatigue, hypotension, hyperkalemia.
Precautions: Reduce dose in renal failure.

❖ ADENOSINE
(Adenocard, Adenoscan)
Class: Antiarrhythmic
Indications: Regular narrow-complex tachycardias, PSVT, and wide-complex tachycardia only if regular and monomorphic.
Dose: 6 mg IV in the antecubital or other large vein given rapidly over 1–3 seconds followed by a 20-mL bolus of normal saline. If the rhythm does not convert, give 12 mg by IV in 1–2 minutes if needed. A third dose of 12 mg IV may be given in another 1–2 minutes, maximum total dose 30 mg.
Contraindications: Hypersensitivity, sick sinus syndrome, second- or third-degree AV block (unless a functional pacemaker is present), drug- or poison-induced tachycardia.
Side Effects: Flushing, dizziness, headache, dyspnea, bronchospasm, chest pain or tightness, discomfort in neck, throat, or jaw, bradycardia, AV block, asystole, ventricular ectopic beats, VF.
Precautions: Ineffective in treating A-fib, A-flutter, or VT. Avoid in patients receiving dipyridamole, theophylline, carbamazepin, or caffeine.

❖ AMIODARONE
(Cordarone, Pacerone)
Class: Antiarrhythmic, Class III
Indications: Management of life-threatening shock-refractory VF or VT, VF or recurrent hemodynamically-unstable VT. Conversion of atrial fibrillation, SVT. Control of rapid ventricular rate in pre-excited atrial arrhythmias. Control of hemodynamically stable VT, polymorphic VT with normal QT interval, or wide-complex tachycardia of uncertain origin.
Dose: *Cardiac arrest* 300 mg IV/IO; consider additional 150 mg IV/IO in 3–5 minutes. *Wide- and narrow-complex tachycardia (stable)* 150 mg IV over first 10 minutes (15 mg/min)—may repeat infusion of 150 mg IV every 10 minutes as needed; slow infusion of 360 mg IV over next 6 hours (1 mg/min); maintenance infusion of 540 mg over next 18 hours (0.5 mg/min). Maximum cumulative dose 2.2 g IV in 24 hours.
Contraindications: Hypersensitivity, cardiogenic shock, symptomatic bradycardia or second-or third-degree AV block without functioning pacemaker, severe sinus node dysfunction.
Side Effects: Vasodilation, hypotension, bradycardia, proarrhythmic effects, visual impairment, hepatotoxicity,

259

pulmonary toxicity, CHF. May prolong QT interval, producing torsade de pointes.

Precautions: Avoid concurrent use with procainamide. Correct hypokalemia and hypomagnesemia, if possible, before use. Draw up amiodarone through a large-gauge needle to reduce foaming. For slow or maintenance IV infusion, mix the medication only in a glass bottle containing D5W or NS and administer through an in-line filter. Use with caution in patients with thyroid disease or patients on warfarin.

❖ **ASPIRIN (Acetylsalicylic Acid)**
Class: Antiplatelet
Indications: Acute coronary syndrome, symptoms suggestive of cardiac ischemia, post percutaneous coronary interventions, atrial fibrillation, stroke, peripheral arterial disease.
Dose: Acute coronary syndrome: 160–325 mg PO. Chewing the tablet is preferable; use non–enteric coated tablets for antiplatelet effect. Give within minutes of onset of ischemic symptoms. Other indications: 81–325 mg PO daily.
Contraindications: Known allergy to aspirin, third trimester of pregnancy, bleeding.
Side Effects: Anorexia, nausea, epigastric pain, anaphylaxis.
Precautions: Active ulcers and asthma, bleeding disorders or thrombocytopenia.

❖ **ATROPINE SULFATE**
Class: Anticholinergic
Indications: Symptomatic sinus bradycardia, junctional escape rhythm, or second-degree type I block. Not likely to be effective in second-degree type II or third-degree AV block with wide QRS complex.
Dose: 0.5mg IV given every 3–5 minutes as needed, maximum total dose 3 mg (0.04 mg/kg).
Contraindications: Atrial fibrillation, A-flutter, glaucoma, asthma, obstructive uropathy.
Side Effects: Tachycardia, headache, dry mouth, dilated pupils, flushing, hypotension.
Precautions: Use caution in myocardial ischemia and hypoxia. Avoid in hypothermic bradycardia and in second-degree (Mobitz type II) and third-degree AV block with wide QRS complex, asystole, bradycardia PEA, colon disease, hepatic or renal impairment, hyperthyroidism.

❖ **BETA BLOCKERS**
Class: Antihypertensive, Antiarrhythmic, Antianginal
Common Agents: Atenolol, Esmolol, Labetalol, Metoprolol, Propranolol.
Indications: Myocardial infarction, unstable angina, PSVT, A-fib, A-flutter, HTN, CHF.

Dose: See individual order and drug for route and dosage.
Contraindications: Heart rate less than 50 bpm, systolic BP less than 100 mm Hg, second- or third-degree AV block or sick sinus syndrome without functioning pacemaker, severe decompensated left ventricular failure, cardiogenic shock. Nonselective beta blockers are contraindicated in patients with bronchospastic disease.
Side Effects: Hypotension, dizziness, bradycardia, headache, nausea and vomiting.
Precautions: Concurrent use with calcium channel blockers, such as verapamil or diltiazem, can cause hypotension. Use beta-1 selective agents with caution in patients with a history of bronchospasm. Use caution in patients with thyroid disease, patients with peripheral arterial disease, and with diabetic patients (monitor blood glucose levels frequently).

❖ **CALCIUM CHLORIDE**
Class: Minerals, Electrolytes, Calcium Salt
Indications: Hyperkalemia, hypocalcemia, hypermagnesemia; antidote to calcium channel blockers and beta blockers.
Dose: *Hyperkalemia and antidote to calcium channel blocker*
500–1,000 mg (5–10 mL of a 10% solution) over 2–5 minutes IV; may be repeated as needed.
Contraindications: Hypercalcemia, VF, digoxin toxicity, renal calculi.
Side effects: Bradycardia, hypotension, hypomagnesemia, VF, nausea and vomiting.
Precautions: Incompatible with sodium bicarbonate (precipitates).

❖ **DIGOXIN (Lanoxin)**
Class: Antiarrhythmic, Cardiac Glycoside
Indications: To slow ventricular response in A-fib or A-flutter, as a positive inotrope in CHF.
Dose: Loading dose of 0.5 mg IV over 5 minutes, 0.25 mg IV in 6–8 hours times two. Maintenance dose determined by body size and renal function.
Contraindications: Hypersensitivity, uncontrolled ventricular arrhythmias, AV block without functioning pacemaker, idiopathic hypertrophic subaortic stenosis (IHSS), constrictive pericarditis, atrial fibrillation with Wolff-Parkinson-White syndrome.
Side Effects: Accelerated junctional rhythm, atrial tachycardia with block, AV block, asystole, VT, VF, ventricular bigeminy and trigemity, dizziness, weakness, fatigue; nausea and vomiting; blurred or yellow vision; headache; hypersensitivity; hypokalemia.
Precautions: Avoid electrical cardioversion of stable patients. If the patient's condition is unstable, use lower current settings such as 10–20 J. Use cautiously in elderly patients and patients with renal impairment and hypothyroidism. Correct electrolyte

abnormalities, monitor digoxin levels, monitor for clinical signs of toxicity. Hypokalemia, hypomagnesemia, and hypercalcemia may precipitate digitalis toxicity. Reduce digoxin dose by 50% in patients on amiodarone.

❖ DIGOXIN IMMUNE FAB (Fragment Antigen Binding) (DigiFab)

Class: Antidote to digoxin and digitoxin
Indications: Symptomatic digoxin toxicity or acute ingestion of unknown amount of digoxin.
Dose: Depends on serum digoxin levels. One 40-mg vial binds to approximately 0.5 mg of digoxin. Dose is typically administered over 30 minutes.
Contraindications: Allergy only, otherwise none known. Allergy to sheep proteins or other sheep products.
Side Effects: Worsening of CHF, rapid ventricular response in patients with A-fib, hypokalemia, postural hypotension, increased serum digoxin levels due to bound complexes (clinically misleading since bound complex cannot interact with receptors).
Precautions: Heart failure, renal impairment.

❖ DILTIAZEM (Cardizem)

Class: Calcium Channel Blocker, Antiarrhythmic
Indications: To control ventricular rate in A-fib and A-flutter, to terminate PSVT (reentry SVT) refractory to adenosine with narrow QRS complex and adequate BP.
Dose: 15–20 mg (0.25 mg/kg) IV given over 2 minutes. May repeat in 15 minutes at 20–25 mg (0.35 mg/kg) IV given over 2 minutes. Start maintenance drip at 5–15 mg/hr and titrate to HR.
Contraindications: Drug- or poison-induced tachycardia, wide-complex tachycardia of uncertain origin, rapid A-fib and A-flutter with Wolff-Parkinson-White syndrome, sick sinus syndrome, second- or third-degree AV block (unless a functional pacemaker is present), hypotension with systolic BP less than 90 mm Hg.
Side Effects: Hypotension, bradycardia (including AV block), chest pain, ventricular arrhythmias, peripheral edema, flushing.
Precautions: Severe hypotension in patients receiving beta blockers, hepatic injury, renal disease.

❖ DOPAMINE (Intropin)

Class: Vasopressor, Inotrope, Adrenergic Agonist
Indications: Symptomatic bradycardia and hypotension, cardiogenic shock.
Dose: Continuous infusions (titrate to patient response): Low dose 1–5 µg/kg/min; moderate dose 5–10 µg/kg/min (cardiac doses); high dose 10–20 µg/kg/min (vasopressor doses). Mix 400 mg/250 mL in normal saline, lactated Ringer's solution, or D5W (1600 µg/mL).

Contraindications: Hypersensitivity to sulfites, pheochromocytoma, VF.
Side Effects: Tachyarrhythmias, angina, hypotension, palpitations, vasoconstriction, dyspnea, nausea and vomiting.
Precautions: Hypovolemia, MI. Adjust dosage in elderly patients and in those with occlusive vascular disease. Ensure adequate hydration prior to infusion. Taper slowly. Do not mix with sodium bicarbonate. Use care with peripheral administration; infiltration can cause tissue necrosis. A central line is preferred.

❖ EPINEPHRINE (Adrenalin)

Class: Adrenergic Agonist
Indications: Cardiac arrest: PEA, asystole, pulseless VT, VF; hypotension with severe bradycardia.
Dose: *Cardiac arrest* 1 mg IV/IO (10 mL of 1:10,000 solution) given every 3–5 minutes as needed; follow each dose with 20 mL IV flush. Give 2.0–2.5 mg diluted in 10 mL normal saline or sterile water if administering by ET tube. *Profound bradycardia or hypotension* 2–10 µg/min IV; add 1 mg (1 mL of a 1:1000 solution) to 500 mL normal saline or D5W.
Contraindications: Hypersensitivity to adrenergic amines, hypovolemic shock, coronary insufficiency. No contraindication in cardiac arrest.
Side Effects: Angina, HTN, tachycardia, VT, VF, nervousness, restlessness, tremors, weakness, headache, nausea.
Precautions: Use caution in HTN and increasing heart rate (may cause increased myocardial oxygen demand). Higher doses can contribute to post-arrest cardiac impairment, but they may be required to treat poison- or drug-induced shock. Avoid mixing with alkaline solutions.

❖ FIBRINOLYTIC AGENTS

Class: Thrombolytic, Fibrinolytic
Common Agents: Alteplase **(Activase, t-PA)**, Reteplase **(Retavase)**, Streptokinase **(Streptase)**, Tenecteplase **(TNKase)**.
Indications: Acute ST elevation MI within the last 12 hours. Alteplase is the only fibrinolytic agent approved for acute ischemic stroke and must be started less than 3 hours from the onset of symptoms.
Dose: See individual order and drug for route and dosage.
Contraindications: Active internal bleeding within 21 days (except menses), neurovascular event within 3 months, major surgery or trauma within 2 weeks, aortic dissection, severe (uncontrolled) HTN, bleeding disorders, prolonged CPR, lumbar puncture within 1 week. History of any intracranial bleed, oral anticoagulation therapy, severe stroke.
Side Effects: Hypotension, reperfusion and arrhythmias, heart failure, headache, increased bleeding time,

deep or superficial hemorrhage, flushing, urticaria, anaphylaxis.

Precautions: Use cautiously in patients with severe renal or hepatic disease. Initiate bleeding precautions. Monitor patient for bleeding complications.

❖ FUROSEMIDE (Lasix)

Class: Diuretic, Loop Diuretics

Indications: Congestive heart failure with acute pulmonary edema, hypertensive crisis, post-arrest cerebral edema, hepatic or renal disease.

Dose: 0.5–1.0 mg/kg IV given over 1–2 minutes; may repeat at 2 mg/kg IV given over 1–2 minutes.

Contraindications: Hypersensitivity (cross-sensitivity with thiazides and sulfonamides may occur), uncontrolled electrolyte imbalance, hepatic coma, anuria, hypovolemia.

Side Effects: Severe dehydration, hypovolemia, hypotension, hypokalemia, hyponatremia, hypochloremia, hyperglycemia, dizziness, ototoxicity.

Precautions: Use cautiously in severe liver disease accompanied by cirrhosis or ascites, electrolyte depletion, diabetes mellitus, pregnancy, lactation, severe renal disease, gout. Risk for otoxicity with increased dose or rapid injection. Monitor electrolytes closely.

❖ IBUTILIDE (Corvert)

Class: Antiarrhythmic, Class III

Indications: Supraventricular tachycardia, including A-fib and A-flutter; most effective for conversion of A-fib or A-flutter of short duration (≤48 hrs).

Dose: *Patients weighing 60 kg or more* 1 mg IV given over 10 minutes; may repeat the same dose in 10 minutes if arrhythmia does not terminate. *Patients weighing less than 60 kg* 0.01 mg/kg IV given over 10 minutes; may repeat the same dose in 10 minutes if arrhythmia does not terminate.

Contraindications: Known hypersensitivity, history of polymorphic VT, QTc greater than 440 msec.

Side Effects: Nonsustained or sustained monomorphic or polymorphic VT, torsade de pointes, AV block, CHF, HTN, headache, hypotension, nausea and vomiting.

Precautions: Monitor ECG for 4–6 hours after administration, with a defibrillator nearby. Correct electrolyte abnormalities prior to use. If A-fib has lasted longer than 48 hours, anticoagulation is required before cardioversion with ibutilide. Monitor QT$_c$.

❖ ISOPROTERENOL (Isuprel)

Class: Sympathomimetic, Beta-Adrenergic Agonist

Indications: Medically-refractory symptomatic bradycardia when transcutaneous or transvenous pacing is not available, refractory torsade de pointes unresponsive to magnesium, bradycardia in heart transplant patients, beta blocker poisoning.

Dose: IV infusion: mix 1 mg/250 mL in normal saline, lactated Ringer's solution, or D5W, run at 2–10 μg/min, and titrate to patient response. In torsade de pointes, titrate to increase heart rate until VT is suppressed.

Contraindications: Hypersensitivity to drug or sulfites, digitalis intoxication, angina, tachyarrhythmias, concurrent use with epinephrine (can cause VF or VT).

Side Effects: Arrhythmias, cardiac arrest, hypotension, angina, anxiety, tachycardia, palpitations, skin flushing.

Precautions: May increase myocardial ischemia, tachycardia, restlessness, distributive shock, hyperthyroidism, diabetes. High doses are harmful except in beta blocker overdose.

❖ LIDOCAINE (Xylocaine)

Class: Antiarrhythmic, Local Anesthetic

Indications: Alternative to amiodarone in ventricular fibrillation or pulseless VT. Use in stable VT, wide-complex tachycardia of uncertain origin.

Dose: *Cardiac arrest from VF or VT* 1.0–1.5 mg/kg IV/IO (or 2–4 mg/kg via ET tube); may repeat 0.5–0.75 mg/kg IV/IO every 5–10 minutes, maximum dose 3 mg/kg. *Stable VT, wide-complex tachycardia of uncertain origin* use 0.50–0.75 mg/kg and up to 1.0–1.5 mg/kg; may repeat 0.50–0.75 mg/kg every 5–10 minutes, maximum total dose 3.0 mg/kg. If conversion is successful, start an IV infusion of 1–4 mg/min (30–50 μg/kg/min) in normal saline or D5W.

Contraindications: Prophylactic use in acute MI, advanced AV block without functioning pacemaker, hypotension, Wolff-Parkinson-White syndrome, hypersensitivity to amide local anesthetics.

Side Effects: Confusion, agitation, anxiety, tinnitus, tremors, hallucinations, seizures, hypotension, bradycardia, cardiovascular collapse, respiratory arrest, slurred speech.

Precautions: Congestive heart failure, respiratory depression, shock. Reduce maintenance dose (not loading dose) in presence of impaired liver function or left ventricular dysfunction or in the elderly. Stop infusion if signs of CNS toxicity develop.

❖ MAGNESIUM SULFATE

Class: Electrolyte, Antiarrhythmic

Indications: Torsade de pointes, hypomagnesemia, life-threatening ventricular arrhythmias due to digitalis toxicity.

Dose: *Torsade de pointes (cardiac arrest)* 1–2 g IV (2–4 mL of a 50% solution) diluted in 10 mL of D5W over 1–2 minutes. *Torsade de pointes (non–cardiac arrest)* load with 1–2 g mixed in 50–100 mL of D5W infused over 5–60 minutes IV, then infuse 0.5–1.0 g/hr IV (titrate to control torsade).

Contraindications: Hypermagnesemia, hypocalcemia, AV block, toxemia of pregnancy 2 hours prior to delivery.

Side Effects: Hypotension, bradycardia, cardiac arrest, respiratory depression, altered LOC, flushed skin, diaphoresis, hypocalcemia, hyperkalemia, hypophosphatemia.

Precautions: Renal insufficiency, occasional fall in BP with rapid administration. Monitor serum magnesium levels.

❖ MORPHINE SULFATE

Class: Opiate Narcotic Analgesic

Indications: Chest pain unrelieved by nitroglycerin, CHF and dyspnea associated with pulmonary edema.

Dose: 2–4 mg IV (given over 1–5 min), administer every 5–30 minutes if hemodynamically stable; may repeat dose of 2–8 mg at 5- to 15-minute intervals.

Contraindications: Hypersensitivity, heart failure due to chronic lung disease, respiratory depression, hypotension, bowel obstruction, asthma, acute or severe hypercarbia. Avoid in patients with RV infarction.

Side Effects: Respiratory depression, hypotension, nausea and vomiting, bradycardia, altered LOC, seizures, somnolence, dizziness, diaphoresis.

Precautions: Administer slowly and titrate to effect. Reverse with naloxone (0.4–2.0 mg IV), if necessary. Use caution in cerebral edema and pulmonary edema with compromised respiration. Use caution with hypovolemic patients; be prepared to administer volume. Use caution in renal and hepatic impairment, seizure disorder, shock.

❖ NITROGLYCERIN (Nitrostat, Nitrolingual [Pump spray])

Class: Antianginal, Nitrate, Vasodilator

Indications: Acute coronary syndrome, angina, CHF associated with acute MI, hypertensive urgency with ACS.

Dose: Sublingual route, 0.3–0.4 mg (1 tablet); repeat every 3–5 minutes, maximum 3 doses/15 min. Aerosol, spray for 0.5–1.0 sec at 3- to 5-minute intervals (provides 0.4 mg/dose), maximum 3 sprays/15 min. Intravenous bolus administration at 12.5–25.0 µg (if no sublingual or spray used). Intravenous infusion: mix 25 mg/250 mL (100 µg/mL) in D5W, run at 5–20 µg/min, and titrate to desired response.

Contraindications: Hypersensitivity, systolic BP less than 90 mm Hg, pericardial tamponade, constrictive pericarditis; severe bradycardia or severe tachycardia associated with hypotension; sildenafil (**Viagra**), vardenafil (**Levitra**) within 24 hours, tadalafil (**Cialis**) within 48 hours; right ventricular infarction, increased intracranial pressure, hypertrophic cardiomyopathy with outflow tract obstruction.

Side Effects: Hypotension with reflex tachycardia, syncope, headache, flushed skin, dizziness.

Precautions: Do not mix with other medications; titrate IV to maintain systolic BP above 90 mm Hg. Mix only in glass IV bottles and infuse only through tubing

provided by manufacturer; standard polyvinyl chloride tubing can bind up to 80% of the medication, making it necessary to infuse higher doses. Do not shake aerosol spray (affects metered dose).

❖ OXYGEN

Class: Gas

Indications: Cardiopulmonary emergencies with shortness of breath and chest pain, cardiac or respiratory arrest, hypoxemia. Used to optimize oxygen saturation that is <94%.

Dose: Nasal cannula 1–6 L/min (21%–44% oxygen), Venturi mask 4–12 L/min (24%–50% oxygen), simple mask 5–8 L/min (40%–60% oxygen), partial rebreathing mask 6–10 L/min (35%–60% oxygen), non-rebreathing mask 6–15 L/min (60%–100% oxygen), bag-valve-mask 15 L/min (95%–100%).

Contraindications: None reported.

Side Effects: Drying of respiratory mucosa, possible bronchospasm if oxygen is extremely cold and dry. Oxygen supports combustion and can fuel a fire. Hypoventilation in patients with severe COPD, pulmonary fibrosis, oxygen toxicity.

Precautions: Respiratory arrest in patients with hypoxic respiratory drive. The patient needs an air-way and adequate ventilation before oxygen is effective.

❖ PROCAINAMIDE (Pronestyl)

Class: Antiarrhythmic

Indications: Recurrent VT or VF, PSVT refractory to adenosine and vagal stimulation, rapid A-fib with Wolff-Parkinson-White syndrome, stable wide-complex tachycardia of uncertain origin, maintenance after conversion. Stable monomorphic VT with normal QT_c and preserved LV function.

Dose: 20 mg/min IV infusion or up to 50 mg/min under urgent conditions, maximum 17 mg/kg loading dose. Maintenance IV infusion: mix 1 g/250 mL (4 mg/mL) in normal saline or D5W, run at 1–4 mg/min.

Contraindications: Second- and third-degree AV block (unless a functioning pacemaker is in place), prolonged QT interval, torsade de pointes, hypersensitivity, systemic lupus erythematosus.

Side Effects: Hypotension, widening QRS, headache, nausea and vomiting, flushed skin, seizures, ventricular arrhythmias, AV block, cardiovascular collapse, arrest.

Precautions: Monitor BP every 2–3 minutes while administering procainamide. If QRS width increases by 50% or more, or if systolic BP decreases to less than 90 mm Hg, stop the drug. Monitor for prolonged PR interval and AV block. Monitor for QT prolongation. May precipitate or exacerbate CHF. Reduce the total dose to 12 mg/kg and maintenance infusion to 1–2 mg/min if cardiac or renal dysfunction is present. Use cautiously in myasthenia gravis, in hepatic or renal disease, and with drugs that prolong the QT interval (e.g., amiodarone, sotalol).

❖ SODIUM BICARBONATE
Class: Alkalinizing Agent, Buffer
Indications: Known preexisting hyperkalemia, bicarbonate-responsive acidosis, prolonged resuscitation with effective ventilation.
Dose: 1 mEq/kg IV; may repeat 0.5 mEq/kg every 10 minutes.
Contraindications: Metabolic and respiratory alkalosis, hypocalcemia, hypokalemia, hypercarbic acidosis, hypernatremia, severe pulmonary edema.
Side Effects: Hypokalemia, hypocalcemia, hypernatremia, metabolic alkalosis, edema, seizures, tetany, exacerbation of CHF.
Precautions: Congestive heart failure, renal disease, cirrhosis, toxemia, concurrent corticosteroid therapy. Not recommended for routine use in cardiac arrest patients because adequate ventilation and CPR are the major "buffer agents" in cardiac arrest. Incompatible with many drugs; flush the line before and after administration.

❖ VASOPRESSIN (Pitressin)
Class: Vasopressor, Hormone
Indication: Cardiac arrest: an alternative to epinephrine in shock-refractory VF and pulseless VT, PEA, and asystole.
Dose: *Cardiac arrest:* 40 units IV/IO single dose to replace first or second dose of epinephrine as an alternative.
Contraindications: Hypersensitivity.

Side Effects: Bradycardia, HTN, angina, MI, arrhythmias, dizziness, headache, nausea and vomiting, abdominal cramps, diaphoresis, bronchoconstriction, anaphylaxis.
Precautions: Coronary artery disease (may precipitate angina or MI), renal impairment; patients with seizure disorders, asthma, vascular disease.

❖ VERAPAMIL (Calan, Isoptin)
Class: Calcium Channel Blocker, Antiarrhythmic, Antihypertensive
Indications: Paroxysmal supraventricular tachycardia (with narrow QRS and adequate BP) refractory to adenosine, rapid ventricular rates in A-fib, A-flutter, or MAT.
Dose: 2.5–5.0 mg IV over 2 minutes; may give second dose, if needed, of 5–10 mg IV in 15–30 minutes, maximum dose 20 mg. An alternative second dose is 5 mg IV every 15 minutes, maximum dose 30 mg.
Contraindications: Atrial fibrillation with Wolff-Parkinson-White syndrome, wide-complex tachycardia of uncertain origin, second- or third-degree AV block (unless a functioning pacemaker is in place), sick sinus syndrome, hypotension, severe CHF, cardiogenic shock concurrent IV beta blocker, VT.
Side Effects: Hypotension, exacerbation of CHF with left ventricular dysfunction, bradycardia, AV block, constipation, peripheral edema, headache.
Precautions: Concurrent oral beta blockers, CHF, impaired hepatic or renal function, hypertrophic cardiomyopathy with outflow tract obstruction; may decrease myocardial contractility. In geriatric patients administer slowly over 3 minutes.

Appendix D

Emergency Medical Skills

DEFIBRILLATION

Indications: Ventricular fibrillation or pulseless VT.

Energy Levels: Use an adult biphasic energy level at 120–200 J (use the manufacturer's device-specific energy level) or deliver 360 J for a monophasic energy level. Continue at a biphasic energy level of 120–200 J for further shocks or a monophasic energy level of 360 J.

Application: Dry moisture off skin; shave excessive hair, if necessary. Use remote adhesive pads or hand-held paddles (Fig. D–1). Always use a conducting gel with paddles and apply firm pressure (15–25 pounds per paddle) to the chest to ensure good skin contact.

Methods: Manual or automated.

Precautions: Place pads or paddles several inches away from an implanted pacemaker or ICD.

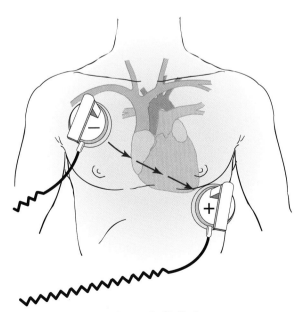

Fig. D.1 ■ Defibrillation.

♥ *Clinical Tip:*

Defibrillation may be used on infants younger than 1 year old and on children (1 yr to puberty). Always use pediatric pads or paddles and follow pediatric protocols.

Manual Defibrillation

A manual defibrillator is used to restore a normal heart rhythm. For a patient experiencing sudden cardiac arrest, first assess for responsiveness, respiration, and pulse. Begin CPR. Verify that the rhythm is either VF or pulseless VT, and then manually deliver an electric shock to the heart.

Procedure

1. Verify that the patient is in cardiac arrest, with no pulse or respiration. Have someone provide CPR while the defibrillator is obtained and placed next to the patient or left on crash cart.
2. Turn on the defibrillator; verify that all cables are connected.
3. Turn "lead select" to "paddles" or "defibrillator."
4. Pads: Place in locations specified for paddles. Roll pads on from top to bottom edges to prevent air pockets.
   Paddles: Use conducting gel or gel pads and place on the apex (lower left chest, midaxillary) and sternum (right of sternum, midclavicular).
5. Remove oxygen away from patient and immediate vicinity.
6. Select the initial energy level for an adult to a biphasic energy level of 120–200 J (use the manufacturer's device-specific energy levels) or a monophasic energy level of 360 J.
7. Verify rhythm as VF or pulseless VT.

8. Say, "Charging defibrillator, stand clear!"
9. Charge the defibrillator.
10. Say, "I'm going to shock on three. One, I'm clear; two, you're clear; three, everybody's clear." Perform a visual sweep to ensure all rescue personnel are clear of the patient, bed, and equipment and oxygen is removed.
11. Discharge the defibrillator, reassess the rhythm, and refer to appropriate advanced cardiac life support protocol.

Automated External Defibrillator

An automated external defibrillator (AED) is a small, lightweight device used by both professionals and laypersons to assess heart rhythm by computer analysis. Using voice and visual prompts, it administers an electric shock, if necessary, to restore a normal rhythm in patients with sudden cardiac arrest. A shock is administered only if the rhythm detected is VF or pulseless VT.

Automated external defibrillators are available from medical device manufacturers and local pharmacies. Although the AEDs all operate in basically the same way, external features vary from model to model. Be sure to follow the manufacturer's recommendations.
Indications: Ventricular fibrillation or pulseless VT in adults, children, and infants.
Dose: The AED will automatically select the energy dose for each defibrillation. Some devices are equipped with pediatric systems that include a pad–cable system or a key to reduce the delivered energy to a suitable dose for children.

Procedure

1. Verify that the patient is in cardiac arrest, with no pulse or respiration. Have someone provide CPR while the AED is obtained and placed next to the patient.
2. Power on the AED. Follow the voice prompts and visual messages.
3. Open the package of adhesive electrode pads and attach pads to the patient's bare chest.
4. Use adult pads for an adult and child pads for a child. If there are no child pads available, you may use adult pads on a child, but be sure the pads do not touch.
5. Attach one pad to the right sternal border (superior–anterior right chest) and place the second pad over the left apex (inferior–lateral left chest). Alternatively, follow the diagrams on each of the AED electrodes.
6. Connect the pad cables to the AED.
7. Clear the patient and stop CPR. Remove oxygen, if applicable.

8. The AED may automatically analyze the patient's rhythm or may be equipped with an "analyze" button.
9. If a shock is advised, say, "I'm going to shock on three. One, I'm clear; two, you're clear; three, everybody's clear." Perform a visual sweep to ensure rescue personnel are not touching the patient or equipment. Remove oxygen, if applicable. Press the shock button.
10. Once the shock is delivered, continue CPR beginning with chest compression.
11. After about 2 minutes of CPR the AED will prompt you with further verbal and visual cues.

♥ *Clinical Tip:*

A fully automated AED analyzes the rhythm and delivers a shock, if one is indicated, without operator intervention once the pads are applied to the patient.

♥ *Clinical Tip:*

A semiautomated AED analyzes the rhythm and tells the operator that a shock is indicated. If it is, the operator initiates the shock by pushing the shock button.

CARDIOVERSION (SYNCHRONIZED)

Indications: Unstable tachycardias ≥150 bpm with a perfusing rhythm. The patient may present with an altered LOC, dizziness, chest pain, or hypotension.
Energy Levels: Regular narrow QRS complex tachycardias (supraventricular tachyarrhythmia)—generally requires less energy, 50 to 100 J either biphasic or monophasic is often sufficient; narrow irregular rhythm (atrial fibrillation)—120 to 200 J biphasic or 200 J monophasic. If the initial cardioversion shock fails, the energy should be increased in a stepwise fashion. Regular wide QRS complex tachycardias (monomorphic ventricular tachycardia)—responds well to biphasic or monophasic initial energies of 100 J. If there is no response to the first shock, it may be reasonable to increase the dose in stepwise fashion. Synchronized cardioversion must not be used for treatment of VF because the device is unlikely to sense a QRS wave, and thus, a shock may not be delivered. Synchronized cardioversion should also not be used for pulseless VT or polymorphic VT (irregular VT). These rhythms require delivery of high-energy unsynchronized shocks (i.e., defibrillation doses).
Application: Use remote adhesive pads or handheld paddles. Always use a conducting gel with

paddles. For conscious patients, explain the procedure and use medication for sedation and analgesia. Consider 2.5–5.0 mg of midazolam (**Versed**) or 5.0 mg diazepam (**Valium**) or fentanyl, 1–2 mcg/kg/min IV, or anesthesia, if available.

Methods: Remove oxygen, if applicable. Place defibrillator in synchronized (sync) mode. Observe marker on R wave to confirm proper synchronization. Charge to appropriate level. Say, "I'm going to shock on three. One, I'm clear; two, you're clear; three, everybody's clear." Perform a visual sweep and ensure oxygen is removed. Press and hold shock button until shock is delivered. If using paddles, press and hold both discharge buttons simultaneously until shock is delivered. Reassess the patient and treat according to the appropriate advanced cardiac life support protocol.

Precautions: Reactivate the "sync" mode after each attempted cardioversion; defibrillators default to the unsynchronized mode. Place pads or paddles several inches away from an implanted pacemaker or implantable cardioverter defibrillator (ICD).

Clinical Tip:

The "sync" mode delivers energy synchronizing with the timing of the QRS complex to avoid stimulation during the refractory, or vulnerable, period of the cardiac cycle when a shock could potentially produce VF.

TRANSCUTANEOUS PACING

Indications: A temporizing measure for symptomatic bradycardia (with a pulse) unresponsive to atropine, bradycardia with ventricular escape rhythms, symptomatic second-degree AV block Type II, or third-degree AV block.

Pacing Modes: *Demand-mode (synchronous)* pacemakers sense the patient's heart rate and pace only when the heart rate falls below the level set by the clinician. *Fixed-mode (asynchronous)* pacemakers cannot sense the heart rate and always operate at the rate set by the clinician. Rate selections vary between 30 and 180 bpm. Output is adjustable between 0 and 200 mA. Pulse duration varies from 20–40 ms.

Application: Pacemaker pads work most effectively if placed in an anterior-posterior position on the patient. For correct pad placement, see Figure D–2.

Contraindications: Not effective in VF, pulseless VT, or asystole.

Side Effects: Chest muscle contraction, burns, and chest discomfort.

Precautions: Make sure pads have good skin contact to achieve capture and avoid burns.

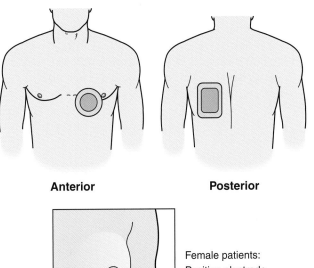

Anterior　　　　**Posterior**

Female patients: Position electrode under breast

Fig. D.2 ■ Placement of anterior-posterior pacemaker pads.

CAROTID SINUS MASSAGE (Vagal Maneuver)

Indications: Can increase vagal nerve stimulation and slow SVT, or even convert SVT to NSR, without severe hemodynamic compromise. **Should be performed only by qualified physicians due to the risk for stroke.**

Method: Place the patient in a supine position, head tilted to either side with the neck hyperextended. Place your index and middle fingers over the carotid artery just below the angle of the jaw, as high on the neck as possible. Massage the artery for 5–10 sec by pressing it firmly against the vertebral column and rubbing (Fig. D–3).

Contraindications: Unequal carotid pulses, carotid bruits, cervical spine injury, or history of cerebrovascular accident or carotid atherosclerosis.

Side Effects: Slow HR or AV block, PVCs, VT, VF, syncope, seizure, hypotension, nausea or vomiting, stroke.

Precautions: Be sure the patient is receiving oxygen and an IV is in place. Never massage both arteries simultaneously. Resuscitation equipment must be readily available.

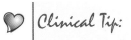*Clinical Tip:*

Performed only by qualified physicians. Each carotid artery should be palpated and auscultated before the procedure to evaluate for contraindications to carotid sinus massage.

♡ | *Clinical Tip:*

Alternate vagal maneuvers include encouraging
the patient to cough, bear down, blowing
through an obstructed straw, ice to the face,
or hold his or her breath.

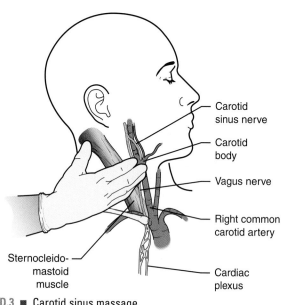

Carotid
sinus nerve

Carotid
body

Vagus nerve

Right common
carotid artery

Sternocleido-
mastoid
muscle

Cardiac
plexus

Fig. D.3 ■ Carotid sinus massage.

Abbreviations Used in Text

AED	Automated external defibrillator		IV	Intravenous
A-fib	Atrial fibrillation		LOC	Level of consciousness
A-flutter	Atrial flutter		MAT	Multifocal atrial tachycardia
AV	Atrioventricular		MI	Myocardial infarction
BBB	Bundle branch block		NSR	Normal sinus rhythm
BP	Blood pressure		PAC	Premature atrial contraction
bpm	Beats per minute		PAT	Paroxysmal atrial tachycardia
BUN	Blood urea nitrogen		PEA	Pulseless electrical activity
CHF	Congestive heart failure		PJC	Premature junctional contraction
CO	Cardiac output		PO	Per os (by mouth)
COPD	Chronic obstructive pulmonary disease		PSVT	Paroxysmal supraventricular tachycardia
CPR	Cardiopulmonary resuscitation		PVC	Premature ventricular contraction
EMD	Electromechanical dissociation		SA	Sinoatrial
ET	Endotracheal		SC	Subcutaneous
HTN	Hypertension		SVT	Supraventricular tachycardia
IHSS	Idiopathic hypertrophic subaortic stenosis		VF	Ventricular fibrillation
			VT	Ventricular tachycardia
IM	Intramuscular		WAP	Wandering atrial pacemaker
IO	Intraoral		WPW	Wolff-Parkinson-White (Syndrome)

Selected References

1. American Heart Association: Basic Life Support for Healthcare Providers (Student Manual), Dallas, TX, 2006.
2. American Heart Association: Guidelines for Cardiopulmonary Resuscitation and Emergency Cardiovascular Care (supplement to Circulation 112: 24, December 13, 2005).
3. Deglin, JH, Vallerand, AH: *Davis's Drug Guide for Nurses*, ed 9. F.A. Davis, Philadelphia, 2006.
4. Deglin, JH, Vallerand, AH: *Med Notes*. F.A. Davis, Philadelphia, 2004.
5. Jones, SA: *ECG Notes*. F.A. Davis, Philadelphia, 2005.
6. Jones, SA: Author's personal collection.
7. Myers, E: *RNotes*. F.A. Davis, Philadelphia, 2003.
8. Myers, E, Hopkins, T: *MedSurg Notes*. F.A. Davis, Philadelphia, 2004.
9. *Physicians' Desk Reference*, ed 60. Thomson Healthcare, Montvale, NJ, 2006.
10. Scanlon, VC, Sanders, T: *Essentials of Anatomy and Physiology*, ed 4. F.A. Davis, Philadelphia, 2003.
11. *Taber's Cyclopedic Medical Dictionary*, ed 20. F.A. Davis, Philadelphia, 2005.

Illustration Credits

The ECG strips in Chapters 3–9 and 11–16 are from Jones: Author's personal collection, with permission. The unnumbered figure in Appendix A is from Jones: *ECG Notes*. Philadelphia: F.A. Davis, 2005, p 115, with permission. The cover and, unit page photographs are from Jones: Author's personal collection, with permission.

Fig. 1.1 ■ From Jones: *ECG Notes*. Philadelphia: F.A. Davis, 2005; p 1, with permission.

Fig. 1.2 ■ From Scanlon and Sanders: *Essentials of Anatomy and Physiology*, ed 4. Philadelphia: F.A. Davis, 2005; p 260, with permission.

Fig. 1.3 ■ From Scanlon and Sanders: *Essentials of Anatomy and Physiology*, ed 4. Philadelphia: F.A. Davis, 2005; p 263, with permission.

Fig. 1.4 ■ From Scanlon and Sanders: *Essentials of Anatomy and Physiology*, ed 4. Philadelphia: F.A. Davis, 2005; p 262, with permission.

Fig. 1.5 ■ From Jones: *ECG Notes*. Philadelphia: F.A. Davis, 2005; p 5, with permission (adapted from Scanlon and Sanders: *Essentials of Anatomy and Physiology*, ed 4. Philadelphia: F.A. Davis, 2005; p 263.

Fig. 1.6 ■ From Scanlon and Sanders: *Essentials of Anatomy and Physiology*, ed 4. Philadelphia: F.A. Davis, 2005; p 279, with permission.

Fig. 1.7 ■ From Scanlon and Sanders: *Essentials of Anatomy and Physiology*, ed 4. Philadelphia: F.A. Davis, 2005; p 283, with permission.

Fig. 1.8 ■ From Scanlon and Sanders: *Essentials of Anatomy and Physiology*, ed 4. Philadelphia, F.A. Davis, 2005, p 284, with permission.

Fig. 1.10 ■ From Jones: *ECG Notes*. Philadelphia: F.A. Davis, 2005; p 10, with permission (adapted from Myers and Hopkins: MedSurg Notes. Philadelphia: F.A. Davis, 2004, p 184.

Fig. 2.1 ■ From Myers and Hopkins: *MedSurg Notes*. Philadelphia, F.A. Davis, 2004, p 186, with permission.

Fig. 2.2 ■ From Jones: *ECG Notes*. Philadelphia, F.A. Davis, 2005; p 13, with permission.

Fig. 2.3 ■ From Jones: *ECG Notes*. Philadelphia, F.A. Davis, 2005; p 14, with permission.

Fig. 2.4 ■ From Jones: *ECG Notes*. Philadelphia, F.A. Davis, 2005; p 15, with permission.

Fig. 2.5 ■ From Myers and Hopkins: *MedSurg Notes*. Philadelphia, F.A. Davis, 2004; p 185, with permission.

Fig. 2.6 ■ From Jones: *ECG Notes*. Philadelphia, F.A. Davis, 2005; p 17, with permission.

Fig. 2.7 ■ From Jones: *ECG Notes*. Philadelphia, F.A. Davis, 2005; p 17, with permission.

Fig. 2.8 ■ From Jones: *ECG Notes*. Philadelphia, F.A. Davis, 2005; p 18, with permission.

Fig. 2.9 ■ From Jones: *ECG Notes*. Philadelphia, F.A. Davis, 2005; p 18, with permission.

Fig. 2.10 ■ From Jones: *ECG Notes*. Philadelphia, F.A. Davis, 2005; p 19, with permission (adapted from Myers and Hopkins: *MedSurg Notes*. Philadelphia, F.A. Davis, 2004; p 185).

Fig. 2.11 ■ From Jones: *ECG Notes*. Philadelphia, F.A. Davis, 2005; p 20, with permission.

Fig. 2.12 ■ From Jones: *ECG Notes*. Philadelphia, F.A. Davis, 2005; p 21, with permission.

Fig. 2.13 ■ From Jones: *ECG Notes*. Philadelphia, F.A. Davis, 2005; p 21, with permission.

Fig. 2.14 ■ From Jones: *ECG Notes*. Philadelphia, F.A. Davis, 2005; p 23, with permission.

Fig. 2.15 ■ From Jones: Author's personal collection, with permission.

Fig. 10.1 ■ From Myers and Hopkins: *MedSurg Notes*. Philadelphia: F.A. Davis, 2004; p 185, with permission.

Fig. 10.2 ■ From Jones: *ECG Notes*. Philadelphia, F.A. Davis, 2005; p 74, with permission.

Fig. 10.3 ■ From Jones: *ECG Notes*. Philadelphia, F.A. Davis, 2005; p 75, with permission.

Fig. 10.4 ■ From Jones: *ECG Notes*. Philadelphia, F.A. Davis, 2005; p 75, with permission.

Fig. 10.5 ■ From Jones: *ECG Notes*. Philadelphia, F.A. Davis, 2005; p 75, with permission.

Fig. 10.6 ■ From Jones: *ECG Notes*. Philadelphia, F.A. Davis, 2005; p 76, with permission.

Fig. 10.7 ■ From Jones: *ECG Notes*. Philadelphia, F.A. Davis, 2005, p 77, with permission.

Fig. 10.8 ■ From Jones: *ECG Notes*. Philadelphia, F.A. Davis, 2005, p 77, with permission.

Fig. 10.9 ■ From Jones: *ECG Notes*. Philadelphia, F.A. Davis, 2005; p 77, with permission.

Fig. 10.10 ■ From Jones: *ECG Notes*. Philadelphia, F.A. Davis, 2005; p 78, with permission.

Fig. 10.11 ■ From Jones: *ECG Notes*. Philadelphia, F.A. Davis, 2005; p 79, with permission.

Fig. 10.12 ■ From Jones: *ECG Notes*. Philadelphia, F.A. Davis, 2005; p 80, with permission.

Fig. 10.13 ■ From Jones: *ECG Notes*. Philadelphia, F.A. Davis, 2005; p 81, with permission.

Fig. 10.14 ■ From Jones: *ECG Notes*. Philadelphia, F.A. Davis, 2005; p 82, with permission.

Fig. 10.15 ■ From Jones: *ECG Notes*. Philadelphia, F.A. Davis, 2005; p 83, with permission.

Fig. 10.16 ■ From Jones: *ECG Notes*. Philadelphia, F.A. Davis, 2005; p 84, with permission.

Fig. 10.17 ■ From Jones: *ECG Notes*. Philadelphia, F.A. Davis, 2005; p 85, with permission.

Fig. A.1 ■ From Jones: *ECG Notes*. Philadelphia: F.A. Davis, 2005, p 110, with permission.

Fig. A.2 ■ From Jones: *ECG Notes*. Philadelphia: F.A. Davis, 2005; p 111, with permission (adapted from Myers and Hopkins: MedSurg Notes. Philadelphia: F.A. Davis, 2004, p 11).

Fig. D.1 ■ From Myers and Hopkins: *MedSurg Notes*. Philadelphia: F.A. Davis, 2004, p 15, with permission.

Fig. D.2 ■ From Jones: *ECG Notes*. Philadelphia: F.A. Davis, 2005, p 103, with permission.

Fig. D.3 ■ From Jones: *ECG Notes*. Philadelphia: F.A. Davis, 2005, p 105, with permission.

Index

Note: Page numbers in **boldface** refer to definition of rhythms; page numbers followed by f refer to figures and rhythm strips; page numbers followed by t refer to tables.